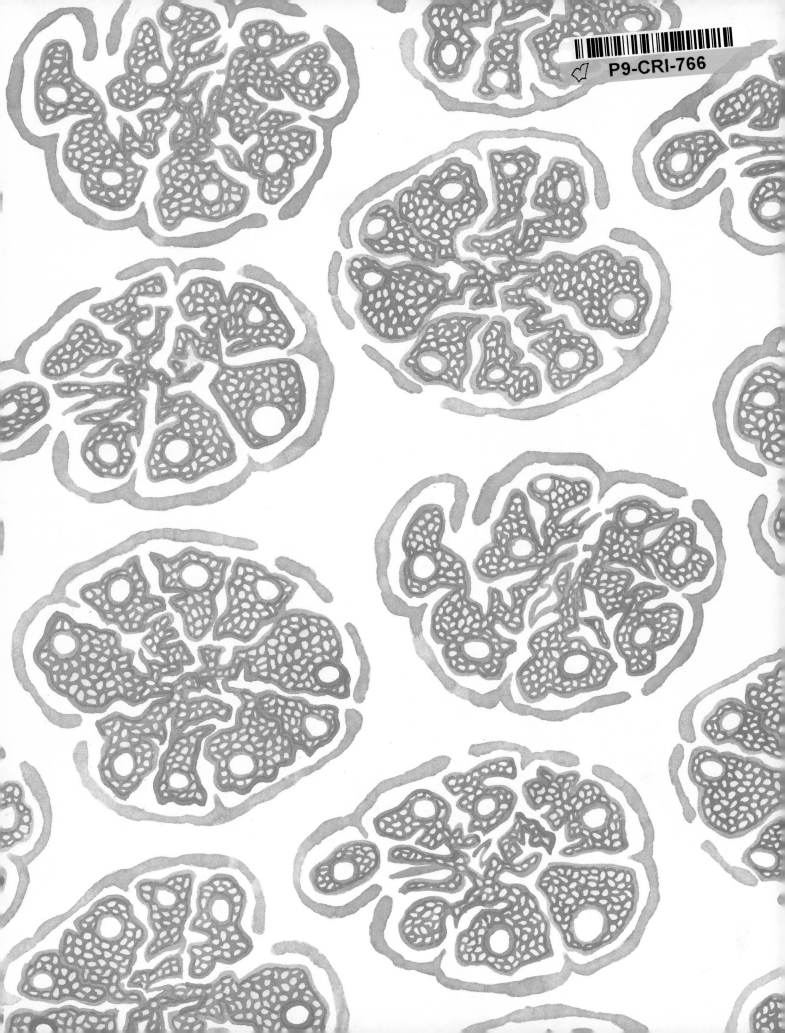

NURSE'S CLINICAL LIBRARY ™

# IMMUNE DISORDERS

*NURSING85* BOOKS ™
SPRINGHOUSE CORPORATION
Springhouse, Pennsylvania

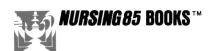
**NURSING85 BOOKS™**

## Nurse's Clinical Library™

**Editorial Director**
Helen Klusek Hamilton

**Clinical Director**
Minnie Bowen Rose, RN, BSN, MEd

**Art Director**
Sonja E. Douglas

### Clinical staff
**Contributing Clinical Editors**
Margaret Belcher, RN, BSN;
Marlene M. Ciranowicz, RN, MSN;
Deena Damsky Dell, RN, MS

**Drug Information Manager**
Larry Neil Gever, RPh, PharmD

**Acquisitions**
Susan Hatch Brunt

### Editorial staff
**Senior Editors**
H. Nancy Holmes, Peter Johnson,
Patricia Minard Shinehouse

**Managing Editor**
Jill Lasker

**Editors**
Lisa Z. Cohen, June Norris, Loralee
Choman Moclock

**Contributing Editors**
Laura Albert, Barbara Hodgson,
Patricia E. McCulla, Frederick Nohl,
Elaine Schott-Jones, Joan Twisdom-
Harty, Patti Urosevich, Rebecca S.
Van Dine, Marylou Webster

**Copy Editors**
David R. Moreau (supervisor), Traci A.
Deraco, Diane M. Labus, Jo Lennon,
Carolyn Mortimer, Doris Weinstock

**Production Coordinator**
Sally Johnson

**Editorial Assistants**
Maree DeRosa, Caroline M. Swider

### Design staff
**Senior Designer**
Jacalyn Bove

**Contributing Designers**
Carol Cameron-Sears, Linda
Franklin, Peter Gerritsen,
Christopher Laird, Matie Patterson

**Illustrators**
Michael Adams, Philip H. Ashley,
Maryanne Buschini, David Cook,
John Cymerman, Design
Management, Marie Garafano, Jean
Gardner, Peter Gerritsen, Lars and
Lois Hokanson, Robert Jackson,
Adam Mathews, Mark Musy, George
Retseck, Eileen Rudnick, Thomas
Schneider, Dennis Schofield

### Production staff
**Art Production**
Robert Perry (manager), Eileen
Hunsicker, Donald Knauss, Kate
Nichols, Sandra Sanders, Joan
Walsh, Robert Wieder

**Typography**
David C. Kosten (manager),
Amanda C. Erb, Ethel Halle, Diane
Paluba, Nancy Wirs

**Manufacturing**
Deborah C. Meiris, Wilbur D.
Davidson (managers), T.A. Landis

Special thanks to Matthew Cahill;
Diane Cochet, RN, BSN; Bernadette
Glenn; Diana Potter; and Dorothy L.
Tengler, who assisted in preparation
of this volume.

## Special Advisor
John J. O'Shea, Jr., MD

**Library of Congress Cataloging in Publication Data**
Main entry under title:
Immune disorders.
    (Nurse's clinical library)
    "Nursing85 books."
    Includes bibliographies and index.
    1. Immunologic diseases.
    2. Immunologic diseases—Nursing.
    I. Series. [DNLM: 1. Immunologic
    Diseases—physiopathology—nurses'
    instruction.
    2. Immunologic Diseases—therapy—
    nurses' instruction.    WD 300 I315]
RC582.I46 1985    616.97    85-2699
ISBN 0-916730-76-X

*Cover:* Color-enhanced soft tissue scan
of arthritic patient.
Photograph by Howard Sochurek.

*Inside front and back covers:* Lymph
nodes.

# CONTENTS

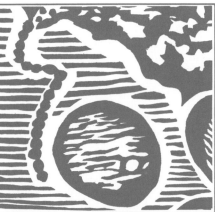
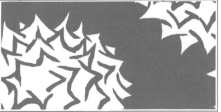
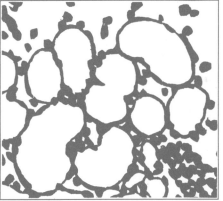
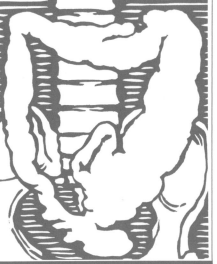

# CONTRIBUTORS AND CLINICAL CONSULTANTS

## Contributors

*At the time of publication, the contributors held the following positions:*

**Diane M. Breckenridge, RN, MSN,** Instructor, Abington Memorial Hospital School of Nursing, Abington, Pa.

**Marlene McNemar Ciranowicz, RN, MSN,** Nursing Instructor, LaSalle University, Philadelphia

**Diane Cochet, RN, BSN,** Clinical Monitor, Biosonics Incorporated, Philadelphia

**Jeffrey C. Delafuente, MS, RPh,** Assistant Professor of Pharmacy and Medicine, Colleges of Pharmacy and Medicine, University of Florida, Gainesville

**Joyce Eddy, RN,** Oncology Research Nurse, National Cancer Institute, National Naval Medical Center, Bethesda, Md.

**Janice Magnor Feldman, RN, MPH,** Chief, Allergy and Infectious Diseases Nursing Service, Clinical Center, National Institutes of Health, Bethesda, Md.

**Christine Grady, RN, MSN,** Clinical Nurse Specialist, Immunology, Allergy and Infectious Disease, National Institutes of Health, Bethesda, Md.

**Clare E. Hastings, RN, BSN,** Head Nurse, Ambulatory Care; Arthritis, Allergy, Immunology, and Child Health; Clinical Center Nursing, National Institutes of Health, Bethesda, Md.

**Diane Kaschak, RN, BSN,** Transplant Nurse Clinician, Albert Einstein Medical Center, Philadelphia

**Lynne Kreutzer-Baraglia, RN, MS,** Assistant Professor, West Suburban College of Nursing, Oak Park, Ill.

**Molly Jean Moran, RN, MS,** Hematology Clinical Nurse Specialist, Ohio State University Hospitals, Columbus

**Beverly A. Post, RN, MS,** Quality Assurance Specialist, West Suburban Hospital Medical Center, Oak Park, Ill.

**Judy Ann Ptak, RN, MSN, CIC,** Infection Control Clinical Specialist, Veterans Administration Medical Center, White River Junction, Vt.

**Basia Belza Tack, RN, MSN, ANP,** Clinical Nurse Educator, Allergy and Infectious Diseases Nursing Service, Clinical Center, National Institutes of Health, Bethesda, Md.

## Clinical Consultants

*At the time of publication, the clinical consultants held the following positions:*

**Barbara A. Ankenbrand, RN, BS, MA,** Assistant Professor of Nursing, Mt. Mercy College, Cedar Rapids, Iowa

**Susan B. Baird, RN, MPH,** Chief, Cancer Nursing Service, Clinical Center, National Institutes of Health, Bethesda, Md.

**Therese E. Bowman, RN, BSN, MS,** Nurse Clinician, Comprehensive Epilepsy Program, University of Minnesota, Minneapolis

**Linda Butterworth, RN, BSN,** Clinical Nurse, Allergy and Infectious Diseases Nursing Service, Clinical Center, National Institutes of Health, Bethesda, Md.

**Donna Calliari, RN, BSN, MN,** Head Nurse, Allergy and Infectious Diseases Nursing Service, National Institutes of Health, Bethesda, Md.

**Leonard Crowley, MD,** Clinical Assistant Professor, Department of Laboratory Medicine and Pathology and Department of Family Practice, University of Minnesota, Minneapolis; Pathologist, St. Mary's Hospital, Minneapolis

**Thomas R. Cupps, MD,** Assistant Professor of Medicine, Department of Medicine, Division of Rheumatology, Immunology, and Allergy, University of Georgetown Medical Center, Washington, D.C.

**Marguerite Donoghue, RN, MN,** Oncology Clinical Nurse Specialist, Cancer Nursing Service, Clinical Center, National Institutes of Health, Bethesda, Md.

**Sister Rebecca Fidler, MT (ASCP), PhD,** Chairperson of Health Sciences and Professor of Medical Technology, Salem (W. Va.) College

**Anne Marie Flaherty, RN, BSN,** Administrative Nurse Clinician, Adult Day Hospital, Memorial Sloan-Kettering Cancer Center, New York

**Joel Glucroft, PhD,** President-Technical Director, Antigen Supply House, Northridge, Calif.

**Max Hamburger, MD,** Assistant Professor of Medicine, State University of New York at Stony Brook

**James A. Hoxie, MD,** Assistant Professor of Medicine, Hematology/Oncology Section, Hospital of the University of Pennsylvania, Philadelphia

**Mary Beth Kingston, RN, MSN,** Evening Clinical Coordinator, Department of Medical Nursing, Hospital of the University of Pennsylvania, Philadelphia

**Joanne Lopes, RN, BS, MS,** Clinical Nurse Specialist, Medicine, University Hospital Stony Brook (N.Y.)

**Hans H. Neumann, MD,** Director of Preventive Medicine, Department of Health, New Haven, Conn.

**John O'Shea, Jr., MD,** Chief Medical Staff Fellow, Clinical Immunology Section, Laboratory of Clinical Investigation, National Institute of Allergy and Infectious Diseases, National Institutes of Health, Bethesda, Md.

**Mark David Pescovitz, MD,** Senior Fellow, National Cancer Institute, Immunology Branch, Transplantation Section, Bethesda, Md.

**Janice Selekman, RN, MSN, PhD,** Associate Professor, Thomas Jefferson University, Philadelphia

**Lois E. Top, BSN, MEd,** Clinical Nurse, Clinical Center, National Institutes of Health, Bethesda, Md.

**David J. Volkman, PhD, MD,** Senior Investigator, Laboratory of Immunoregulation, National Institute of Allergy and Infectious Diseases, National Institutes of Health, Bethesda, Md.

**James N. Woody, MD, PhD,** Director, Transplantation Research Program Center, Naval Medical Research Institute, Bethesda, Md.

# FOREWORD

Immunology, one of the few disciplines with a full range of involvement in all aspects of health and disease, is one of the most rapidly expanding fields in medicine today.

The sheer volume of new immunologic information generated by clinical researchers makes keeping current difficult indeed. Yet, this information has practical implications across the whole range of nursing practice; immunologic concepts apply in every clinical area from pediatrics to geriatrics.

Obviously, nurses need reliable and comprehensive knowledge about immunologic functions. To provide effective health care, they require in-depth knowledge of immune-related diseases, diagnostic measures, and treatments. The escalating complexity of immunologic care requires nurses to have comprehensive scientific and psychosocial knowledge to identify problems correctly, to report observations, and to intervene appropriately. Also, since patients themselves are becoming better informed health-care consumers, nurses must be prepared to play a greater role in patient and family education.

These professional needs obviously require access to reliable and comprehensive reference information that focuses strongly on clinical applications and implications. IMMUNE DISORDERS, a volume in the Nurse's Clinical Library series, provides just such reliable and comprehensive information.

The book is divided into two main parts. In the first, *Fundamental Immune Facts,* four chapters present a wealth of detailed information on the basic concepts of immunology. The first chapter provides a clear overview of the immune system: its organs and structure; cellular characteristics; physiologic mechanisms; and the complex interactions of the humoral, cell-mediated, and combined immune responses in normal and abnormal function. Other chapters in this section describe and offer practical guidelines for nursing assessment, diagnostic tests, and immunotherapeutic methods.

The second part discusses specific immune disorders, including the latest information on acquired immunodeficiency syndrome and graft-versus-host disease. Each of these ten disorder chapters contains three major sections. *Pathophysiology* covers the origins of each disorder, so far as this is known; characteristic signs and symptoms; and effects on interactive body systems. *Medical management* summarizes appropriate diagnostic tests and findings, current treatments, and prognosis. And *Nursing management* provides detailed information for planning nursing care, all presented according to the nursing process. The discussion includes suggestions for getting a detailed patient history, conducting the nursing assessment, and providing appropriate nursing diagnoses. Expanding on these diagnoses, it summarizes the goals of patient care, suggests nursing interventions needed to achieve them, and, finally, offers a guide to evaluation.

An especially useful feature of this book are the numerous clear drawings, diagrams, and charts, many in color, that augment and illustrate the text. Special graphic devices call the reader's attention to patient-teaching aids, to practical guidelines for managing emergencies such as anaphylaxis and hemorrhage, and to brief summaries of key points in each chapter.

Clearly, the combined expertise and talents of leading clinical experts in the field of immunology have produced in IMMUNE DISORDERS a concise, up-to-date, and clinically applicable reference book for nurses at all professional levels.

JANICE MAGNOR FELDMAN, RN, MPH
Chief, Allergy and Infectious Diseases Nursing Service,
Clinical Center, National Institutes of Health,
Bethesda, Md.

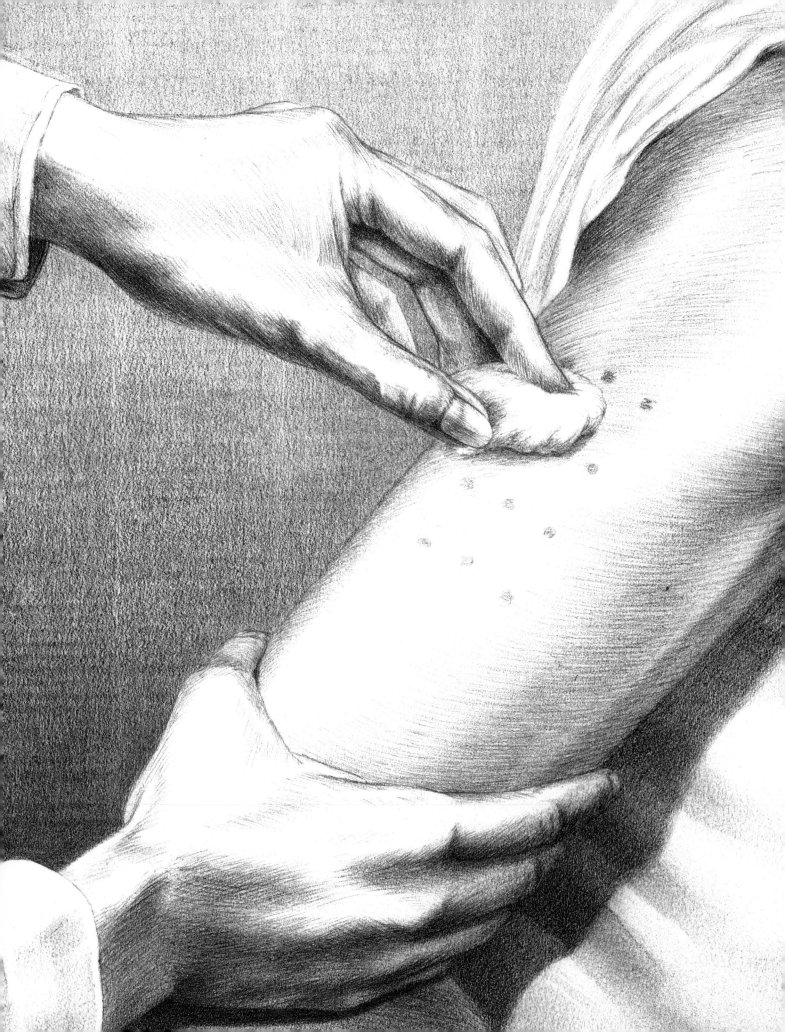

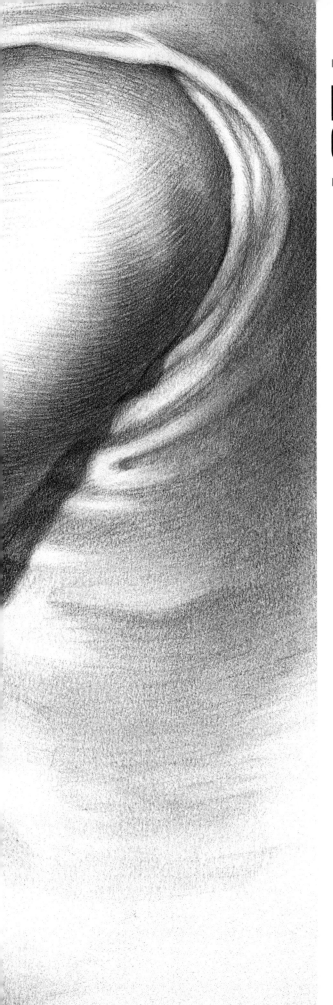

# FUNDAMENTAL CONCEPTS

# 1 REVIEWING BASIC PRINCIPLES

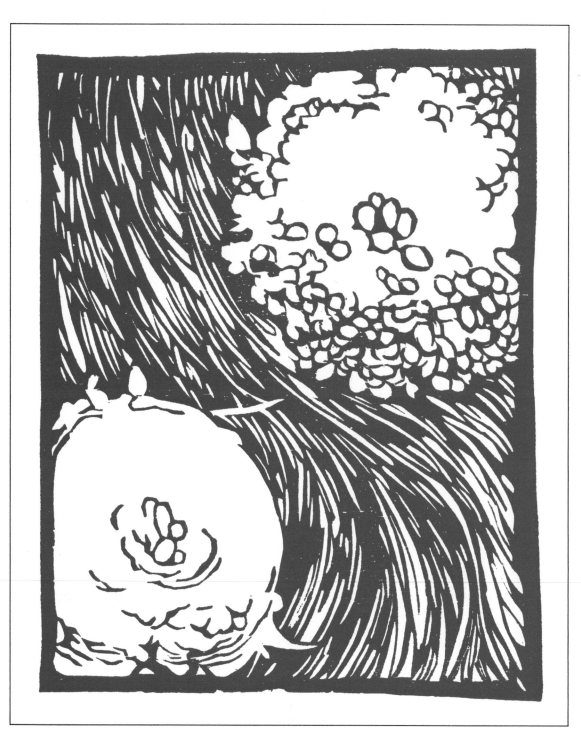

T and B cells

**A**lmost daily, research tells us something new about the immune system—that complex network of cells and their products which interact to shield the body against harmful agents. How to keep current with this information explosion and effectively care for patients with immune disorders may seem overwhelming. But it's a challenge you're likely to meet no matter what your nursing specialty. Whether you're a pediatric nurse considering immunization schedules for childhood infectious diseases or a medical-surgical nurse caring for the patient with a recent kidney transplant, you'll be expected to understand the immune system's normal function and its mechanisms of dysfunction. For example, you should understand what happens when some of its essential cells are lacking (in immunodeficiency disorders) and know what symptoms result when this elaborate defense system turns against the body (in autoimmune disorders). Understanding the immune system and its disorders will help you to recognize the effects of immune dysfunction and to manage them confidently.

### Lines of defense
*Immunity,* derived from the Latin *immunitas* (exemption), denotes protection against infectious organisms. The major suppliers of this protection are the nonimmunologic host defense mechanisms, the inflammatory response, the mononuclear phagocyte system, and the immune system itself. Singly and in tandem, all play a part in defending against pathogenic invasion.

**Host defenses.** Nonimmunologic host defenses—such as the skin, cilia, mucous membranes, and antimicrobial factors in tears and saliva—represent the frontier between body surfaces and the exterior. Once a pathogen penetrates this initial barrier, it's met by a more complex internal system, the mononuclear phagocyte system.

**Inflammation.** The inflammatory response to pathogenic invasion involves vascular and cellular changes that eliminate dead tissue, microorganisms, toxins, and inert foreign matter. Inflammation may result from immunologic or nonimmunologic mechanisms or a combination of both.

Through interaction with components of the immune system (see below), the inflammatory response can focus quickly, efficiently, and effectively on a specific target. The immune response can intensify an inflammatory response, even to the point of excess and self-destruction, or can suppress or supplant an inflammatory response. (See Chapter 10).

**Mononuclear phagocyte system.** Also called the reticuloendothelial system, this system removes pathogens from blood and tissue through phagocytosis. Its chief cell, the macrophage (or mononuclear phagocyte), also reacts to stimulation from activated lymphocytes.

**Immune system.** By circulating its component cells and substances, the immune system maintains an early warning system against both exogenous microorganisms and endogenous cells that have become neoplastic, and it can mount an attack wherever necessary. With only a handful of cell types, it can produce a variety of reactions and can magnify or restrain the response to match the danger. In this manner, the immune system protects the body *(self)* from antigens *(nonself).*

## ANTIGEN-ANTIBODY INTERACTIONS
Key to an understanding of the complex immune system are the interactions of antigen and antibody.

### Antigen
Any substance—exogenous or even endogenous—capable of eliciting an immune response is an antigen. Generally, it's a protein, polysaccharide, or lipid with a high molecular weight (10,000 daltons or more). Microorganisms such as bacteria and viruses contain such antigenic proteins and polysaccharides on their surfaces or in their cell walls; enzymes and toxins secreted by bacteria are also antigenic.

Substances of low molecular weight (less than 10,000 daltons), such as most drugs, cannot elicit an immune response by themselves. Called haptens, they can, however, combine with a higher-weight carrier molecule, usually a serum protein. This hapten-carrier complex is then able to elicit an immune response.

### Antibody
Antibodies are serum proteins that bind to specific antigens and begin the processes that induce lysis or phagocytosis of an offending antigen. They're produced by plasma cells, which differentiate from B lymphocytes (B cells) in response to recognition of that specific antigen. Antibodies are associated primarily with gamma globulin, one of several serum protein fractions, although some antibodies are also found in serum alpha- and

beta-globulin fractions. These protein molecules that function as antibodies are also called immunoglobulins (see page 16).

## ORGANS OF THE IMMUNE SYSTEM

The lymphoid system includes organs and tissues in which lymphocytes predominate, as well as cells that circulate in peripheral blood. Central (primary) organs include the bone marrow and thymus; peripheral (secondary) organs include the lymph nodes and vessels, spleen, tonsils, and intestinal lymphoid tissue (Peyer's patches and the appendix).

This system has four chief functions: to bring B and T cells to maturity, to concentrate antigens from throughout the body into a few lymphoid organs, to circulate lymphocytes through these organs so that any antigen is quickly exposed to the full battery of antigen-specific lymphocytes, and to carry antigen-specific lymphocytes and antibodies to the blood and tissues.

### Central lymphoid organs

The bone marrow and the thymus play a role in developing the immune system's principal cells: B and T cells. Both types of cells appear to originate in the bone marrow.

In the chicken, research has identified the bursa of Fabricius as the site of B-cell differentiation from stem cells. In humans, although a similar site hasn't been positively identified, the bone marrow appears to be the bursa equivalent.

The thymus, site of T-cell differentiation, is a bilobular endocrine gland located in the upper mediastinum. It grows steadily during fetal and neonatal periods, achieves full size in early puberty, and then progressively shrinks. The thymus consists of a cortex and medulla. The larger cortex houses many tightly packed thymocytes and epithelial cells, which then travel to the medulla before leaving the gland and entering the circulation. Along with epithelial cells, the medulla contains less densely packed thymocytes, many of which have matured and are ready to leave the gland.

### Peripheral lymphoid organs

Both B and T cells are distributed throughout the tissue of the peripheral lymphoid organs, with the lymph nodes and spleen holding the principal concentrations.

**Lymph nodes.** Small, bean-shaped lymph nodes occur throughout the body but are most abundant in the head and neck, axillae, abdomen, and groin. They serve to filter lymph-borne antigens. (See *The lymph nodes: Immune control center.*) Afferent lymphatic vessels, originating in the interstitial spaces of body tissues, drain lymph into the lymph nodes. Lymph diffuses through the nodal sinuses and leaves by the efferent lymphatic vessels, finally draining into major lymphatic vessels such as the thoracic duct, and thence into venous circulation.

Structurally, the lymph node consists of an outer cortex, which divides into the superficial cortex and the deep cortex, and an inner core, the medulla. In the superficial cortex, lymphocytes lie closely packed in primary follicles; since most of the cells are B cells, this area of the cortex is called thymus-independent. When a lymph-borne antigen stimulates an immune response, primary follicles enlarge and develop into secondary follicles with germinal centers that proliferate B cells.

In the deep cortex (and between superficial cortical follicles) lie layers of lymphocytes passing from the blood to the lymph. Since most of the cells here are T cells, this area of the cortex is called thymus-dependent. Many lymphocytes, predominantly T cells, circulate constantly between the blood and lymph, and cortical tissue serves as the chief cross-over point from the venous system to the lymphatic system.

The lymph node filters antigens that are transported in lymph. In the deep cortex and the lining of the walls of the cortical and medullary sinuses lie phagocytic cells (macrophages and specialized reticular cells), which seize and hold passing antigens. Once an immune response begins, follicles located in the superficial cortex also trap and process antigens.

**Spleen.** The chief site of the immune response to antigens, the spleen filters and concentrates blood-borne antigens and other particles. This organ divides into white pulp and red pulp. The white pulp, composed of lymphoid tissue massed around small arteries and arterioles, subdivides into thymic-dependent and thymic-independent areas. The thymic-dependent area, composed of T cell–rich lymphoid tissue, surrounds the arterioles and is called the periarteriolar lymphatic sheath; the thymic-independent area, composed of B-cell follicles, surrounds the T-cell areas.

The red pulp is a network of splenic cords (tissue filled with lymphocytes, macrophages, and plasma cells), which filter incoming

# The lymph nodes: Immune control center

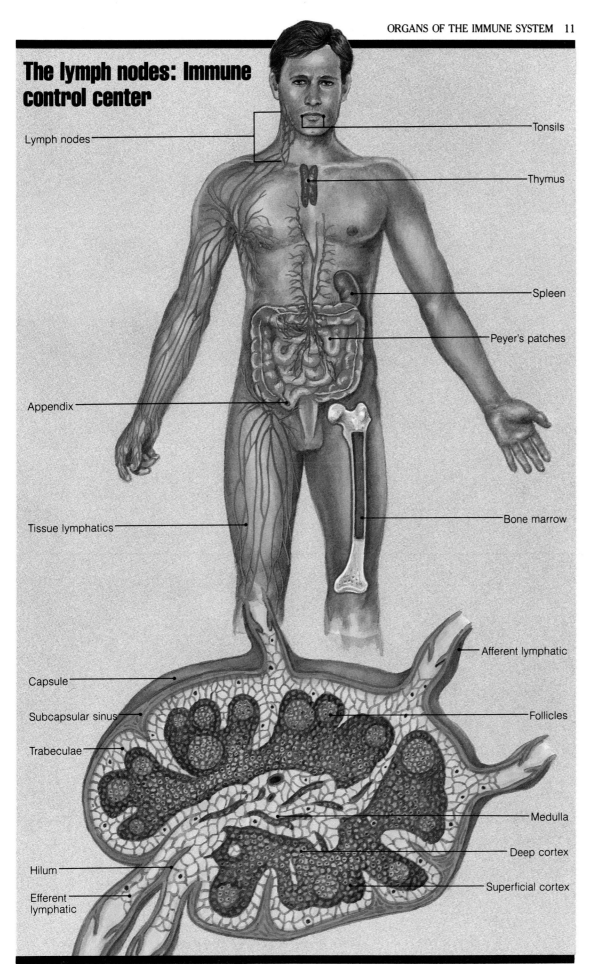

Lymph nodes
Tonsils
Thymus
Spleen
Peyer's patches
Appendix
Bone marrow
Tissue lymphatics
Afferent lymphatic
Capsule
Subcapsular sinus
Follicles
Trabeculae
Medulla
Hilum
Deep cortex
Efferent lymphatic
Superficial cortex

Lymph nodes, which are most abundant in the head, neck, axillae, abdomen, pelvis, and groin, store B and T cells, key participants in immune responses. The lymph nodes help remove and destroy antigens circulating in the blood and lymph. Here's how:

Each small, bean-shaped lymph node is enclosed by a fibrous *capsule*. Bands of connective tissue (*trabeculae*) that extend deep inside the node from the capsule divide the node into compartments. These nodal compartments are further divided into three regions:
• The outer region (*superficial cortex*) contains follicles made up predominantly of B cells. During an immune response, the follicles enlarge and develop a central area with large proliferating cells—the germinal center.
• The interfollicular areas consist mostly of T cells, as does the *deep cortex*. These cells are in transit from the bloodstream to the lymph vessels.
• The innermost region (*medulla*) is the last collecting place for lymphocytes before they exit the node through the efferent lymph vessels. During an immune response, the medulla contains numerous plasma cells that actively secrete immunoglobulins.

Multiple afferent lymph vessels carry lymph into the node to the subcapsular sinus. From there, it flows through cortical sinuses and smaller radial medullary sinuses. Phagocytic cells in the deep cortex and lining the sinuses avidly take up the antigen. The antigen may also be trapped in the follicles of the superficial cortex when the immune response has been initiated and antibody is available to form antigen-antibody complexes.

Cleansed lymph leaves the node through efferent lymph vessels at the hilum.

Structurally and functionally, the spleen, appendix, Peyer's patches, tonsils, and other lymphoid tissues resemble the lymph nodes.

# Hematopoiesis: Differentiation of the stem cell

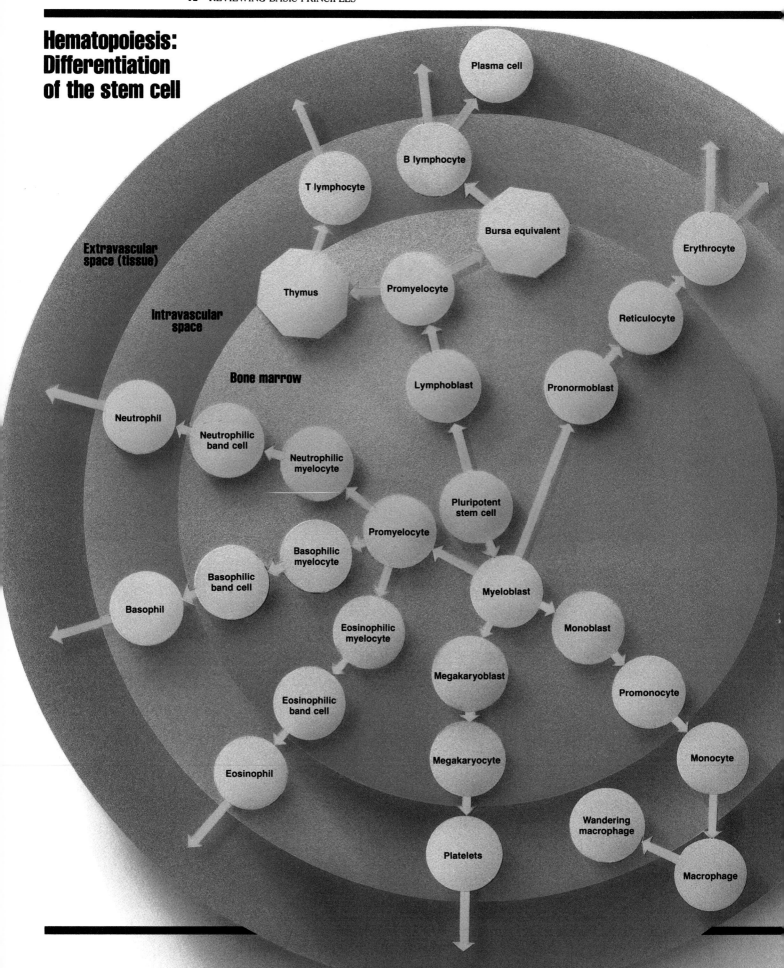

Hematopoiesis supplies all the body's blood cells, including those essential for immunologic defense, which are described below. These cells originate from pluripotent *stem cells* in the bone marrow, represented by the inner ring in this illustration. The middle ring represents the intravascular space; the outer ring, the extravascular space, which includes body tissues.

**Erythrocytes** (red blood cells) circulate in the blood for about 120 days. As they age, these cells become fragile, rupture, and are removed by the spleen.

**Leukocytes** (white blood cells) include five cell types: *neutrophils, eosinophils, basophils, monocytes, and lymphocytes.* Neutrophils, eosinophils, and basophils are collectively known as *granulocytes* because of their granular cytoplasm. A few slightly immature granulocytes, called *band cells* for their band-shaped nuclei, also normally appear in peripheral blood.

*Neutrophils* (polymorphonuclear cells), the most abundant granulocytes, are intensely phagocytic.

*Eosinophils* may participate in phagocytosis. They also may be involved in modulating allergic responses and participate in host defenses against parasites.

*Basophils* have no phagocytic function; they release histamine and other inflammatory agents in acute allergic reactions. Basophils are similar to tissue-based mast cells.

*Monocytes* and *lymphocytes* are mononuclear cells. Monocytes differentiate into highly phagocytic *macrophages.* Lymphocytes include *T cells,* which mature in the thymus, and *B cells,* which appear to mature in the bone marrow.

*Platelets* (thrombocytes) protect vascular surfaces and aggregate to promote blood clotting and stop bleeding.

blood, and sinuses carrying erythrocyte-rich venous blood from the spleen.

**Accessory organs.** The remaining peripheral lymphoid organs—tonsils, Peyer's patches, and appendix—are masses of lymphoid tissue containing lymphocytes, plasma cells, germinal centers, and thymus-dependent areas. Lymphoid tissue, consisting of embedded lymphocytes and macrophages, also lies in the fibrous connective tissue immediately beneath the mucous membrane.

## CELLS AND MEDIATORS OF THE IMMUNE SYSTEM

The major cellular components of the immune system—the lymphocytes (B and T cells) and the macrophages—originate in the hematopoietic system. These highly differentiated cells derive from the original undifferentiated stem cells of the bone marrow. During embryogenesis, stem cells proliferate in the wall of the fertilized ovum's yolk sac and in the liver, spleen, and bone marrow. In adults, stem cells may proliferate in the bone marrow.

The stem cell can develop into a wide assortment of cells. (See *Hematopoiesis: Differentiation of the stem cell.*)

### Lymphocytes

To defend against the huge number of possible antigens, lymphocytes differ structurally and functionally. Structurally, many groups of specialized lymphocytes exist, with each group genetically programmed to respond only to a distinct range of physically similar antigens. Within a group, individual lymphocytes have identical receptors on the cell membrane that are specific for binding sites (called antigenic determinants) on structurally related antigens. One lymphocyte group differs from another in the structure of its receptors and, thus, in the types of antigens that will activate it.

Functionally, two major lymphocyte groups exist: B cells, the precursors of antibody-producing plasma cells; and T cells, whose various subclasses either promote or suppress the immune response, kill antigens directly, or participate in other immune responses such as delayed hypersensitivity. Both B and T cells may also exist as long-lived memory cells. (See *How B and T cells mature,* pages 14 and 15.) A third group is composed of lymphocytes that perform several cytotoxic functions. Among these, natural killer (NK) cells destroy certain tumor cells, but the mechanism whereby they recognize those cells re-

*(continued on page 16)*

# How B and T cells mature

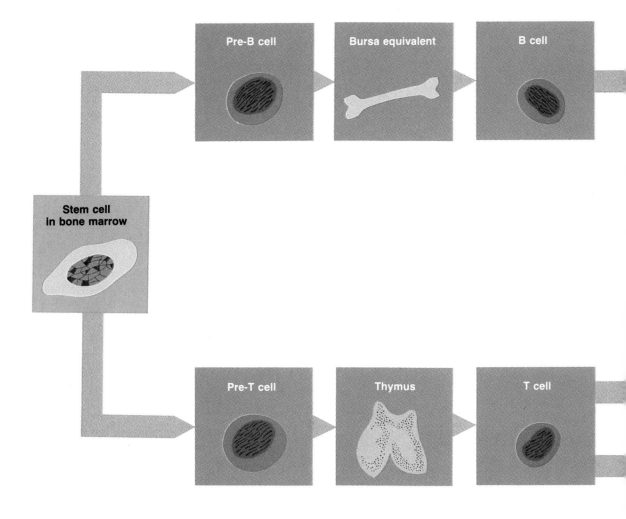

Although both derive from bone marrow stem cells, B and T cells mature differently. *B-cell ontogeny* was first detected in the chicken's central lymphoid organ, the bursa of Fabricius. In humans, the bone marrow presumably serves as the bursa equivalent; here, pre-B cells are believed to mature to B cells. These B cells then migrate to peripheral lymphoid organs, such as the lymph nodes and spleen, for storage. When an antigen-presenting cell (APC) presents an antigen to a B cell, with T-cell help, the B cell is activated and proliferates. Many of these cells then differentiate into antibody-secreting plasma cells. Others remain in the lymphatic tissue as memory B cells and, upon reexposure to the same antigen, quickly differentiate into antibody-secreting plasma cells for an accelerated immune response.

In *T-cell ontogeny,* T-cell precursors (pre-T cells) travel to the thymus, where they mature to T cells. These T cells then leave the thymus to circulate in the blood or become constituents of the peripheral lymphoid organs.

When an APC presents an antigen in the presence of the major histocompatibility complex antigen, the T cell activates and differentiates into various subsets with overlapping functions. Helper T cells interact with B cells to stimulate B-cell proliferation and differentiation into antibody-secreting cells. Suppressor T cells appear to control the amount of T-cell help available to stimulate antibody production. Other T cells produce lymphokines, soluble mediators involved in delayed hypersensitivity and other immune reactions.

Cytotoxic (or killer) T cells directly destroy the antigenic agent, whereas memory T cells remain in circulation and in lymphatic tissue to recognize and promptly attack that same antigen in any subsequent appearance.

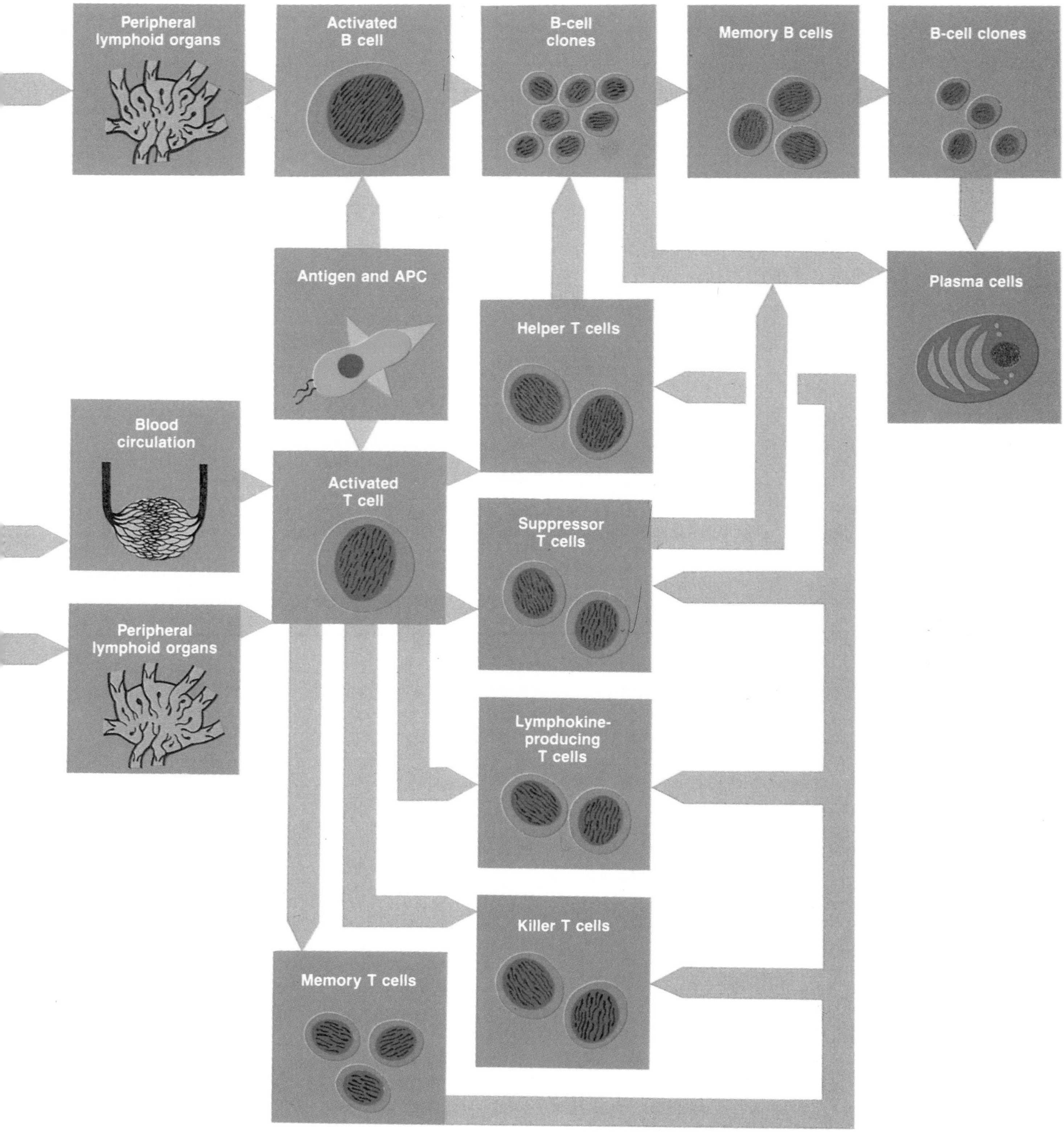
Peripheral lymphoid organs
Activated B cell
B-cell clones
Memory B cells
B-cell clones
Antigen and APC
Plasma cells
Helper T cells
Blood circulation
Activated T cell
Suppressor T cells
Peripheral lymphoid organs
Lymphokine-producing T cells
Killer T cells
Memory T cells

## Immunoglobulins: Variations on a Y-shaped monomer

Immunoglobulins, large protein molecules, consist of four polypeptide chains: two long, heavy (H) chains and two short, light (L) chains. Each L chain is linked to an H chain, and the two H chains are linked to each other by disulfide bonds.

The basic structure (monomeric unit) of an immunoglobulin is Y-shaped. The two arms of the Y contain the *antigen-binding fragment* (Fab). Thus, immunoglobulin monomers are bivalent, having two antigen-binding sites, one at the end of each arm.

The outer portion of the Fab region, where variable sequences of polypeptide chains reside, defines the character of the antigen-binding site and is known as the *variable* (V) region. The inner Fab region is known as the *constant* (C) region because of the constancy of the amino acid sequence.

The stem of the Y is known as the *fragment, crystallizable* (Fc) region. This area, which is also part of the C region, contains the disulfide bond that links the H chains. The Fc region participates in effector functions of immunoglobulins, such as activation of complement, and provides a binding site for Fc receptors on phagocytic cells. The major structural differences among IgG, IgM, IgA, IgE, and IgD are in the H chains, which are specific for each class.

**IgM**

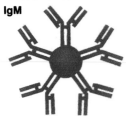

**Secretory IgA**

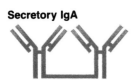

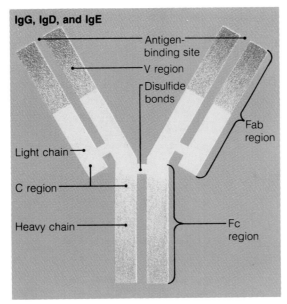

**IgG, IgD, and IgE**

Antigen-binding site
V region
Disulfide bonds
Fab region
Light chain
C region
Heavy chain
Fc region

mains unclear. Other lymphocytes in this group, which may also be or include the NK cells, destroy target cells through antibody-dependent cellular cytotoxicity. These lymphocytes (and sometimes other cell types) kill antibody-coated target cells after recognizing the fragment, crystallizable (Fc) portion of the antibody bound to those cells.

**B cells.** Precursors to antibody-secreting plasma cells, B cells derive from hematopoietic stem cells. Although the exact developmental sequence of B cells is unknown, studies on mice indicate that the immediate precursors of B cells (called pre-B cells) can be found in the mammalian fetal liver 3 to 4 days before B cells appear. These pre-B cells are large lymphoid cells that lack membrane-bound antigen receptors but contain an antibody (IgM) in the cytoplasm. As the fetus develops, the number of pre-B cells in the liver decreases, while the number in the bone marrow and spleen increases. After birth and in the adult, pre-B cells appear only in the bone marrow, making this the likely site for maturation of pre-B cells to B cells.

As they mature, B cells develop antigen receptors on their surface membranes. Serving as these receptors are molecules of antigen-specific immunoglobulin secreted by the B cell. These surface immunoglobulins—IgM, IgD, and, to a lesser extent, IgG—function in B-cell activation.

Memory B cells play an important part in developing rapid secondary (anamnestic) antibody responses upon reexposure to the

same antigen. Regulatory B cells that can amplify or suppress lymphocyte responses may also exist.

Recognition of an antigen activates B cells to proliferate and differentiate. Proliferation expands the number of cells able to respond to the antigen, since the number of B cells specific for any individual antigen is very low before the first exposure. The proliferative phase of B-cell responses is driven, at least in part, by a T-cell product called B-cell growth factor. Proliferated cells differentiate into either antibody-secreting plasma cells (the cells that synthesize and secrete immunoglobulin molecules) or memory B cells, similar to the original precursor and able to respond more promptly to subsequent attack by the same antigen.

**Immunoglobulins.** The products of these antibody-producing plasma cells are the immunoglobulin molecules (see *Immunoglobulins: Variations on a Y-shaped monomer*). Based on their structure and function, immunoglobulins are divided into five classes: IgG, IgM, IgA, IgD, and IgE. IgG, IgM, and IgA have identifiable subclasses.

*IgG.* The major immunoglobulin in the blood, IgG constitutes approximately 75% of the serum immunoglobulin fraction. It's also found in the extravascular fluids of the body: lymph, cerebrospinal fluid, synovial fluid, and peritoneal fluid. The IgG molecule is the smallest of the immunoglobulins; its bivalent, Y-shaped monomeric structure allows only two antigen-binding sites, one on each arm of the Y.

IgG is the only immunoglobulin that crosses the placenta and provides temporary natural passive immunity until the infant's own humoral immune system becomes functional. In breast-fed infants, the presence of IgG in colostrum and breast milk enhances IgG levels.

IgG is the second immunoglobulin (after IgM) to respond to an antigen in a primary immune response, but it's the major immunoglobulin to respond after reexposure to the antigen (secondary, or anamnestic, antibody response). After IgG combines with an antigen, the immunoglobulin's Fc portion (stem of the IgG monomer) can bind to $C1\overline{qrs}$, the first component of the classical complement pathway. This activates the complement cascade (see below), which leads to cytolysis.

*IgM.* Found mainly in the blood, IgM constitutes approximately 10% of the serum immunoglobulin fraction. The fetus usually begins to produce IgM after the fifth or sixth month,

# The major histocompatibility complex

**A**lso known as the human leukocyte antigen (HLA) system, the *major histocompatibility complex* (MHC) is a group of genes located on the short arm of chromosome 6. These genes code for surface antigens on many kinds of cells. They're critical to recognition of "self" versus "nonself," since the MHC defines what is "self." Thus, HLA antigens are important in tissue cross-matching procedures and are partially responsible for tissue transplant rejection, which occurs when donor MHC and recipient MHC don't match. They also have been associated with over 60 diseases, such as ankylosing spondylitis, insulin-dependent diabetes, nontropical sprue (celiac disease), and rheumatoid arthritis.

The MHC genes occupy five recognized positions (loci) on chromosome 6: HLA-A, HLA-B, HLA-C, HLA-D, and HLA-DR (HLA-D-related).

Based on their tissue distribution and structure, HLA antigens have been divided into three classes. Class I antigens include the HLA-A, -B, and -C antigens. Class II antigens include HLA-D and -DR. Class III antigens include certain complement proteins, such as Factor B and C4.

Class I antigens are found on virtually every cell. During tissue graft rejection, they are the principle antigens recognized by the host. In cell-mediated cytolysis, Class I antigens serve as target antigens recognized by killer T cells. The true physiologic role of Class I histocompatibility is probably related to histocompatibility restriction of cell-mediated lysis of virus-infected cells. When killer T cells are exposed to a viral antigen, they recognize it in the context of a Class I antigen.

Class II antigens are found chiefly on cells of the immune system, including B cells, some T cells, and macrophages. These antigens elicit a mixed lymphocyte response, in which helper T cells proliferate and help activate killer T cells and antibody-producing B cells. Class II antigens are also involved in antigen presentation by macrophages to T cells, and in tissue graft rejection, as well as in aiding efficient collaboration between immunocompetent cells. The T-cell antigen receptor recognizes antigen in the context of Class II antigens.

The individual's ability to respond to many relatively simple antigens is determined by the polymorphic form of Class II genes (or, sometimes, Class I genes) in an individual. Research suggests that the process controlled by immune response (Ir) genes within the MHC reflects general phenomena critical to the individual's ability to make T cell–dependent immune responses to all antigens. Ir-gene-determined responsiveness may represent a special case of the corecognition of antigenic determinants and structures on Class II antigens. The Ir genes determine whether individuals of one MHC type can respond to an antigen, while those of another cannot.

---

when protective maternal IgG has dissipated. Therefore, increased levels of IgM in the neonate's umbilical blood may indicate intrauterine infection.

IgM is the largest immunoglobulin. Its structure incorporates five Y-shaped monomeric units (arranged radially in a star-shaped molecule known as a pentamer) with a small polypeptide chain called a J chain. Therefore, each IgM molecule contains 10 potential antigen-binding sites. However, not all the sites appear able to bind with equal efficiency, and up to half may be inoperative.

IgM is temporally the first immunoglobulin to respond to an antigen and is the major antibody involved in the primary immune response.

IgM functions like IgG but is even more effective in activating the complement system. One of IgM's major functions is to bind with viral and bacterial antigens in the circulation, thereby activating the complement cascade. IgM and IgG function together as specific antitoxins in response to diphtheria, tetanus, anthrax, botulism, and snake venom.

*IgA.* This immunoglobulin exists in two types: serum IgA and secretory IgA. Serum IgA constitutes between 10% and 15% of the serum immunoglobulin fraction and usually consists of one Y-shaped monomeric unit. Secretory IgA, the immunoglobulin's predominant form, consists of two IgA molecules and a J chain bound to a secretory component by disulfide bonds. This type concentrates in the exocrine secretions, such as colostrum, milk, tears, sweat, and saliva, and in secretions of the respiratory, gastrointestinal, and urogenital tracts. At these potential antigen sites of entry, it provides specific antibody protection against pathogens.

*IgD.* This immunoglobulin constitutes less than 1% of the serum immunoglobulin fraction. It's found on the surface of B cells and may be involved in their differentiation.

*IgE.* Normally present in only trace amounts of the serum immunoglobulin fraction, IgE levels are usually elevated in allergic disorders and certain parasitic infections. Most IgE-producing cells are located in the respiratory and intestinal mucosa. This immunoglobulin operates primarily in allergic reactions; its Fc region binds with high affinity to mast cells and basophils, leaving its Fab region free to bind with an allergen (an antigen that can produce an allergic reaction). (See Chapter 6.) Binding of two or more IgE molecules to an allergen triggers the mast cells or basophils to release histamine, kinins, serotonin, leukotrienes (also known as SRS-A, the slow-reacting substance of anaphylaxis), and neutrophil chemotactic factor. These chemical mediators, in turn, produce the characteristic wheal-and-flare allergic reaction of the skin, allergic (extrinsic) asthma, and allergic seasonal rhinitis (hay fever). IgE may also provide protection against some parasitic worms.

*Immunoglobulin genes.* One of the most extraordinary attributes of the immune system is its ability to generate diversity. Since the body must recognize a phenomenal number of distinct antigens and since an individual is genetically programmed to generate between 1 million and 100 million distinct antibody (Ig) molecules, understanding the mechanism that accomplishes this diversity has become a cornerstone of immunology. At the embryonic level, genetic material provides the potential to produce this extraordinary number of related but distinct Ig molecules by permitting relatively few constant region genes to associate with numerous variable region genes in a multitude of permutations to form the wide range of immunoglobulin molecules. Upon B-cell activation, further rearrangement of deoxyribonucleic acid may occur: even the class of immunoglobulin can vary.

**T cells.** Derived from hematopoietic stem cells, many T-cell precursors enter the thymus. Within the thymus, the cells learn to distinguish "self" from "nonself," a function of the major histocompatibility complex (MHC). (See *The major histocompatibility complex,* page 17.) Although many cells are destroyed during this process, some continue to mature and exit the gland. Once matured into T cells, they migrate to the peripheral lymphoid tissues.

T-cell subgroups include the regulatory helper and suppressor T cells, which respectively enhance or suppress the development of immune responses, particularly antibody production. These two activities are paramount among T-cell regulatory functions. Helper T cells stimulate B-cell proliferation and differentiation into antibody-secreting plasma cells. To do this, the helper T cell recognizes antigen determinants on antigen bound to the B cell and corecognizes the Class II major histocompatibility complex molecule, usually on the surface of a specialized antigen-presenting cell. The underlying mechanism is still unclear, but B cells would be unable to respond to most protein antigens without this help; these antigens are called thymus-dependent antigens. Antigens (such as certain polysaccharides and certain bacteria) capable of stimulating B cells directly, without the helper T cells, are called thymus-independent antigens.

Helper T cells also aid in B-cell activation by producing soluble, nonspecific mediators called lymphokines, some of which are also MHC-restricted in their function.

Suppressor T cells reduce the immune response, apparently by limiting the amount of T-cell help available to activate B cells. This process may involve other cells.

Other T cells include cytotoxic, or killer, T cells, which kill antigens directly; memory T cells, which recognize antigens on reexposure and quickly proliferate; and T cells that produce lymphokines and other mediators, initiate various inflammatory responses, and participate in delayed hypersensitivity.

**Lymphokines**
Lymphokines are soluble mediators that are produced by activated lymphocytes (except for interleukin-1, which is produced by macrophages). They facilitate intracellular communication between macrophages, B cells, T cells, and nonlymphoid cells. Among the identified lymphokines are chemotactic factor (CF), macrophage activating factor (MAF), macrophage (or migration) inhibiting factor (MIF), transfer factor (TF), blastogenic factor (BF), lymphotoxin, B-cell growth factor (BCGF), T-cell replacing factor (TRF), interleukin-1 (IL-1, also known as lymphocyte activating factor), interleukin-2 (IL-2, also known as T-cell growth factor), and interferon.

CF, MIF, and MAF stimulate and maintain macrophage activity at the antigen site. CF promotes migration of macrophages, polymorphonuclear leukocytes, and sensitized T cells to the antigen site. MIF inhibits migration of macrophages away from the reaction site, so that they remain active there. MAF transforms local macrophages into active phagocytes.

TF probably converts nonsensitized T cells to sensitized T cells. BF initiates proliferation of the sensitized T cells. Lymphotoxin causes lysis of certain target cells.

BCGF regulates B-cell proliferation in response to stimulation by an antigen. TRF causes proliferating B cells to differentiate into antibody-secreting cells.

IL-1 stimulates the growth of thymocytes and T cells, sustains chronic inflammatory reactions (in damaged joints), and is involved in the production of fever. IL-2 stimulates the growth of T cells.

Interferons may have a variety of functions, including taking part in host defenses against viruses. This type of interferon halts intracellular proliferation of viruses by producing antiviral protein in infected cells. Interferons also appear to stimulate cytotoxic cells, particularly T cells and NK cells, which may explain their performance against tumor cells.

## Macrophages

Originating in the stem cell, monocytes differentiate into macrophages, which circulate in the blood. Some of these free (wandering) monocytes move to the tissues to mature, and the resulting fixed macrophages are named according to these tissue sites: histiocytes (connective tissue), alveolar macrophages (lung), Kupffer's cells (liver), and pleural and peritoneal macrophages (spleen, lymph nodes, bone marrow, and serous cavities). Additional cells that may be of macrophage origin include osteoclasts (bone tissue) Langerhans' cells (skin), and microglial cells (nervous system).

Macrophages are the chief cells of the mononuclear phagocyte system. One of their functions is phagocytosis—engulfing and ingesting bacteria, fungi, dead tissue, antigen-antibody complexes, and tumor cells. Wandering macrophages perform final cleanup of a damaged site before tissue repair. Fixed macrophages engulf and destroy foreign material in their environments. As they mature, their phagocytic ability increases.

Macrophages also perform other functions essential to the immune response. They play a role in antigen processing and presentation, ensuring B-cell and T-cell activation. They also release mediators (including IL-1), which have diverse effects on T cells, fibroblasts, and neutrophils (see below), and are also responsible for producing fever.

## Associated cell types

In addition to the major immune cells—B and T cells and macrophages—other cells participating in immunologic reactions include

## Steps of phagocytosis

Microorganisms and other foreign material (antigens) that invade the skin and mucous membranes are removed by phagocytosis, a defense mechanism carried out by macrophages (mononuclear leukocytes) and neutrophils (polymorphonuclear leukocytes). Here's how macrophages accomplish phagocytosis:

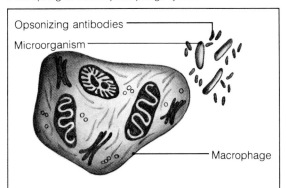

Opsonizing antibodies
Microorganism
Macrophage

**Chemotaxis**
Chemotactic factors attract macrophages to the antigen site.

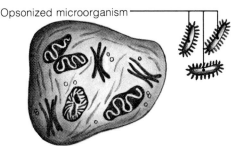

Opsonized microorganism

**Opsonization**
Antibody (IgG) or complement fragment (C3b) coats the microorganism, enhancing macrophage binding to this antigen.

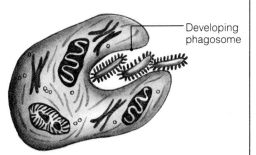

Developing phagosome

**Ingestion**
The macrophage extends its membrane around the opsonized microorganism, engulfing it within a vacuole (phagosome).

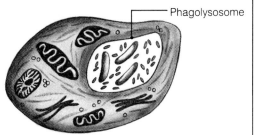

Phagolysosome

**Digestion**
As the phagosome shifts away from the cell periphery, it merges with lysosomes, forming a phagolysosome, where antigen destruction occurs.

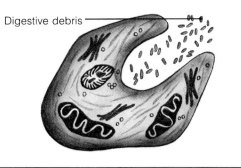

Digestive debris

**Release**
Once digestion is complete, the macrophage expels digestive debris, including lysozymes, prostaglandins, complement components, and interferon, which continue to mediate the immune response.

# Complement cascade: Two pathways of antigen destruction

The complement system plays an indispensable role in the humoral immune response. Activation of this system, the complement cascade, follows one of two pathways: the *classical pathway*, initiated by antigen-antibody complexes, or the *alternative pathway*, triggered by IgA; some IgG molecules; and certain polysaccharides, lipopolysaccharides, and trypsin-like enzymes.

*Classical:* Upon activation of the classical pathway by antigen-antibody complexes, C1$\overline{qrs}$ generates an enzyme that cleaves C4 and C2, producing C$\overline{142}$ (the classical pathway C3 convertase). C$\overline{142}$ then cleaves C3 into C3a (anaphylatoxin) and C3b. This forms C$\overline{1423b}$, the classical pathway C5 convertase.

*Alternative:* C3b, spontaneously cleaved from C3 continuously in the blood, is inactivated by Factors I and H. However, in the presence of certain activators (such as polysaccharides), Factors I and H are less able to inactivate C3b. This initiates the alternative pathway. Factor B combines with C3b in the presence of Factor D to form the alternative pathway C3 convertase, C3bBb. C3bBb, in turn, acts on C3 to form C3bBbC3b, the alternative pathway C5 convertase. Properdin stabilizes both C3bBb and C3bBbC3b. C3bBbC3b induces cleavage of C5, producing C5a and C5b.

The binding of C5b to C6,7 initiates the membrane attack complex. C5b,6,7 causes leakage of intracellular fluid. Leakage increases dramatically when C5b,6,7 binds with C8. Rapid cytolysis occurs when the final complement component, C9, binds to C5b,6,7,8.

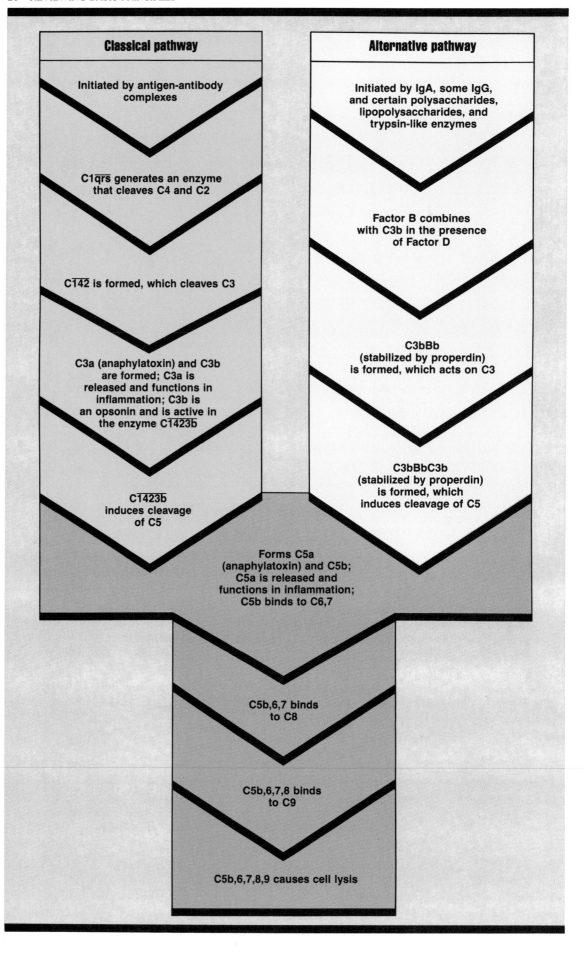

**Classical pathway**

Initiated by antigen-antibody complexes

C1$\overline{qrs}$ generates an enzyme that cleaves C4 and C2

C$\overline{142}$ is formed, which cleaves C3

C3a (anaphylatoxin) and C3b are formed; C3a is released and functions in inflammation; C3b is an opsonin and is active in the enzyme C$\overline{1423b}$

C$\overline{1423b}$ induces cleavage of C5

**Alternative pathway**

Initiated by IgA, some IgG, and certain polysaccharides, lipopolysaccharides, and trypsin-like enzymes

Factor B combines with C3b in the presence of Factor D

C3bBb (stabilized by properdin) is formed, which acts on C3

C3bBbC3b (stabilized by properdin) is formed, which induces cleavage of C5

Forms C5a (anaphylatoxin) and C5b; C5a is released and functions in inflammation; C5b binds to C6,7

C5b,6,7 binds to C8

C5b,6,7,8 binds to C9

C5b,6,7,8,9 causes cell lysis

# Combined immune response

Most antigens do not activate an independent humoral or cell-mediated response; instead they activate a combination of both responses.

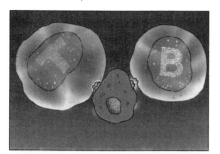

Once an antigen is recognized as foreign, the antigen-presenting cell (APC) captures, processes, and presents it to immunocompetent B and T cells, thus activating them.

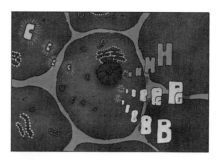

The complement cascade attracts macrophages by chemotaxis and triggers the release of histamine, prostaglandins, and bradykinin. These chemical mediators increase capillary permeability and promote vasodilation, facilitating macrophage movement.

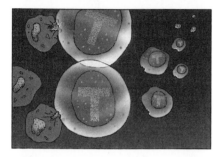

Stimulated immunocompetent T cells can attack the antigen (in this case, a transplanted cell) directly (killer T cells); can secrete lymphokines that recruit other cells, such as macrophages; or can influence B-cell activation (helper and suppressor T cells).

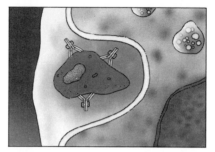

Complement also promotes opsonization—antibody coating of the antigen—which speeds phagocytosis of the antigen by macrophages and neutrophils.

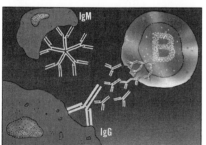

Meanwhile, stimulated immunocompetent B cells release first IgM, then IgG antibodies, which bind to the antigen at specific sites (humoral response).

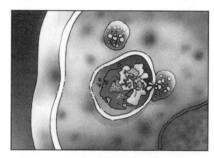

After forming a phagolysosome, the secretion of lysosomal enzymes breaks down the cell's protein and lipids.

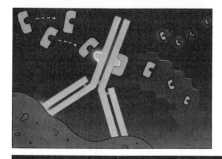

Antigen-antibody binding then activates the complement cascade.

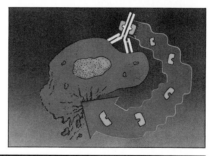

More cellular damage occurs during the membrane attack phase of the complement cascade. In this phase, C5b, 6, 7, 8, and 9 bind to the cell membrane, causing cytolysis.

granulocytes and mast cells. Granulocytes (neutrophils, eosinophils and basophils) arise from the stem cell. Mast cells may arise from a bone marrow precursor.

The granulocytes share certain developmental similarities; however, at maturation, they show distinguishable characteristics, such as the formation of granules with different staining properties. Mature neutrophils are actively phagocytic. Eosinophils play an important role in allergic reactions. Basophils and mast cells are essential for the function of an antibody (IgE) response that's important in anaphylactic reactions.

## IMMUNE MECHANISMS
Having reviewed the concepts of immunity and the anatomy and physiology of the organs and cells of the immune system, we're ready to consider the specific immune mechanisms: humoral, cell-mediated, and combined.
*(continued on page 24)*

# Gell and Coombs classification of hypersensitivity reactions

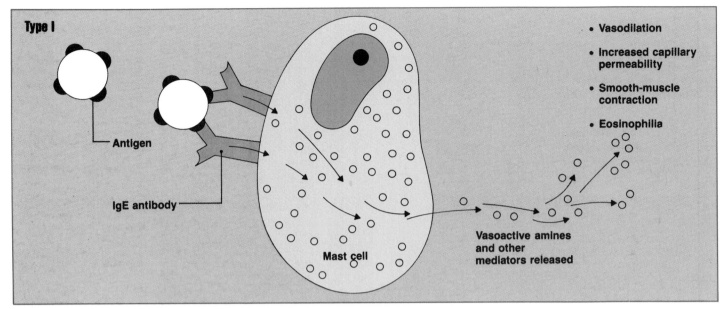

**Type I**

Antigen

IgE antibody

Mast cell

Vasoactive amines and other mediators released

- Vasodilation
- Increased capillary permeability
- Smooth-muscle contraction
- Eosinophilia

**Reactions**
Anaphylactic (immediate, atopic, IgE-mediated, reaginic)

**Pathophysiology**
IgE antibodies bind to certain cells; antigen binding causes release of vasoactive amines and other mediators, resulting in vasodilation, increased capillary permeability, smooth-muscle contraction, and eosinophilia.

**Signs and symptoms**
Systemic: angioedema; hypotension; bronchial, GI, or uterine spasm; stridor
Local: urticaria

**Clinical examples**
Extrinsic asthma, seasonal allergic rhinitis, systemic anaphylaxis, reactions to stinging insects, some food and drug reactions, some cases of urticaria, infantile eczema

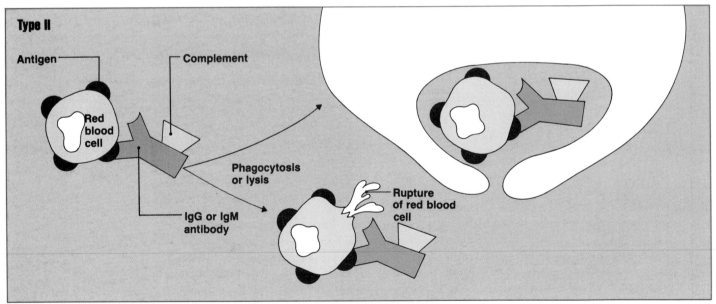

**Type II**

Antigen

Red blood cell

Complement

Phagocytosis or lysis

Rupture of red blood cell

IgG or IgM antibody

**Reactions**
Cytotoxic (cytolytic, complement-dependent cytotoxicity, cell-stimulating)

**Pathophysiology**
IgG or IgM antibodies bind to cellular or exogenous antigens. This can result in activation of complement components through C3 with phagocytosis or opsonization of the cell or activation of the full complement system with cytolysis or tissue damage.

**Signs and symptoms**
Varies with disease; can include dyspnea, hemoptysis, fever

**Clinical examples**
Goodpasture's syndrome, autoimmune hemolytic anemia, thrombocytopenia, pemphigus, pemphigoid, pernicious anemia, hyperacute graft rejection of transplanted kidney, transfusion reaction, hemolytic disease of the newborn, some drug reactions

## Gell and Coombs classification of hypersensitivity reactions (continued)

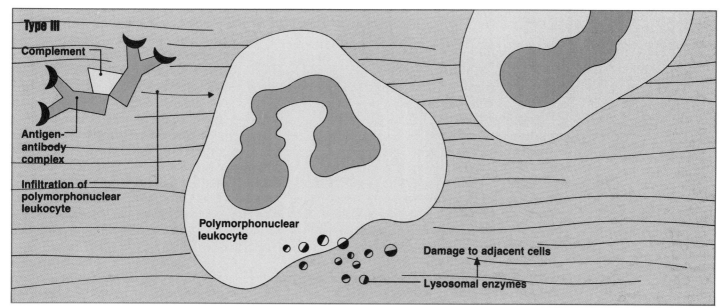

**Reactions**
Immune complex (soluble complex, toxic complex)

**Pathophysiology**
IgG or IgM antigen-antibody complexes are deposited in tissue where they activate complement. This reaction is marked by infiltration of polymorphonuclear leukocytes and by release of lysosomal proteolytic enzymes and permeability factors in tissues, which produce an acute, inflammatory reaction.

**Signs and symptoms**
Urticaria; multiform, scarlatiniform, or morbilliform rash; adenopathy; joint pain; fever; serum sickness–like syndrome

**Clinical examples**
Systemic: serum sickness due to serum, drugs, or viral hepatitis antigen; acute glomerulonephritis; systemic lupus erythematosus; rheumatoid arthritis; polyarteritis; cryoglobulinemia
Local: Arthus reaction

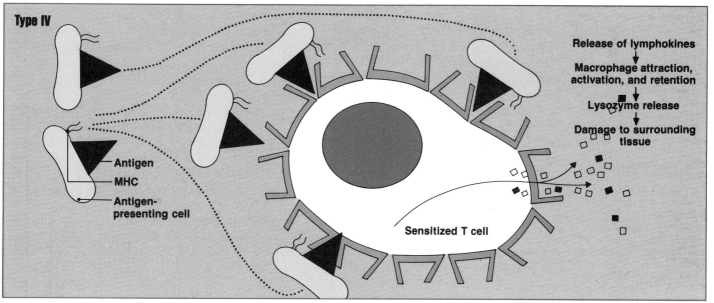

**Reactions**
Delayed (cellular, cell-mediated, tuberculin-type)

**Pathophysiology**
An antigen-presenting cell presents antigen to T cells in presence of MHC. The sensitized T cells release lymphokines, which stimulate macrophages; lysozymes are released; and surrounding tissue is damaged.

**Signs and symptoms**
Varies with disease; can include fever, erythema, and-itching.

**Clinical examples**
Contact dermatitis, graft-versus-host disease, allograft rejection, granuloma due to intracellular organisms, some drug sensitivities, Hashimoto's thyroiditis, tuberculosis, sarcoidosis

## Phagocytosis

In phagocytosis, two classes of phagocytic cells engulf microorganisms and other particles. The first and by far the most important class includes the polymorphonuclear leukocytes and macrophages. These cells are known as professional phagocytes because their membranes possess specialized receptors for the Fc portion of IgG molecules and for activated C3 complement component. Thus equipped, these cells easily ingest microorganisms coated with IgG or activated C3.

The second class of cells, called nonprofessional, or facultative phagocytes, includes endothelial and epithelial cells, fibroblasts, and other cells that ingest microorganisms under specialized conditions. Unlike professional phagocytes, these cells lack membrane receptors for IgG or C3.

Generally, phagocytosis involves five steps: in *chemotaxis,* the phagocytic cells move toward the antigen; in *opsonization,* the antigen becomes coated with opsonins that enhance macrophage binding; in *ingestion,* the opsonized antigen is engulfed in a vacuole (phagosome); in *digestion,* the phagosome merges with a lysosome to form a phagolysosome, where the antigen is destroyed; and in *release* (excretion), the digested antigen is expelled from the phagolysosome. (See *Steps of phagocytosis,* page 19.)

## The immune response

The body's response to antigens may be via two distinct mechanisms, *humoral* and *cell-mediated* immune responses, which work together in a *combined response* to combat immunologic threats.

**Humoral immunity.** This immune response produces specific antibodies against antigens such as bacteria, some viruses, and microbial toxins. It consists of two parts. The *primary* humoral response occurs when an antigen, such as a bacterium, is processed by a macrophage and presented to antigen-specific B cells. When stimulated by helper T cells, these B cells proliferate and differentiate; most of them develop into plasma cells that synthesize and release specific antibodies, and some differentiate into memory cells. Plasma cell antibodies then activate the complement system (see below), and the bacterium is either phagocytized or lysed.

In the *secondary* humoral response and in subsequent humoral responses, *memory cells* respond more rapidly and strongly to antigenic challenges.

*Complement pathways.* The complement system is the primary humoral activator of inflammation. It consists of approximately 20 distinct complement components, plasma proteins that normally circulate as functionally inactive molecules. These components are capable of interacting with each other, with antibody, and with cell membranes to mediate inflammatory reactions and to facilitate phagocytosis or cytolysis.

Complement activation follows one of two "cascading" sequential pathways: the *classical* pathway, activated by antigen-antibody complexes, and the *alternative* (properdin) pathway, activated by IgA; some IgG molecules; and certain complex polysaccharides, lipopolysaccharides, and trypsin-like enzymes. (See *Complement cascade: Two pathways of antigen destruction,* page 20.)

The activated complement system mediates inflammatory processes through two components, C5a and C3a, also known as anaphylatoxins. They cause chemotaxis and the release of vasoactive amines, such as histamine from mast cells; induce smooth-muscle contraction and increase vascular permeability; and cause granulocytes to aggregate and to release lysosomal enzymes.

Complement functions as an opsonin, binding to microorganisms and making them more susceptible to phagocytosis. It also causes cytolysis of various cells, bacteria, and viruses by depositing C5 to C9 on their surfaces. Known as the *membrane attack complex,* this deposition of C5 to C9 occurs by activation of the terminal portion of the complement sequence.

**Cell-mediated immunity.** This mechanism resists such antigens as fungi, viruses and rickettsiae, tuberculosis bacteria, transplanted tissues, and tumor cells. It also has primary and secondary components.

In a primary cell-mediated response, an antigen, such as tuberculosis bacterium, is processed by a macrophage and presented to immunocompetent T cells. (The macrophage is acting as an APC—an antigen-presenting cell.) The T cells become sensitized and flood the circulation; some locate antigens and destroy them. Other T cells become fixed (noncirculating) and release lymphokines that activate macrophages, thereby enhancing antigen destruction. Helper, suppressor, and memory T cells are also formed.

The memory cells recognize and promptly attack specific antigens long after the initial sensitization.

**Combined immune response.** Most antigens do not activate an independent humoral or cell-mediated response; instead they activate both, which involves interactions between macrophages and B and T cells.

The combined response begins when macrophages capture an antigen, process it, and present it to immunocompetent B and T cells. Either killer T cells attack and destroy the antigen directly, or certain lymphocytes may secrete lymphokines that recruit other cells such as macrophages. Other T cells (helper or suppressor) influence B-cell activation. (See *Combined immune response,* page 21.)

## PATHOPHYSIOLOGIC MECHANISMS
Immune disorders involve dysfunction of the immune response mechanism, causing over-responsiveness, or blocked, misdirected, or limited responsiveness to antigens. These disorders may result from a developmental defect, infection, malignancy, trauma, a metabolic disorder, or drug use. Immunologic disorders may be classified as immunodeficiency, hypersensitivity, autoimmune, and immunoproliferative disorders.

### Immunodeficiency disorders
These disorders result from impaired development of the immune system's structural components (cells) or defective expression of the immune response. Either can increase susceptibility to infection. (See Chapter 5.)

Immunodeficiency is classified as primary or secondary. Primary immunodeficiency results from a genetic or developmental defect of T cells, B cells, or tissues (such as the thymus). Since cells and tissues of the immune system develop sequentially, the stage at which the defect or interference occurs determines the type and severity of the disorder. Most immunodeficiency disorders involve an abnormal B- or T-cell response, or both. But abnormalities can also occur in phagocytic cells or in the complement system. Secondary immunodeficiency results from an underlying disease or factor that interferes with the immune system, depressing or altering the immune response.

### Hypersensitivity disorders
Instead of protecting the host, an exaggerated immune response (manifesting itself as hypersensitivity) can produce severe and even fatal results. (See Chapter 6.)

Hypersensitivity reactions generally do not occur after initial exposure (the sensitizing dose) to an antigenic stimulant (allergen); they follow reexposure after sensitization in a predisposed individual. Sensitization allows for synthesis of antibodies (humoral response) or proliferation of sensitized T cells (cell-mediated response). A classification of hypersensitivity reactions was devised by Gell and Coombs. (See *Gell and Coombs classification of hypersensitivity reactions,* pages 22 and 23.) Type I, II, and III reactions are mediated by antibodies (humoral response), whereas type IV reactions are mediated by T cells (cell-mediated response). Roitt has also proposed a fifth type, called stimulatory hypersensitivity, in which antibodies are directed against cellular receptors. Clinical examples of this reaction include myasthenia gravis and Graves' disease.

### Autoimmune disorders
Autoimmunity results from an inability to distinguish self from nonself, causing the immune system to direct immune responses against normal self tissue. (See Chapter 7.)

Autoimmune disorders may be classified as organ-specific diseases and generalized (systemic) diseases. Organ-specific diseases involve autoimmune reactions limited to one organ, as in thyroiditis. Generalized autoimmune diseases involve reactions in various body organs and tissues, as in systemic lupus erythematosus.

Immune response mechanisms that distinguish self from nonself are believed to be homeostatically regulated and are probably related to T-subset disorders or defective recognition of Class I antigens.

### Immunoproliferative disorders
An appropriate immune response hinges on B-cell proliferation into antibody-secreting cells and T-cell proliferation into sensitized T cells. Abnormal proliferation may cause an immunoproliferative disorder such as leukemia or lymphoma. (See Chapter 11.)

### Opportunities for dysfunction
The complexity of the immune system allows many opportunities for dysfunction. Fortunately, this intricate system has built-in safeguards of flexibility and duplication. When one defense mechanism falters, another may rally to combat antigens. However, when the immune system cannot compensate for dysfunction, the outcome may be devastating, since the body is then vulnerable to the attack of harmful antigens.

**Points to remember**

• The function of the immune system is to protect the body (self) from foreign materials, or antigens (nonself).
• The immune response to specific antigens is usually the result of an exquisitely well-regulated interplay between both humoral and cell-mediated responses. The humoral response involves B cells, which differentiate into plasma cells and produce antibodies to attack specific antigens. The cell-mediated response involves killer T cells, which, when sensitized, directly attack specific antigens; helper T cells, which spur B-cell proliferation and differentiation into plasma cells; suppressor T cells, which can limit antibody production; other T cells, which produce mediators such as lymphokines; and memory T cells, which can mount a quick response upon reexposure to the same antigen.
• Alteration of immune mechanisms can result in immunodeficiency, hypersensitivity, autoimmune, or immunoproliferative disorders.
• Knowledge and understanding of recent and continuing advances in immunology can help you deal effectively with disorders of this complex system.

# 2 ASSESSING IMMUNE FUNCTION

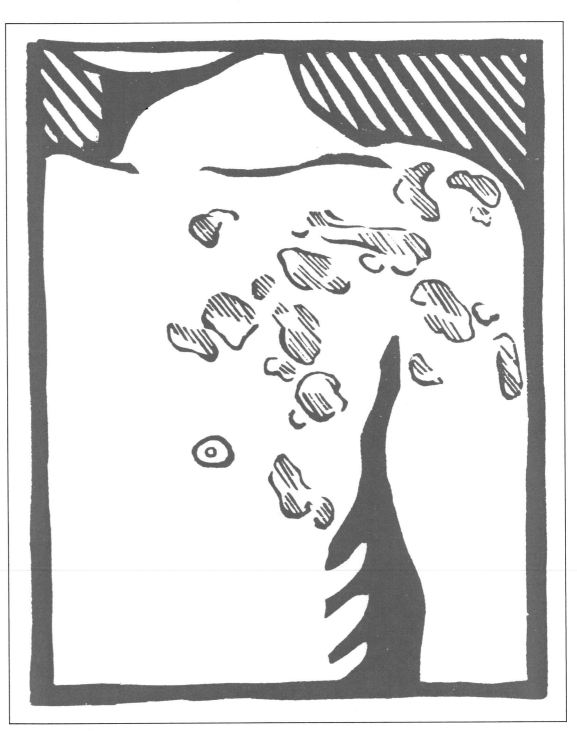

Extensive urticaria

As a nurse, you're bound to know the great difficulty involved in assessing patients with immune disorders. No other area of nursing assessment is so clinically confusing and requires you to keep so many different points of clinical reference in your mind at the same time.

Since immune disorders produce multisystemic effects, immune assessment requires a thorough nursing history, a total physical assessment, and the ability to recognize immune-related symptoms.

Consider, for example, a patient who complains of heartburn, looks tired and extremely underweight, and says he has trouble swallowing. Does he have a primary GI disorder? Not necessarily. Your nursing history reveals that his joints ache, that his skin shows changes in pigmentation, and that his hands become paralyzed in cold weather. Recognizing these as possible immune-related signs and symptoms and as a pattern of an autoimmune disorder, you may reasonably suspect scleroderma in preference to a nonimmune disorder.

This chapter will help you achieve such accurate assessments by guiding you in collecting a comprehensive data base and by helping you understand the classification of immune disorders.

### Immune classification
Throughout your assessment, keep in mind the following classification of immune dysfunction.
• *immunodeficiency disorders,* such as severe combined immunodeficiency (SCID) and acquired immunodeficiency syndrome (AIDS)
• *hypersensitivity disorders,* including asthma, infantile eczema, urticaria, and GI reactions to specific foods
• *autoimmune disorders,* including such diverse disorders as systemic lupus erythematosus (SLE), rheumatoid arthritis, progressive systemic sclerosis (PSS), myositis, ankylosing spondylitis, Reiter's syndrome, psoriatic arthritis, and arthritis associated with chronic inflammatory bowel disease
• *immunoproliferative disorders,* such as leukemias, lymphomas, and plasma cell dyscrasias.

### Prepare the environment
Make sure to conduct your examination in a well-lit, warm room. Set the examining table at a convenient height for examining the patient when he's lying down *and* when he's sitting up. Then check your equipment. You'll need the following: otoscope; ophthalmoscope; nasal speculum; penlight; tongue blade; sphygmomanometer; stethoscope; tape measure (calibrated in millimeters and centimeters); reflex hammer; cotton-tipped applicator; cotton; pins with sharp and dull ends; tuning fork; and soap for testing the sense of smell.

### Prepare the patient
As for any physical assessment, begin by introducing yourself to the patient and explaining what you are about to do. Try to put him at ease, and give him a chance to ask questions about the examination.

Even at this early stage, begin to form impressions of the patient's physical and mental status.

### HISTORY AND OBSERVATION
As you know, signs and symptoms of immune disorders can appear in any body system, so you need to obtain a complete history. This complete history will help you correctly identify such nonspecific symptoms as fatigue or shortness of breath, as part of a pattern of an immune disorder.

As you talk with the patient, pay attention to his general appearance and record any signs of possible illness. For example, does he look emaciated or older than his stated age? Does he appear tired, anxious, depressed, or in pain?

### Determine the chief complaint
Ask the patient his chief complaint—why he is seeking medical help. Record his complaint in his own words. Obtain further information about his present illness by asking appropriate follow-up questions.

**Abnormal bleeding.** Ask the patient about any unusual bleeding (such as frequent nosebleeds) or frequent, unexplained bruises. (Easy bruising can indicate a platelet or clotting mechanism deficiency.)

A platelet or clotting mechanism deficiency can occur in certain immunodeficiencies and immune disorders and also during antineoplastic drug therapy and drug therapy to prevent rejection of transplanted body parts.

Ask the patient if he experiences prolonged bleeding after accidentally cutting himself and if he ever starts bleeding for no apparent reason. Has he passed black stools or bloody urine? If your patient is female, has she experienced unusually heavy menstrual periods, possibly indicating Hashimoto's disease? Also remember that excessive bleeding can cause anemia.

**Lymphadenopathy.** If the patient has noticed any swelling in his neck, armpits, or groin, ask when he first noticed it; whether the swollen areas are sore, hard, or red; and whether they're on one or both sides. Swollen lymph nodes may mean inflammation, infection, or the elevated lymphocyte production characteristic of certain leukemias. Primary lymphatic tumors typically aren't painful, but red, tender, enlarged lymph nodes may accompany Hodgkin's disease.

Also find out whether the patient has ever had a biopsy of an enlarged lymph node and if he has a history of malignancy.

**Fatigue and weakness.** Ask the patient who complains of fatigue if he feels tired all the time or only after exertion. How much sleep does he get at night? Does he take naps during the day? Find out if he has a history of anemia.

If the patient complains of weakness, ask whether it began recently or has been developing for some time. Is it persistent, or does it come and go? Ask him to describe his ability to perform activities of daily living, such as taking care of personal hygiene, doing his laundry, cooking, or driving a car.

Fatigue and weakness—present in most patients with immune disorders—can have various causes, depending on the specific disorder. Occurring with exertion, fatigue and weakness may suggest moderate anemia; extreme or constant fatigue and weakness may suggest severe anemia or neuropathy from an autoimmune disease.

**Fever.** Ask the patient with fever when his fever began, whether it's constant or intermittent, and what his highest temperature has been. If his temperature fluctuates, ask over what period of time. A fever that recurs every few days (Pel-Ebstein fever) characterizes Hodgkin's disease, whereas temperatures that rise and fall within a 24-hour period may indicate an infection such as gonococcal endocarditis. Frequently recurring fevers may indicate an impaired immune system or rapid cell proliferation. In a patient with serum sickness or allergy, temperature may reach 103° to 105° F. (39.4° to 40.5° C.); in a patient with thyrotoxicosis or malignancy without infection, however, temperature elevation may be slight, in the 99.5°-to-100.5° F. (37.5°-to-38.1° C.) range.

**Joint pain.** If the patient has joint pain, ask which joints are affected. Pain in any joint may suggest an autoimmune disorder. Ask if the pain occurs bilaterally; if it's accompanied by redness, swelling, warmth, nausea, or dizziness; and if he feels any bone pain. Is his pain continuous, intermittent, or transient? How long has it persisted? Ask him to rate his pain level on a scale of 0 to 10.

Assess his degree of disability from pain. What activities increase his pain? Does he feel pain at rest? Do his joints feel stiff in the morning? How does he relieve the pain? Does pain affect his outlook on life, his attitude toward others, and his eating habits (appetite or ability to eat)?

### Review medical history

Review the patient's medical history to help you identify conditions or diseases that may affect his present illness.

**General health.** Keep in mind that patients with immune disorders often report poor general health, and patients with immunodeficiency syndrome or immunosuppression experience recurrent infections.

**Allergies.** Ask the patient if he has a history of allergies or if he has ever come in contact with a substance that caused itching, rash, swelling, fever, or difficulty breathing. Have him describe the reaction, including how long it lasted and any treatment he received for it. If he has asthma or you suspect asthma, ask about precipitating factors. Ask if he has a pet: animal dander is a common allergen. Also ask the patient to describe any allergic drug reaction he has experienced. He may be mistaking an adverse effect for a drug allergy.

**Drug use.** Obtain a history of drugs the patient has taken, including over-the-counter remedies, prescription drugs, and illicit drugs, if any. This information can be critically significant, because many drugs can enhance or suppress the immune system. For example, antibiotics, corticosteroids, and chemotherapeutic agents commonly depress immune function. Patients who use illegal drugs, such as heroin, intravenously may be at risk for contracting acquired immunodeficiency syndrome (AIDS) and hepatitis.

**Diseases and past therapies.** Ask the patient about any preexisting health problems, especially if the patient has ever been diagnosed as having cancer or an autoimmune disease. (Remember, having one autoimmune disease predisposes a patient to other autoimmune diseases.) Ask about past radiation treatments that can cause diminished blood-cell production. For example, radiation of the thymus during childhood is significant. Past surgeries are also significant, especially thymectomy and organ transplants, such as kidney transplants.

**Immunizations.** Obtain a complete immunization history (pertussis, diphtheria, measles, polio, tetanus); this is especially important if your patient is a child.

## Discuss family history

Attempt to obtain a detailed history of immune disorders occurring in the patient's family. Pernicious anemia and hemolytic anemia are examples of immune disorders that can be inherited.

## Take an occupational history

Focus on exposure to irritating or toxic materials, radiation, or infectious agents, and on any allergic responses to substances in the work environment. Be sure to consider any hazardous exposure through military service, such as exposure to Agent Orange.

## Consider psychosocial factors

Certain aspects of a patient's life-style can increase his risk of developing an immune disorder. Ask about the following:

**Stress.** Persistently high levels of stress can reduce resistance to infection. Ask the patient if there have been any major changes in his life in the past 2 years (deaths, job changes, divorce, marriage). Does he have a stressful job or home situation?

**Diet.** Ask the patient what he eats and drinks in a typical day and whether he restricts his diet according to religious, cultural, or personal beliefs. Remember that protein intake is necessary for immunoglobulin production; this means that a severely protein-deficient diet can result in lymphoid tissue atrophy, diminished antibody response, reduction in T-cell circulation, and impaired cell-mediated immunity. Ask the patient whether he uses any dietary supplements, such as vitamins or caloric supplements? Find out about his appetite and any unintentional weight gain or loss. (Weight loss is typical in patients with AIDS, rheumatoid arthritis, or cancer.) Ask about alcohol intake, which can cause nutritional deficiency.

Also ask the patient whether he has reactions to any common food allergens—shellfish, strawberries, milk, chocolate, or eggs. Ask him to describe the reaction so you can distinguish between food intolerance and true allergic reaction. Food intolerance may cause

a mild GI disturbance. Its severity doesn't increase with repeated exposure. Allergic reaction increases in severity with repeated ingestion and may cause laryngeal edema, wheals, and severe nausea and vomiting.

**Sexual preference.** Homosexuality may be a factor increasing the risk of contracting AIDS. So be sure to ask the patient about his sexual preference.

**Self-image.** Ask the patient to describe himself and how he feels about himself; then try to assess his self-image. Keep in mind that a chronic autoimmune disorder (such as rheumatoid arthritis), with accompanying body changes, can profoundly affect a patient's self-image. Ask him about body changes he's noticed since his illness began and how those changes have affected him. Ask what his roles and responsibilities were before his illness— have they changed? If so, how?

**Family and social environment.** If he has a family, ask the patient whether they support and comfort him—and each other. Can he describe how his family perceives his illness? If he doesn't have a family or receives little support from them, find out if he has any close friends or is involved in any social group that can provide support. If necessary, refer him to a supportive agency.

**Coping ability.** Immunodeficiency diseases, such as AIDs, and chronic autoimmune disorders, such as multiple sclerosis, can be devastating. Inquire about stressful events in the patient's family history. What did he and his family members do to cope with these events? Has there been a change in his family's coping abilities related to his present illness? If necessary, refer the family to a supportive agency.

## Conduct a systems review

Proceeding according to body systems, ask the patient about signs and symptoms related to immune dysfunction.

**Skin.** Question whether the patient has noticed any changes in his skin's texture and pigmentation. A patient with scleroderma, for example, typically has hard, thickened, and rigid skin with pigmented patches. Has he noted any itching or rashes, characteristic of allergic reactions? Is his skin dry, as in Hashimoto's disease?

Does he have a history of Raynaud's phenomenon in which his fingers turned blue, white, then red and felt tingly or numb? Emotional upset and exposure to cold may trigger these attacks. Has your patient experienced

## Assessing ocular muscle strength

**Six cardinal fields of gaze.** To perform this test, hold a pencil, tongue depressor, or your finger in front of the patient's eyes. Ask her to hold her head still and to follow the movement of the object with her eyes. Then move the object clockwise through the six cardinal fields.

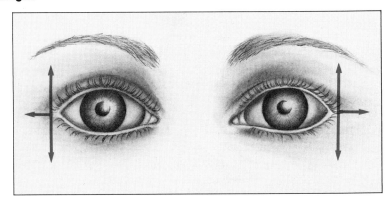

**Convergence test.** To perform the convergence test, hold the object in front of the patient and move it slowly toward the bridge of her nose. Her eyes should converge and remain that way until the object is approximately 2″ to 3″ (5 to 8 cm) away.

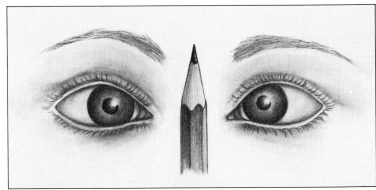

either recently? What effect does exposure to sunlight have on his skin? A patient with SLE may complain of photosensitivity to sunlight.

Also ask the patient whether he's noticed unusually slow healing in any cuts or sores; this may indicate a malignancy or immunodeficiency.

**Eyes.** Ask about recent vision problems, such as double vision or increased sensitivity to light, that can indicate Graves' disease or SLE.

**Ears.** Ask the patient if he's noticed any recent hearing loss or discharge from his ears. Find out when his last hearing test was done. Keep in mind that ear infections and Hashimoto's disease can decrease hearing.

**Cardiopulmonary system.** Ask the patient if he's experienced any wheezing, rhinitis, or difficulty breathing; if so, consider the possibility of an allergic reaction. Dyspnea may suggest anemia, connective tissue disease, or infection.

Find out if he has experienced chest pain, which may signal pericarditis in a patient with SLE. Has he noticed any irregular or rapid heart beats? Atrial dysrhythmia and tachycardia can occur in patients with Graves' disease. Tachycardia can also mean infection in patients with immunodeficiency disorders, such as AIDS and immunodeficiency syndrome.

**Genitourinary system.** Ask the patient if he's noticed pain on urination, frequency, or a change in the appearance of his urine (hematuria can occur in glomerulonephritis). Has he experienced any incontinence, a common problem in patients with multiple sclerosis (MS) or myasthenia gravis?

Also ask the patient about sexual function. Chronic illness or pain can have a profound effect on sexual performance and satisfaction. Begin by asking about his usual pattern of sexual functioning. Then question him about his present pattern. Specifically ask the male patient if he is experiencing any difficulty with erection or ejaculation.

**Gastrointestinal system.** Has the patient experienced nausea, vomiting, loss of appetite, or bowel changes? These signs and symptoms can signal autoimmune disease. Ask about dysphagia, a characteristic of scleroderma.

**Neurologic system.** Immune disorders can affect sensory and motor functions and mental status. Has he had trouble performing activities of daily living, such as household chores, food shopping, cooking, driving a car, or taking care of personal hygiene? This is common in patients with neurologic disorders such as myasthenia gravis or MS. If he reports a pins-and-needles sensation or has trouble walking, he may have pernicious anemia. Find out if the patient is experiencing emotional instability, irritability, depression, or headaches. These are common in chronic immune disorders.

## THE PHYSICAL EXAMINATION
After you've completed the history, proceed to a detailed, comprehensive, and systematic physical examination, checking for clues to immune dysfunction.

Ask the patient to undress and put on a hospital gown. Make sure to ask him to urinate, too, because you'll be doing deep abdominal palpation.

Now, compare the patient's weight to the normal weight for his height, bone structure, and build. Then obtain vital signs to use as baseline measurements during the patient's care. (Remember that fluctuations in temperature, heart rate, respiratory rate, and blood pressure are common in patients with immune disorders.)

### Observe facial features
Look for facial edema, facial weakness, and grimacing or lack of facial expression. Edema may indicate glomerulonephritis or Hashimoto's disease. Facial weakness occurs in myasthenia gravis, producing either lack of expression or a snarling expression when the patient smiles.

### Inspect the skin
Assess the patient's skin for pallor, cyanosis, or jaundice. Pallor can occur in pernicious anemia. Pallor and jaundice may be present in hemolytic anemia.

Check for areas of erythema, possibly indicating local inflammation. Evaluate the skin's texture, mobility, temperature, and thickness; keep in mind these facts.
• In Hashimoto's disease, the patient may have a sallow complexion and very dry, coarse skin.
• In PSS, the skin is taut.
• In Graves' disease, the patient's skin is typically pink, warm, smooth, and sweaty.

If you suspect your patient has scleroderma or SLE, assess him for the characteristic signs of Raynaud's phenomenon—intermittent vasospasm of digital arterioles, usually of hands but sometimes of the nose or tongue, result in a blanching of the affected part, followed by a reactive hyperemia (blue, white, then red).

Check the skin for petechiae or purpuric lesions, classic signs of autoimmune thrombo-cytopenic purpura. Palpate for subcutaneous nodules characteristic of rheumatoid arthritis. In myxedema and Graves' disease, you may see pretibial edema, from mucopolysaccharide substances infiltrating the skin. Also observe for signs of infection, such as abnormally warm skin, erythema, pain, wound drainage, ulceration, or poor wound healing.

Sometimes rashes accompany immune disorders. Check for the characteristic butterfly rash of SLE and the heliotrope rash of dermatomyositis. Look for allergic skin reactions, such as wheals, eczema, and angioneurotic edema. Wheals are areas of localized skin edema varying in size and shape and accompanied by itching (acute or chronic hives). Eczema is an allergic response characterized by symmetrical lesions, redness, weeping, and dry scales. Angioneurotic edema usually results from food allergy and manifests as local allergic wheals accompanied by subcutaneous or submucosal swelling.

### Inspect the hair and nails
Check the texture and distribution of the patient's hair. Look for patches of alopecia (baldness or hair loss) on his arms, legs, and head and for short, broken hairs above the forehead (lupus hairs)—these are both signs of SLE. In patients with hypothyroidism, hair and eyebrows are dry, coarse, and lifeless. Patients with Graves' disease generally have thin, fine hair.

Inspect the nails for longitudinal striations (characteristic of anemia), platyonychia (abnormally broad or flat nails), and koilonychia (spoon nail). Platyonychia can progress to koilonychia, characteristic of iron deficiency anemia. Check also for onycholysis (separation of nails from nailbeds) and brittleness, common in Hashimoto's disease.

### Examine the eyes
Inspect the eyes for edema, redness, lesions, and position and alignment of the eyeballs. Abnormal protrusion (giving a wide-eyed, staring appearance), upper and lower lid retraction, and lid lag signify Graves' disease. In lid lag, the edge of the sclera appears between the upper lid and the iris. Ptosis (drooping of the eyelids) occurs in myasthenia gravis. Periorbital edema occurs in Graves' disease and glomerulonephritis.

Test for ocular muscle weakness using the six cardinal fields of gaze. (See *Assessing ocular muscle strength.*) Perform this test more than once. Muscle weakness increases with

## Palpating lymph nodes

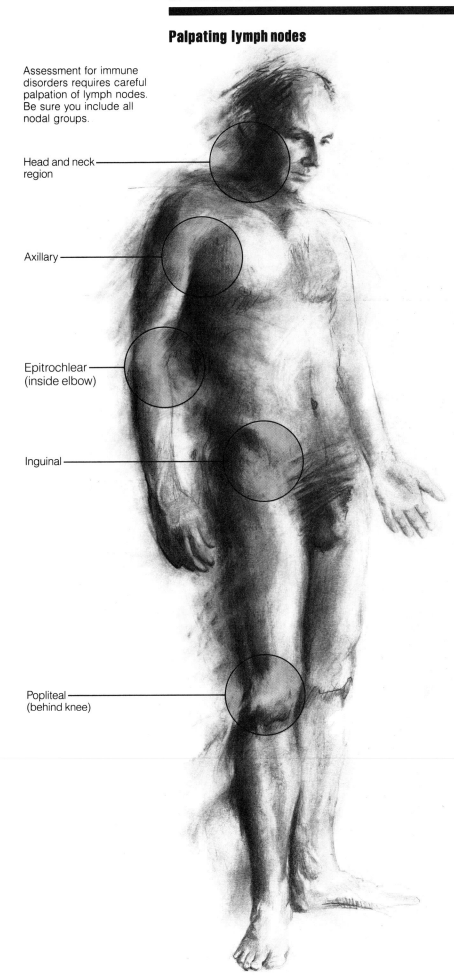

Assessment for immune disorders requires careful palpation of lymph nodes. Be sure you include all nodal groups.

Head and neck region

Axillary

Epitrochlear (inside elbow)

Inguinal

Popliteal (behind knee)

fatigue. Patients with myasthenia gravis experience transient ocular muscle weakness.

Note the convergence of the patient's eyes. Have him follow your finger or pen as you bring it toward the bridge of his nose. Normally, convergence will be sustained to within 5 to 8 cm. Poor convergence can be a symptom of Graves' disease.

Gently pull down the lower lids to check for pallor. Pale conjunctivae may indicate hemolytic anemia or anemia accompanying SLE, or rheumatoid arthritis. Also inspect for conjunctivitis (discharge with lid swelling), a sign of some immunodeficiency infections and hypersensitivity disorders.

Using the ophthalmoscope, examine the retinas for tortuosity, hemorrhage, or infiltration.

### Examine the ears

Using an otoscope, observe the ear canal and tympanic membrane for signs of otitis media, an infection frequently found in patients with immune disorders. In otitis media, the tympanic membrane looks erythematous and possibly bulging; landmarks are indistinct; and the light reflex is displaced. Beware—if the patient has drainage in the ear canal, don't insert the otoscope; this could push the drainage inward. Bloody, then serosanguineous, and finally purulent otorrhea may follow spontaneous perforation of the tympanic membrane.

Use your voice to test auditory acuity. Test one ear at a time, occluding the untested one. Stand 1' to 2' from the patient. To prevent lip reading, stand behind him. Begin whispering numbers and progress to a loud voice as needed. Ask the patient to repeat what he hears. Patients with Hashimoto's disease may show diminished auditory acuity.

### Examine the nose and mouth

Examine the nasal cavity by pushing the tip of the patient's nose upward and shining a penlight into the nostrils. Look for ulceration of the mucous membranes, seen in SLE, and for the pale, boggy turbinates and polyps typical of chronic allergy.

Next, examine the mucous membranes of the mouth, again using a penlight. Check for color variations, ulcers, and white patches of exudate.

Patients with SLE sometimes develop ulcerations of the mouth. Patients receiving chemotherapy and immunodeficient patients may develop oral *Candida* infections characterized by white patches of exudate and ulcerations.

Inspect the patient's tongue. Keep in mind that certain diseases, such as Hashimoto's disease and multiple myeloma, cause tongue enlargement. Check for a fine tremor of the fully extended tongue, which may occur in some patients with Graves' disease. Look also for tonsillar hypertrophy, which occurs in patients with chronic lymphomas.

### Examine the neck
Check for thyroid changes. In certain immune disorders, such as Graves' disease and Hashimoto's disease, the thyroid gland becomes enlarged. To check for this, ask the patient to take a sip of water; then have him extend his neck slightly and swallow. If you can see enlarged thyroid tissue, note its contour and symmetry. Have the patient swallow again and palpate the thyroid for size, firmness, and tenderness. In a patient with Hashimoto's disease, it's smooth or nodular and substantially firmer and more rubbery than normal, and palpation doesn't cause pain. In a patient with Graves' disease, the thyroid feels slightly firmer than normal, and palpation is painless.

**Palpate the lymph nodes.** Use your finger pads to move the patient's skin over each nodal area. Begin with the neck nodes, and proceed to other nodal areas—axillary, epitrochlear, inguinal, and popliteal—as you examine each related area of the body. (See *Palpating lymph nodes.*)

As you palpate the nodes, note their size and firmness and whether they're fixed or movable, tender or painless. When you palpate neck nodes, be sure the patient is sitting. For palpation of the axillary nodes, he should be sitting or lying down, with his right arm relaxed. Use your nondominant hand to support his right arm, and put your other hand as high in his right axilla as possible. Palpate against the chest wall for the lateral, anterior, posterior central, and subclavian nodes. Follow the same procedure for the left axilla. For the epitrochlear nodes, palpate the medial area of the elbow. For the inguinal nodes, palpate below the inguinal ligament and along the upper saphenous vein.

Enlarged nodes indicate acute or chronic inflammation. In acute infection, nodes are large, tender, and discrete. In chronic infection, they become confluent. In metastatic cancer, involved nodes (generally unilateral) are discrete, nontender, and firm or hard. Generalized lymphadenopathy (involving three or more node groups) occurs in certain autoimmune disorders such as SLE, infectious disorders, and neoplastic disorders. In SLE, nodal enlargement may be diffuse or local.

### Assess respiratory function
Immune disorders often result in respiratory difficulty, so assess your patient's respiratory status thoroughly.

**Breathing pattern.** Begin by observing the patient's breathing pattern and looking for signs of respiratory distress, such as dyspnea, wheezing, or cyanosis. Chest expansion may be restricted in patients with scleroderma. In patients with bronchial asthma, breathing may be slow or fast and laborious, with wheezing. (During a bronchial asthma attack, the patient sits up to use every accessory muscle, chest expansion is hardly visible, expiration is more strenuous and prolonged than inspiration, and interspaces bulge on expiration and retract on inspiration.) In patients with pneumonia and *Pneumocystis carinii,* which often occur in AIDS, breathing may be labored, rapid, and shallow.

Assess the patient's cough. Is it productive or nonproductive? If it's productive, note the color, consistency, and odor of the sputum. Frothy, thin, white sputum can result from an asthmatic attack.

**Percussion and auscultation.** Percuss the anterior, lateral, and posterior areas of the patient's chest wall bilaterally, comparing one side to the other and avoiding bony areas. Dullness indicates consolidation, as in pneumonia; hyperresonance could mean trapped air, as in bronchial asthma.

Auscultate symmetrical areas of the lungs, too, following the pattern you used for percussion. During auscultation, ask the patient to breathe through his mouth slowly and more deeply than usual. Carefully listen for pitch, intensity, and duration of both inspiration and expiration.

Also listen for abnormal sounds, such as wheezes, crackles, and pleural rubs, and note their location and when in the breathing cycle they occur (inspiratory or expiratory phase). In a patient with bronchial asthma, breath sounds may be distant; you may hear wheezes, especially during expiration. In a patient with pneumonia and pneumocystitis, you may hear bronchial breath sounds and crackles over the affected lung.

Next, test the patient for egophony, bronchophony, and whispered pectoriloquy, which may be present over areas of consolidation and pleural effusion.

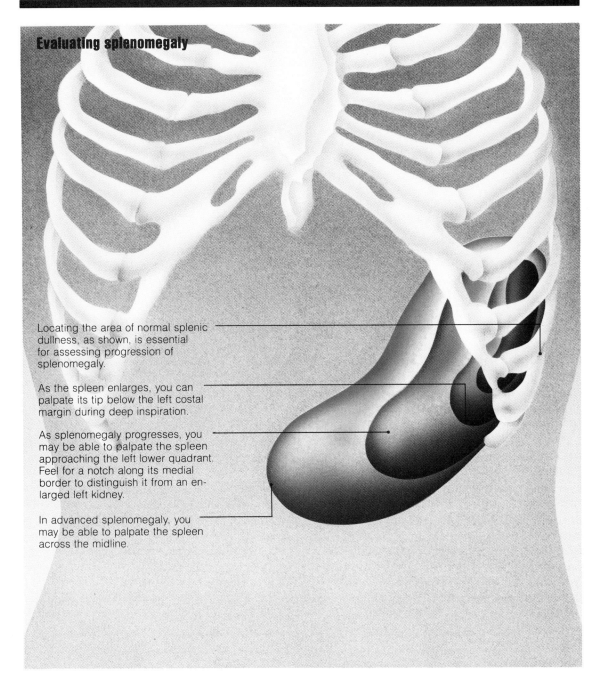

**Evaluating splenomegaly**

Locating the area of normal splenic dullness, as shown, is essential for assessing progression of splenomegaly.

As the spleen enlarges, you can palpate its tip below the left costal margin during deep inspiration.

As splenomegaly progresses, you may be able to palpate the spleen approaching the left lower quadrant. Feel for a notch along its medial border to distinguish it from an enlarged left kidney.

In advanced splenomegaly, you may be able to palpate the spleen across the midline.

**Evaluate cardiovascular changes**
Measure the patient's blood pressure first while he's lying down, then while he's sitting, and then while he's standing. A patient with Graves' disease may exhibit an elevated systolic pressure with a wide pulse pressure or a rapid, irregular pulse, indicating atrial fibrillation or atrial flutter. Tachycardia may accompany anemia or infection.

Listen for pericardial friction rubs. To do so, place the patient in a prone position. Use the diaphragm of the stethoscope to auscultate the precordium during deep expiration. A pericardial friction rub sound is high-pitched and sounds like two pieces of leather rubbing together. You can hear it during the entire cardiac cycle. Pericardial friction rub is associated with endocarditis or pericarditis with effusion. It occurs in approximately 50% of patients with SLE and also in patients with scleroderma.

Check for impaired peripheral circulation by assessing for such signs as Raynaud's phenomenon (severe pallor and paresthesia of the fingers or toes).

**Examine the abdomen**
Inspect the abdomen with the patient in a supine position. Look for pigmentation changes as seen in scleroderma. Also, you'll

be able to more readily see jaundice (from hepatitis) in the abdomen than you would in less exposed areas. Also observe for allergic rashes, wheals, and eczema. Note the presence of any small, hard, painless nodules spread over a wide area.

**Auscultate all four quadrants for bowel sounds.** In some autoimmune disorders that cause diarrhea, such as ulcerative colitis and Crohn's disease, bowel sounds are increased. But in some autoimmune disorders and in scleroderma, bowel sounds are decreased as a result of constipation.

**Percuss the liver and spleen.** Normally, the liver's span is 2.4″ to 4.7″ (6 to 12 cm). The spleen should produce dullness on the left side between the sixth and tenth ribs just posterior to the midaxillary line. Hepatosplenomegaly occurs in many immune disorders, such as idiopathic thrombocytopenic purpura, hemolytic anemia, immunodeficiency disorders, and lymphomas. (See *Evaluating splenomegaly.*)

**Palpate for masses and enlarged organs.** Note the exact location and characteristics of any masses you find. If the liver is enlarged but smooth and tender, suspect hepatitis; if it's enlarged but hard and nodular, suspect a neoplasm. The spleen is not normally palpable; if you can palpate it, it's already at least three times its normal size.

Finally, palpate for abdominal tenderness, an indication of possible infection. Infections are common in patients with immunodeficiency disorders.

### Assess neurologic function
A patient with a suspected or confirmed immune disorder should have a thorough neurologic evaluation. Neurologic effects of immune disorders are common and varied. A patient with SLE, for example, may experience altered mentation, depression, or psychosis; convulsions; cranial nerve palsies; and peripheral neuritis. (Peripheral neuropathy is also the most frequent neurologic complication of rheumatoid arthritis.)

### Determine musculoskeletal limitations
Ask the patient to perform some simple maneuvers, such as walking, standing up, or bending over. Test his range of motion, too, particularly for the joints of the hands, wrists, and knees. Palpate the joints, and test his muscle strength by applying resistance to his movements as he performs active range-of-motion exercises.

In rheumatoid arthritis, joint involvement is symmetrical. In early stages, this disorder affects the small joints of the hands and feet; in later stages, it affects the large joints (knees, hips, elbows, ankles, and shoulders). Severely affected joints become red, deformed, and swollen; joint movement in any direction produces pain. Eventually, the patient experiences muscle weakness and limited mobility.

In patients with SLE, joints may be red, swollen, and painful on movement, but not deformed; muscle weakness is common in patients with dermatomyositis.

In patients with PSS, contracted skin and, possibly, muscle weakness severely limit mobility. The patient may have trouble with such simple motions as opening and closing his jaw, closing his lips over his teeth, and moving his fingers.

In patients with Graves' disease, expect hyperkinesis. Look for a fine tremor when fingers are extended and for proximal muscle weakness.

MS causes extensive muscle weakness and progressive atrophy. If your patient has MS, assess quadriceps involvement by asking him to rise from a chair. A patient with weakened quadriceps pushes on the arms of a chair to stand up.

A patient with myasthenia gravis may have trouble standing up, climbing stairs, combing his hair, or even holding his head up. Muscle weakness (generally proximal) increases with repeated exertion and is more severe at the end of the day. It may or may not be present when the muscles are at rest.

### NURSING DIAGNOSES
After you've completed your assessment, integrate and organize your impressions and data to form appropriate nursing diagnoses and to allow for timely intervention. Keep in mind that nursing diagnoses specify actual or potential health-care problems that nurses can resolve, prevent, or reduce.

Common nursing diagnoses for patients with immune disorders include knowledge deficit, potential for ineffective coping, and disturbance in self-concept. Examples of diagnoses for specific disorders include alterations in comfort: pain and activity intolerance in patients with rheumatoid arthritis and polymyositis; and potential for infections in patients with AIDS or immunodeficiency syndrome. For all immune disorders, keep your diagnoses and care plan relevant with continual immune system assessment.

**Points to remember**

- A thorough history and physical examination can reveal subtle characteristics of immune disorders, which may initially appear to result from other body system dysfunctions.
- Three categories of immune disorders are immunodeficiency disorders, hypersensitivity disorders, and autoimmune disorders.
- The most common chief complaints of patients with immune disorders are abnormal bleeding, lymphadenopathy, fatigue and weakness, fever, and joint pain.
- Significant predisposing factors in immune disorders include a family history of immune disorders, a history of radiation treatments, and a history of drug use including prescription drugs, over-the-counter drugs, or illicit drugs.

# 3 UPDATING DIAGNOSTIC CONCEPTS

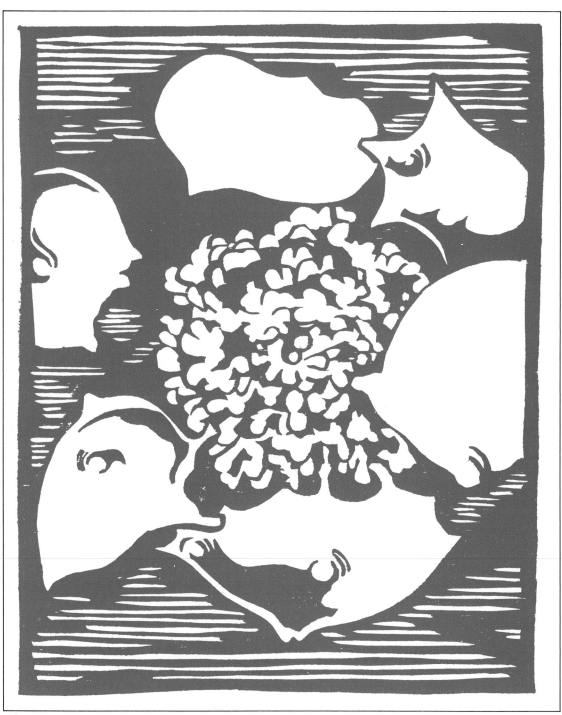

T cell encircled by sheep erythrocytes

Recent advances in understanding the chemistry and biology of immune mechanisms have significantly improved diagnosis of immunologic disorders by refining some traditional tests and replacing others with more accurate methods. Some of the newest tests use monoclonal antibodies, which allow unlimited numbers of completely homogeneous antibodies for typing cells and cell subsets, detecting specific antigens, and differentiating between malignant and nonmalignant cells. (See *Producing monoclonal antibodies,* page 38.)

These changes have enlarged your nursing role beyond the traditional supportive one. Now, in addition to supporting the patient, you must teach him about the tests he'll undergo and monitor his condition throughout the diagnostic workup. These responsibilities require that you understand diagnostic methods and know the implications of their results. This chapter reviews the tests you can expect to be ordered for patients studied for immune dysfunction.

### Basic immunologic methods

Diagnostic immunology uses various in vitro techniques, such as immunodiffusion, agglutination, precipitation, immunofluorescence, and radioimmunoassay.

Agglutination and precipitation reactions form the basis of many tests of humoral immune activity. In *agglutination,* a solid or particulate antigen and a soluble antibody form a lattice. The antigen is part of the surface of some particle—a red blood cell (RBC), bacterium, or inorganic particle. In *precipitation,* a soluble antigen and a soluble antibody form a complex lattice of interlocking aggregate, which may remain soluble or eventually fall to the bottom of the test container. To determine concentrations of antibody in a test sample, a known amount of antigen is added to a solution of antiserum containing an unknown amount of antibody. Clumping indicates agglutination, and cloudiness indicates precipitation. Results are based on standards with known concentrations.

To obtain a sample of lymphocytes for in vitro testing, whole blood is diluted with normal saline solution or another medium, then layered over a Ficoll-Hypaque gradient. This high-molarity solution separates cells according to density. After centrifugation, dense cells (RBCs and granulocytes) settle at the bottom, and lighter cells (lymphocytes, monocytes, and platelets) settle in the middle in a white layer. This second layer is pipetted out, then washed to remove platelets. The remaining lymphocytes are then used for various laboratory studies.

### THE DIAGNOSTIC WORKUP

Laboratory evaluation of the immune system begins with the complete blood count and differential and may also include T- and B-lymphocyte proliferation tests and T- and B-lymphocyte counts.

### Complete blood count and differential

This test provides quantitative values for hemoglobin, hematocrit, platelets, RBCs, and white blood cells (WBCs). Decreased hematocrit and hemoglobin levels indicate anemia, a common finding in Goodpasture's syndrome, rheumatoid arthritis, and systemic lupus erythematosus (SLE). A decreased platelet count (thrombocytopenia) can result from autoimmune disorders. The differential cell count provides values for neutrophils, eosinophils, basophils, monocytes, and lymphocytes. Abnormal WBC counts have a wide range of causes. (See *Understanding the white blood cell differential,* page 39.)

### Proliferation tests

Proliferation tests evaluate lymphocyte function without intradermal injection of antigens. The *lymphocyte transformation test,* performed using nonspecific stimulants, evaluates the mitotic response of T and B cells to a foreign antigen. For example, pokeweed stimulates primarily B lymphocytes; phytohemagglutinin stimulates T lymphocytes. A low proliferative response indicates a decrease in available cells, a functional defect, or an unidentified serum factor that inhibits proliferation.

The *mixed lymphocyte culture test* determines lymphocyte competence to respond to foreign histocompatibility antigens and is useful in matching transplant recipients and donors. In this test, the recipient's lymphocytes are cultured with the donor's for 3 to 4 days to test compatibility.

### T- and B-lymphocyte counts

Counting of T and B cells aids diagnosis of immunodeficiency disease, evaluates immunocompetence in autoimmune disease, and monitors response to therapy. An abnormal T- or B-cell count suggests, but does not confirm, specific diseases; a normal count doesn't always ensure a competent immune system. For

## Producing monoclonal antibodies

Lymphocytes respond to antigen stimulation by rapidly proliferating and producing antibodies against the antigen. Laboratory production of monoclonal antibodies takes advantage of lymphocyte reaction to an antigen. Typically, a selected antigen is injected into a mouse, stimulating its immune response. After a few days, the mouse's spleen is removed, and its antibody-producing cells are then fused with continuously dividing mouse tumor cells, such as myelomas, which don't secrete antibody. The result is hybridomas, which are grown in culture, cloned, and tested for the desired antibody. Finally, selected hybridomas are grown in culture or injected into a mouse to produce monoclonal antibodies, which are purified for future use.

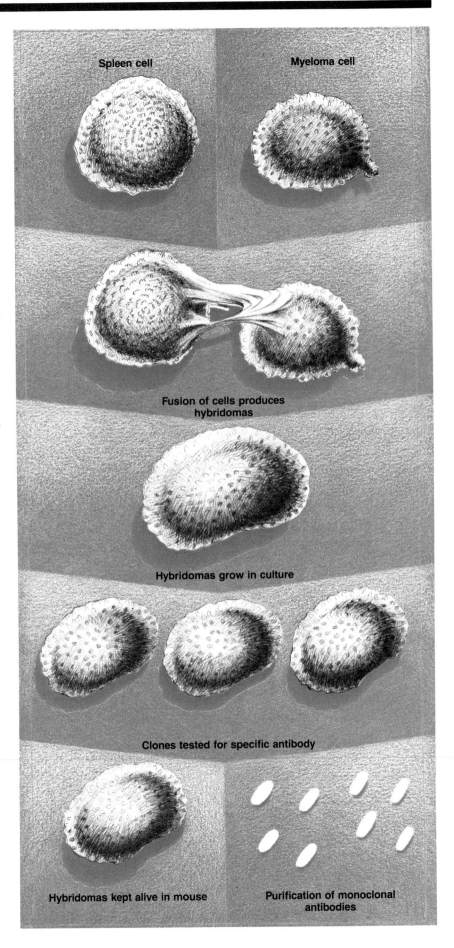

Spleen cell

Myeloma cell

Fusion of cells produces hybridomas

Hybridomas grow in culture

Clones tested for specific antibody

Hybridomas kept alive in mouse

Purification of monoclonal antibodies

example, normal numbers of T and B cells may not function normally in autoimmune diseases or in malignancies.

Normally, T cells constitute about 55% to 75% of circulating peripheral lymphocytes. They increase in infectious mononucleosis, multiple myeloma, and acute lymphocytic leukemia and decrease in DiGeorge's and Wiskott-Aldrich syndromes. B cells, which constitute about 15% to 30% of circulating lymphocytes, increase in chronic lymphocytic leukemia, DiGeorge's syndrome, and multiple myeloma and decrease in acute lymphocytic leukemia and in certain congenital or acquired immunoglobulin deficiency diseases.

## TESTS FOR CELL-MEDIATED IMMUNITY

Unlike B cells, T cells display no surface immunoglobulin but show unique surface antigens and receptor sites (markers). (See *Identifying lymphocyte surface markers,* page 40.) Evaluation of cell-mediated immunity includes tests to identify surface markers, tests for immunodeficiency, proliferation tests, and cytotoxicity tests.

### T-cell surface markers

A rosette test identifies T cells by their tendency to spontaneously form E rosettes after exposure to untreated sheep RBCs at 39.2° F. (4° C.). In addition monoclonal antibodies have been used to detect specific T-cell surface antigens.

### Immunodeficiency

The absolute number of circulating T cells doesn't determine cell-mediated immunity because much cell activity occurs outside of circulation, in tissues. Tests to confirm immunodeficiency must evaluate primary and secondary immune responses to a test antigen. Common test antigens include candidin, mumps, and purified protein derivative of tuberculin, which are used to perform *delayed hypersensitivity skin tests* on older children and adults. Infants and young children may

## Understanding the white blood cell differential

| Cell type | Relative value | Increased by | Decreased by |
|---|---|---|---|
| **Neutrophils** | 50% to 70% | Infection, cancer, poisoning, stress, hemorrhage, myelocytic leukemia | Chemotherapy, radiotherapy, deficiency of vitamin $B_{12}$ or folic acid |
| **Lymphocytes** | 16.2% to 43% | Hepatitis, herpes simplex and zoster, mononucleosis, syphilis, lymphocytic leukemia | Wiskott-Aldrich syndrome; occasionally, systemic lupus erythematosus (SLE) |
| **Monocytes** | 2% to 6% | Tuberculosis, cancer, anemia, rickettsial infection, typhoid, myelocytic leukemia | Rarely decreased |
| **Eosinophils** | 1% to 4% | Allergies, asthma, worm or parasite invasion, inflammation, lymphoreticular malignancy, and many other conditions | SLE, stress, Cushing's syndrome |
| **Basophils** | 0.3% to 2% | Granulocytic leukemia, basophilic leukemia | Occasionally, hyperthyroidism; allergies |

## Identifying lymphocyte surface markers

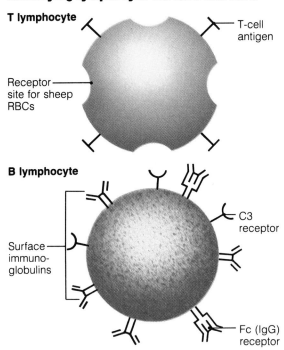

**T lymphocyte**

T-cell antigen

Receptor site for sheep RBCs

**B lymphocyte**

Surface immunoglobulins

C3 receptor

Fc (IgG) receptor

Morphologically uniform under light microscopy, lymphocytes are comprised of two major subclasses—T and B cells—that give rise to the cell-mediated and humoral immune systems. Various techniques distinguish these subclasses by their surface markers.

not respond to such testing because they lack prior sensitization. (See *Testing for delayed hypersensitivity.*)

A *chemical antigen,* such as dinitrochlorobenzene (DNCB), may be used to sensitize patients with suspected anergy—diminished or absent ability to react to antigens. About 7 to 10 days after application of DNCB, a positive reaction to a challenge dose—erythema or induration at the challenge site—indicates the ability to develop cellular immunity to a new antigen. Failure to react indicates abnormal delayed hypersensitivity.

The *migration inhibiting factor (MIF) assay* assesses the ability of lymphokines to inhibit macrophage migration. It may represent an in vitro correlate of the in vivo skin test for delayed hypersensitivity. In this test, human lymphokines are collected and concentrated, then tested for their ability to inhibit migration of macrophages from a capillary tube. The area of cell migration is then measured. Absence of MIF may indicate deficient cellular immunity.

### Proliferation tests

In these in vitro tests for hypersensitivity, a subpopulation of sensitized lymphocytes from patients previously exposed to an antigen is

cultured with the antigen for several hours. Radiolabeled deoxyribonucleic acid (DNA) precursors are then added to the culture tube to detect cell proliferation. A positive response—cellular incorporation of DNA precursors (as measured by uptake of radioactive precursors of DNA)—indicates antigen recognition. A negative response indicates defective cellular immunity or absence of previous exposure to the antigen. In some disorders, these in vitro tests may prove more reliable than skin tests in assessing antigen recognition in cellular hypersensitivity.

### Cytotoxicity tests

Cytotoxicity occurs when sensitized T cells destroy target cells. Primarily used for research, these tests measure the ability of previously sensitized T cells to kill antigen-bearing target cells.

### TESTS FOR HUMORAL IMMUNITY

Tests for humoral immunity identify B-cell surface markers; measure immunoglobulin levels; diagnose immunodeficiency; and evaluate complement, neutrophil, and macrophage function.

### B-cell surface markers

B cells have surface receptors, including a receptor of complement (C3) and the Fc portion of immunoglobulin molecules. A rosette test detects complement receptors on their surfaces. In this test, RBCs are coated with complement components and then mixed with the lymphocyte to be identified. RBCs cluster around B lymphocytes bearing complement receptors to form erythrocyte antibody complement rosettes. Alternatively, erythrocytes coated with immunoglobulin are used to detect Fc receptors on B-cell surfaces. These tests to detect B-cell surface markers are used primarily in research.

### Immunoglobulin levels

Immunoelectrophoresis measures total immunoglobulin concentration; immunodiffusion measures the quantity of specific immunoglobulin that's synthesized and secreted by B lymphocytes. (See *Measuring immunoglobulin concentration,* page 42.) Nephelometry, photometric measurement of light scattering during immunoprecipitation, may also be used to measure relative immunoglobulin concentration. Generally, immunoglobulin levels increase in allergy, infection, and autoimmune disorders and decrease in certain leukemias, cancer, and immunodeficiency disease. However, normal serum concentrations of specific immunoglobulins do not confirm the ability to make other antibodies. (See *Understanding immunoglobulins,* page 43.)

### Immunodeficiency

Tests to diagnose humoral immunodeficiency evaluate ability to form antibodies and include immunohematologic tests, the Schick test, and tests for viral clearing.

**Immunohematologic tests.** Isohemagglutinins—naturally occurring antibodies to RBCs—are present in all immunocompetent persons by age 2 (except those of blood type AB). Type A blood has anti-B isoantibodies; type B, anti-A isoantibodies; type O, both anti-A and anti-B isoantibodies; and type AB, neither. Isohemagglutinin titers should normally be greater than 1:4. Their absence indicates defective B-cell function, especially deficiency of IgM function. Similarly, absence of *Escherichia coli* antibody, another naturally occurring antibody, indicates immunodeficiency.

**The Schick test.** This test evaluates IgG function through subcutaneous injection of diphtheria toxin in previously immunized persons. A positive reaction, marked by redness and swelling at the injection site, indicates inability to neutralize the toxin—an immunodeficiency.

**Viral clearing.** This test evaluates antibody production after administration of the harmless bacteriophage X174. Determined by phage titers, viral clearing typically shows a sharp increase in IgM and a secondary increase in IgG. Absence of antibody production indicates severe combined immunodeficiency or X-linked hypogammaglobulinemia.

### Complement function

Complement fixation—binding of complement to antigen-antibody complexes—may occur during antigen-antibody reactions. Fixed complement is detected by fluorochrome-labeled antibodies.

The complement system works by promoting removal of pathogens or by lysing them. Hemolytic assay, the most commonly used functional assay of complement, measures the lytic capacity of sample plasma. Because lysis requires all nine complement components, this test serves as a screen for defects in any part of the pathway. In this test, immunoglobulin-coated sheep RBCs are added to serial dilutions of a serum sample. A spectro-

### Testing for delayed hypersensitivity

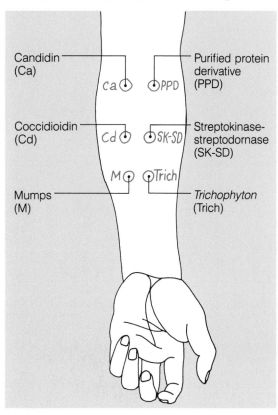

Candidin (Ca)

Coccidioidin (Cd)

Mumps (M)

Purified protein derivative (PPD)

Streptokinase-streptodornase (SK-SD)

*Trichophyton* (Trich)

Delayed hypersensitivity skin testing evaluates cell-mediated immunity in vivo. In these tests, a small amount of antigen (or group of antigens) is injected intradermally at the forearm volar surface with 25G to 27G needles and tuberculin syringes. Antigen injections are spaced at least 2″ (5 cm) apart and circled with a marker or pen. The type and site of each antigen is noted on a schematic drawing. Signs of anaphylaxis—urticaria, respiratory distress, and hypotension—may appear within 15 minutes of injection, requiring epinephrine administration. Delayed hypersensitivity reactions are assessed at 24, 48, and 72 hours. A positive response—5 mm or more of induration at the injection site—indicates that cell-mediated immunity is intact. A negative response indicates abnormal hypersensitivity. For consistency, the same person should apply the antigens and take the skin reaction readings.

photometer measures the resulting free hemoglobin (reflecting the degree of hemolysis) in each dilution. Complement activity, reported in $CH_{50}$ units, is the dilution capable of lysing 50% of available RBCs. Depressed total complement levels (which are clinically more significant than elevations) may result from excessive formation of antigen-antibody complexes, insufficient synthesis of complement, inhibitor formation, or increased complement catabolism and are characteristic of such conditions as SLE, acute poststreptococcal glomerulonephritis, and acute serum sickness. Serial changes in $CH_{50}$ titers help monitor the clinical course of such diseases as SLE and rheumatoid arthritis.

### Neutrophil and macrophage function

In phagocytosis, neutrophils and macrophages engulf and destroy bacteria and foreign particles. Tests for chemotaxis evaluate their ability to migrate to an antigen site. Other tests evaluate their capacity to kill a target antigen.

**Chemotaxis.** *In vitro assessment* of chemotaxis uses a two-part chamber containing bacteria in the lower half and phagocytic cells in the upper half. After a fixed time, migrating cells are counted microscopically. Abnormal chemotaxis occurs in various disorders.

# Measuring immunoglobulin concentration

Electrophoresis, immunoelectrophoresis, and immunodiffusion are commonly used to measure immunoglobulin.

*Electrophoresis* uses an electrical field to separate proteins. *Zone electrophoresis* can be used to estimate total immunoglobulin concentration in serum, urine, or other body fluids after proteins are separated on cellulose acetate or an agar medium by an electrical charge. Five bands of protein appear; when scanned with a densitometer, their band pattern is converted into peaks, which can be measured for approximate protein concentration. Immunoglobulin concentration is represented primarily by the gamma region, the beta region, and, possibly, the alpha region. Abnormal peaks in these regions represent immunoglobulin concentration abnormalities.

*Immunoelectrophoresis* combines electrophoresis and immunodiffusion. Serum is placed in a well on a slide containing agar gel, and an electric current is passed through the gel. Immunoglobulins (and other surface proteins) separate according to their electrical charge. Then, antiserum is placed in a shallow trough alongside the separated proteins, from which it diffuses into the agar. Precipitin arcs form wherever the antiserum reacts with specific serum proteins, identifying immunoglobulins and other proteins.

*Immunodiffusion* relies on the tendency of antigen and antibody particles to diffuse in an agar matrix and to form a precipitation ring or line where they meet. Radial immunodiffusion employs a Petri dish or agar slide containing antibody specific to a certain antigen. A well punched in the agar is filled with the specific antigen. After 24 hours, a precipitation ring forms where maximal binding occurs. The distance between the precipitation ring and the well is directly proportional to the antigen concentration. Serial dilution of known antigen quantities produces rings of varying size to help determine immunoglobulin concentrations in specimens.

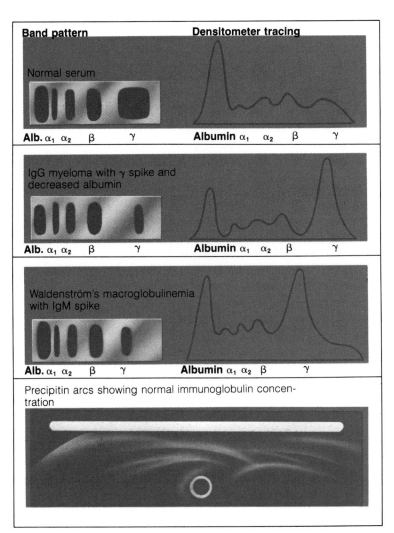

**Band pattern** — **Densitometer tracing**

Normal serum

Alb. $\alpha_1$ $\alpha_2$ $\beta$ $\gamma$    Albumin $\alpha_1$ $\alpha_2$ $\beta$ $\gamma$

IgG myeloma with $\gamma$ spike and decreased albumin

Alb. $\alpha_1$ $\alpha_2$ $\beta$ $\gamma$    Albumin $\alpha_1$ $\alpha_2$ $\beta$ $\gamma$

Waldenström's macroglobulinemia with IgM spike

Alb. $\alpha_1$ $\alpha_2$ $\beta$ $\gamma$    Albumin $\alpha_1$ $\alpha_2$ $\beta$ $\gamma$

Precipitin arcs showing normal immunoglobulin concentration

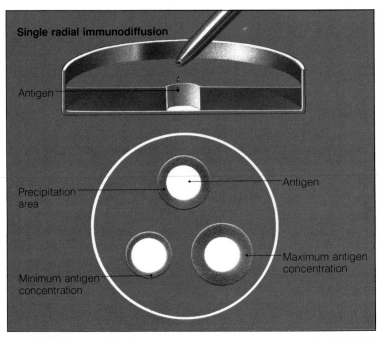

**Single radial immunodiffusion**

Antigen

Precipitation area

Minimum antigen concentration

Antigen

Maximum antigen concentration

The *Rebuck skin window technique* assesses chemotactic ability in vivo. For the Rebuck technique, an abraded area of skin is covered with a sterile coverslip. Normally, leukocytes travel to the site and adhere to the coverslip within a period of several hours. Failure of cells to adhere indicates neutropenia or defective chemotaxis.

**Killing ability.** To assess killing ability of neutrophils, the *nitroblue tetrazolium (NBT) test* relies on neutrophil generation of bactericidal enzymes and toxins during killing, which results in increased oxygen consumption and glucose metabolism. This action reduces colorless NBT to blue formazan, which is then extracted from neutrophils with pyridine and measured photometrically. Failure of NBT reduction indicates chronic granulomatous disease.

## TESTS FOR AUTOIMMUNITY

As the name implies, autoimmune disorders occur when the immune system fails to distinguish self from nonself and misdirects the immune response against the body's own tissues. These disorders are often systemic, but they may focus on a single organ or system. Their diagnosis is usually based on clinical signs and symptoms, with laboratory tests used for confirmation and for assessing the disorder's activity. Tests for autoimmune disorders include those for rheumatoid factor, antinuclear antibodies, anti-DNA antibodies, lupus erythematosus cell preparation, human leukocyte antigen (HLA), abnormal antibodies to blood components; and percutaneous renal biopsy.

### Rheumatoid factor (RF)

This common test confirms rheumatoid arthritis by differentiating it from chronic forms of inflammatory arthritis. Two agglutination tests can detect RF: the sheep cell agglutination test and the latex fixation test. In the *sheep cell agglutination test,* rabbit IgG adsorbed onto sheep RBCs is mixed with serum in serial dilutions; in the *latex fixation test,* human IgG absorbed into latex particles

## Understanding immunoglobulins

| Class | Activity | Normal values | Causes of increased levels | Causes of decreased levels |
|-------|----------|---------------|----------------------------|----------------------------|
| IgG | Provides host defense by activating complement system and functions as opsonin in Fc receptor–mediated clearance | 500 to 2,000 mg/dl | Bacterial infections<br>Hepatitis A<br>Glomerulonephritis<br>IgG myeloma<br>Rheumatoid arthritis<br>Systemic lupus erythematosus (SLE) | Lymphoid aplasia<br>Agammaglobulinemia<br>Type I dysgammaglobulinemia<br>IgA myeloma<br>Chronic lymphocytic leukemia |
| IgA | Protects mucosal surfaces of the respiratory, gastrointestinal, and urogenital tracts | 50 to 400 mg/dl | IgA myeloma<br>Laennec's cirrhosis<br>Rheumatoid arthritis<br>SLE<br>Glomerulonephritis | Immunoglobulin disorders (such as agammaglobulinemia and ataxia-telangiectasia)<br>IgG myeloma<br>Acute and chronic lymphocytic leukemia<br>Hypogammaglobulinemia |
| IgM | Active in viral and bacterial infections | 50 to 200 mg/dl | Hepatitis A and B<br>Glomerulonephritis<br>Waldenström's macroglobulinemia<br>Trypanosomiasis | Lymphoid aplasia<br>Agammaglobulinemia<br>Type II dysgammaglobulinemia<br>IgG myeloma<br>IgA myeloma<br>Chronic lymphocytic leukemia<br>Hypogammaglobulinemia |
| IgD | Activity unknown | 0.5 to 5 mg/dl | Eczema and related skin disorders | Unknown |
| IgE | Triggers mast cell release of mediators in response to allergens | 0.01 to 0.10 mg/dl | Hyperimmunoglobulin E | Hypogammaglobulinemia<br>Ataxia-telangiectasia |

## Understanding percutaneous renal biopsy

For percutaneous renal biopsy, the patient must receive nothing by mouth for 8 hours. He is placed in a prone position, with a sandbag beneath his abdomen for support. After injection of a local anesthetic, the biopsy needle is inserted under ultrasonographic guidance through a small incision midway between the last rib and the iliac crest. The tissue sample is removed and im- · mediately examined under a hand lens to ensure that it contains tissue from the cortex and medulla.

After the procedure, pressure must be applied to the incision site for 3 to 5 minutes, followed by application of a pressure dressing. Vital signs should be checked frequently and the incision site observed for bleeding. The patient should lie flat for 12 hours after this procedure. He should receive extra fluids to initiate mild diuresis, which helps minimize colic and obstruction from blood clots in the renal pelvis.

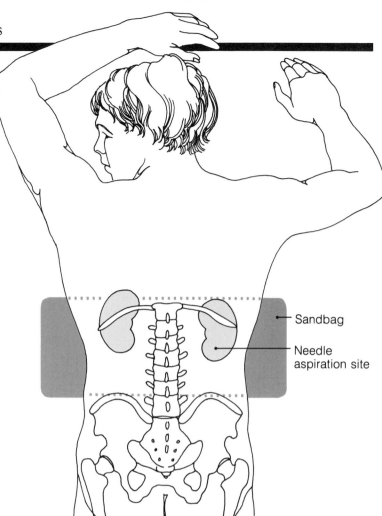

Sandbag

Needle aspiration site

is mixed with the patient's serum. Visible agglutination identifies RF.

### Antinuclear antibodies (ANAs)

This immunofluorescence test detects antibodies against various cell components, including the membrane or nucleoprotein. ANAs are present in many autoimmune disorders and in chronic pulmonary fibrosis or chronic infection. In some immune disorders, this test may produce specific fluorescence patterns, but such test results are not standardized.

The test for ANAs is negative at a titer of 1:32 or below. It may produce false-positive results in patients taking penicillin, isoniazid, oral contraceptives, hydralazine, or procainamide hydrochloride.

### Anti-DNA antibodies

Once ANAs have been identified, anti-DNA antibody testing can confirm diagnosis, particularly of SLE, and monitor response to therapy. In this test, the serum sample is mixed with radiolabeled native DNA. If anti-DNA antibodies are present in the serum, they combine with the native DNA, forming large complexes that are trapped by a membrane filter and can be titrated. If such antibodies are absent, the radiolabeled DNA passes through the filter.

### Lupus erythematosus (LE) cell preparation

This in vitro test helps confirm SLE and monitor its response to treatment. Microscopic examination of blood samples in LE cell preparation tests reveals LE cells in about 50% to 60% of patients with SLE; however, LE cells alone do not confirm SLE. This test is less sensitive and less reliable than ANA or anti-DNA antibody tests but is often used because it requires minimal equipment and reagents.

### HLA test

This test identifies human leukocyte surface antigens for histocompatibility typing of tissue transplant recipients and donors. The major histocompatibility antigens, HLA antigens are present on all nucleated cells and are most easily detected on lymphocytes. In this test, a sample of lymphocytes is tested against antiserums to HLA antigens. Complement added to the sample lyses the cells, allowing dye to enter. HLA antigens are then detected by phase microscopy. High incidences of specific HLA types have been linked with systemic diseases, such as rheumatoid arthritis and multiple sclerosis; however, these findings have little diagnostic significance.

## Abnormal antibodies to blood components

Immunohematologic tests assess antigen-antibody reaction on RBC surfaces and help monitor potential antigen-antibody reaction in blood transfusions, neonatal hemolytic disease, acquired hemolytic anemia, and RBC antigen sensitization. Among the most important such tests are ABO and Rh blood typing, antibody screening, and antiglobulin tests.

**Blood typing.** Typing and cross-matching of donor and recipient blood for ABO and Rh antigens is essential to minimize the risk of transfusion reaction. ABO typing, also performed to detect humoral immunodeficiency, involves forward and reverse methods. In forward typing, the patient's RBCs are mixed with anti-A serum, then with anti-B serum; the presence or absence of agglutination determines the blood group. Reverse typing verifies the results of the forward method by mixing the patient's serum with known group A and group B cells. Blood group determination is confirmed when the results of forward or reverse typing match perfectly.

Rh typing classifies blood by the presence or absence of the $Rh_o(D)$ antigen on the surface of RBCs. In this test, the patient's RBCs are mixed with serum containing anti-D antibodies. Agglutination indicates the presence of the D antigen—blood type Rh-positive; absence of agglutination indicates the absence of the D antigen—blood type Rh-negative.

**Antibody screening.** Also known as the indirect Coombs' test, antibody screening detects antibodies to RBC antigens in the serum and not attached to the cell. It's routinely performed before RBC transfusion and may also detect Rh-positive antibody in maternal blood. In this test, cells of known antigenic content are mixed with serum suspected of containing antibody. Agglutination signals the presence of antibody.

**Antiglobulin test.** Also known as the direct Coombs' test, this test detects immunoglobulins (antibodies) that coat RBCs but fail to complete the action of agglutination. In this test, antiglobulin serum (anti-IgG or anticomplement) is added to saline-washed RBCs. Agglutination (a positive reaction) occurs if immunoglobulin or complement is present,

indicating autoimmune hemolytic anemia, which may result from underlying lymphoma or SLE. This test is also performed on the cord blood of babies of Rh mothers or on any newborns with suspected hemolytic disease caused by maternal antibody. A positive result may follow use of cephalothin and penicillin.

Antibodies against platelets or against coagulation factors, which may cause bleeding disorders, also appear in autoimmune disorders; however, tests for these antibodies are complex and not routinely performed. Diagnosis of bleeding disorders, such as idiopathic thrombocytopenic purpura, is often made without these tests.

## Percutaneous renal biopsy

This procedure is performed to confirm SLE and glomerulonephritis. Preliminary blood and urine studies rule out bleeding disorders. (See *Understanding percutaneous renal biopsy.*) In this test, an excised core of kidney tissue is examined histologically, using light, electron, and immunofluorescent microscopy.

## TESTS FOR ALLERGY

Diagnosis of allergic disorders typically begins with a thorough history and physical examination to identify offending agents. This criti-

### Assessing skin-test reactions

| Type of test | Reaction scale | Reaction appearance |
|---|---|---|
| Prick or scratch test | Negative | No wheal or erythema |
| | 1+ | No wheal; erythema < 20 mm in diameter |
| | 2+ | No wheal; erythema > 20 mm in diameter |
| | 3+ | Wheal and erythema |
| | 4+ | Wheal with pseudopods; erythema |
| Intradermal test | Negative | Same as control |
| | 1+ | Wheal twice as large as control; erythema < 20 mm in diameter |
| | 2+ | Wheal twice as large as control; erythema > 20 mm in diameter |
| | 3+ | Wheal three times as large as control; erythema |
| | 4+ | Wheal with pseudopods; erythema |

## Sites of bone marrow aspiration and biopsy

The posterior iliac crest is the preferred site for bone marrow aspiration and biopsy. The anterior iliac crest and the spinous vertebral processes T10 to L4 may occasionally be used. The sternum may be used for aspiration in adults; it is not recommended for biopsy because of the risk of cardiac and mediastinal perforation. In children, using the sternum is not recommended; the tibia is the preferred site for children under age 1.

These illustrations show biopsy sites in the shaded areas.

**Posterior superior iliac crest**

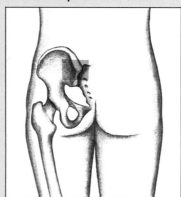

**Anterior iliac crest**

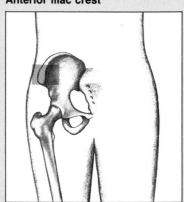

**Spinous process**

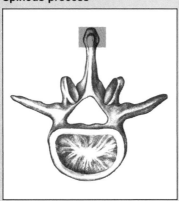

**Sternum**

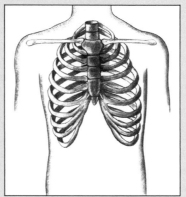

**Tibia**

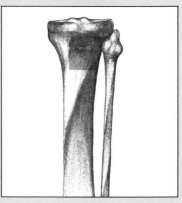

cal first step helps narrow the list of possible allergens and makes the diagnostic workup shorter and less costly. Specific diagnostic tests to detect allergic disorders include traditional skin testing, food allergen testing, bronchial inhalation challenges, nasal cytology, and radioallergosorbent tests.

### Skin testing

This technique, commonly used to identify specific allergens, involves two methods: prick or scratch testing and intradermal testing.

**Prick or scratch test.** This technique introduces extracts of fresh, concentrated pollens; inhalants; and other suspected environmental antigens. For this test, an area of skin on the patient's back or forearm is cleansed with alcohol. Test areas are marked off to allow adequate space for reactions. In the *prick technique,* a sterile needle passes through a single drop of extract on the skin and penetrates the top layer of skin without causing bleeding. Typically, prepared control areas are also pricked with the antigen diluent. In the *scratch technique,* the allergen is applied to a short linear scratch on the skin. After 20 to 30 minutes, the allergen is wiped off and the reaction is recorded.

**Intradermal test.** This technique confirms negative or weak-positive reactions to prick or scratch tests. For this test, 0.02 to 0.05 ml of the extract is injected intradermally; control sites are also usually injected. Using dilute solutions of the extract and injecting them into a peripheral site help minimize the risk of systemic reaction.

Immediate skin-test reactions may be measured on a graduated scale (usually 1 + through 4 + ), based on the size of the wheal or the extent of erythema. (See *Assessing skin-test reactions,* page 45.)

Skin testing is commonly used because it's easy to perform, provides prompt results, and is economical. However, it's contraindicated in pregnant women and in patients with diffuse dermatitis. It should be avoided when patients are taking antihistamines or other drugs that control allergy symptoms. Such drugs inhibit test responses and must be discontinued 24 hours before testing.

## Food allergen testing

When the patient's dietary history indicates that certain foods provoke symptoms, food challenges or elimination diets may identify the allergen.

**Food challenges.** These tests are best conducted in a double-blind procedure (so neither doctor nor patient knows what food is being tested) to ensure objectivity. Typically, patients follow a limited diet of foods not suspected to cause symptoms and ingest the suspected food in disguised or encapsulated form. The degree of suspected hypersensitivity determines the challenge dosage, and the history determines the reaction time. A positive reaction reproduces the patient's original symptoms, which may include sneezing, vomiting, diarrhea, urticaria, angioedema, or rash. Unfortunately, challenge testing is time-consuming because suspected allergens must be administered individually.

**Elimination diets.** Like food challenges, elimination diets aim to identify dietary allergens. Typically, suspected foods are eliminated from the diet for 7 to 14 days. If the patient's symptoms don't improve, food allergy is unlikely. If the limited diet does relieve symptoms, suspected foods are then added at 2-day intervals until symptoms recur. Then, the food most recently added is withdrawn and administered again to confirm its effect. Elimination diets are often deficient in essential vitamins and nutrients and are not recommended for prolonged use.

## Bronchial inhalation challenges

When allergic reactions include respiratory symptoms such as wheezing (bronchoconstriction), a bronchial inhalation challenge may help identify an inhaled allergen. In this test, the patient inhales aerosol preparations of suspected allergens (including suspected occupational allergens) via a special unit-dose nebulizer. Normal saline solution is used as a control. The forced expiratory volume, the total vital capacity, the maximum midexpiratory flow rate, or all three, are measured before, during, and immediately after nebulization of the antigen and control. The same measurements are repeated at 5, 10, and 20 minutes after nebulization. Subjective respiratory distress or a significant decline in any measure of pulmonary function is a positive reaction. Sympathomimetic amines and antihistamines may interfere with test results and should be discontinued 18 hours before the test.

Bronchial inhalation challenge is more definitive than skin testing but has some disadvantages: allergen extracts are not deposited in the same airway portion as naturally inhaled allergenic particles; some extracts may cause nonspecific irritant responses; a positive reaction may provoke severe bronchospasm, requiring immediate measures to control an asthmatic attack; and finally, the test is more cumbersome and time-consuming than skin testing.

## Nasal cytology

In this test, which aids diagnosis of allergic rhinitis or infection, the nostrils' lateral walls are scraped to obtain cells for microscopic examination. An increase in eosinophils, basophils, and mast cells suggests allergic rhinitis; an increase in neutrophils and bacteria suggests an infectious process.

## Radioallergosorbent test

This widely used means of detecting allergens provides a qualitative measure of IgE. For this test, a sample of the patient's serum is exposed to a panel of suspected allergen particle complexes—for example, from grasses, trees, and animals—on cellulose disks. If the sample contains antibodies to certain allergen particle complexes, these antibodies combine with radiolabeled allergens. After centrifugation, radioimmunoassay detects the allergen-specific IgE antibody. Test results are compared with control values. A positive result exceeds control levels by 400%.

This in vitro test eliminates the risk of adverse reaction in skin testing. It's also easier to perform, more specific, and less painful for the patient than skin testing. And in addition to detecting an allergen, this test also indicates the quantity necessary to elicit an allergic reaction; however, it's more costly, slightly less sensitive, and applicable only to allergens that can be chemically coupled to the immunosorbent.

## TESTS FOR LYMPHOPROLIFERATIVE DISORDERS

Increased levels of lymphoid cells and immunoglobulins characterize the lymphoproliferative state in infection and in neoplasms. Although patient history provides the best clues to causes of lymphoproliferation, specific diagnostic tests help confirm diagnosis. For example, the history may indicate infectious mononucleosis marked by cervical lymphadenopathy. A test to detect heterophile antibody

## Biopsy of abnormal lymph node

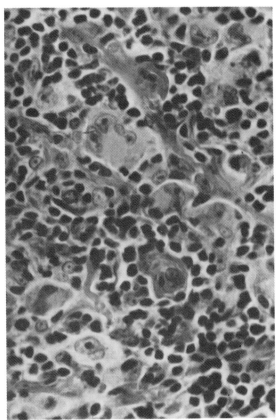

This lymph node biopsy reveals Hodgkin's disease (nodular sclerosing type), which is indicated by the presence of characteristic Reed-Sternberg cells in a matrix of small lymphocytes and collagen bands.

(an IgM molecule identified by its ability to agglutinate sheep RBCs) can confirm infectious mononucleosis and rule out the possibility of malignancy. When lymphoproliferation appears without signs of infection, histologic studies confirm suspected disorders.

Diagnosis of these disorders requires invasive procedures, such as bone marrow aspiration and biopsy, lymph node biopsy, and lymphangiography, and noninvasive procedures, such as computerized tomography (CT) scan and magnetic resonance imaging (MRI).

### Bone marrow aspiration and biopsy

Histologic and hematologic examination of bone marrow—the source of stem cells for all cellular components—helps confirm lymphoproliferative disorders and monitor reponse to treatment.

Aspiration of bone marrow is performed to study cellular components of the marrow; biopsy, to study its structure. These procedures are preceded by coagulation and platelet studies. Despite local anesthesia, they cause discomfort and anxiety for the patient. Thor-

ough patient teaching and allowing the patient to talk with others who've experienced these procedures may help reduce anxiety. Similarly, relaxation exercises reduce muscle tension and encourage the patient to feel in control of his body.

### Lymph node biopsy

Microscopic examination of a biopsy of an enlarged lymph node is essential to confirm malignancy and to evaluate immunocompetence. Lymph node tissue is obtained by needle aspiration or by surgical excision of an entire node. Excision is preferred because it provides a larger specimen. (See *Biopsy of abnormal lymph node.*) Analgesics may be administered for several days following the procedure.

### Lymphangiography

This radiographic study of the lymph system detects and stages lymphomas, identifies metastatic involvement of the lymph nodes, and suggests or evaluates treatment of malignancy. To avoid an adverse reaction to the dye or contrast medium, the patient should be questioned about allergies (especially to shellfish or iodine) and should have a preliminary chest X-ray. Preliminary fasting is not required; in fact, because this test may take longer than 4 hours, the patient may wish to have a light meal just before the test.

Enlarged, foamy-looking nodes are consistent with lymphoma. Filling defects or lack of opacification indicates metastatic involvement of the lymph nodes. The number of nodes affected, extent of unilateral or bilateral involvement, and extent of extranodal involvement help determine staging of lymphoma. However, definitive staging requires additional diagnostic tests, such as CT scan, ultrasonography, selective biopsy, and laparotomy.

Rarely, lymphangiography produces pulmonary complications—shortness of breath, chest pain, cyanosis, or hypotension—resulting from embolization of the oily contrast agent. Report such complications immediately, and take appropriate measures to manage them. Another potential complication is lymphangitis, manifested by chills, high fever, swelling, and pain.

The patient should be advised that his urine and stools may be tinged blue for a few days and that the skin around the incisions may be temporarily stained. He should also be advised to keep the dressings clean and dry and to report signs of infection, such as redness or warmth. He may require analgesics to relieve discomfort.

### CT scan

CT scan is a safe, noninvasive means of diagnosing lymphatic disorders and serially monitoring response to therapy. The CT scan often visualizes upper abdominal lymph nodes and enlarged mesenteric lymph nodes not identified by lymphangiography. It's also helpful for evaluating the kidney in such diseases as SLE. And because a CT scan involves minimal discomfort, it's valuable for monitoring serial response to therapy. Prior to this test, the patient should void. He may be given an analgesic or sedative to ensure that he can lie quietly on the X-ray table for approximately 90 minutes. He should be assured that radiation exposure is minimal and that a technician will watch him during the test and halt the procedure if necessary.

### MRI

Like the CT scan, MRI provides cross-sectional images of the body, but it does so without exposing the body to ionizing radiation. This noninvasive test detects structural and biochemical abnormalities by directing magnetic and radio waves at body tissue to determine the response of a test element. MRI relies on the natural magnetic properties of atoms in the body and uses superconducting or resistive magnets to create an electromagnetic echo. Sensitive receivers then pick up this echo and relay it to computers. MRI distinguishes between normal and malignant tissue but doesn't visualize bone. The magnetic field used in this procedure has the potential disadvantage of displacing small clips, sutures, or other ferrous metal in the body and of converting a cardiac pacemaker from a fixed rate to demand mode. Advances in MRI may soon aid diagnosis of immune disorders.

### TESTS FOR NONSPECIFIC INFLAMMATION

During an inflammatory reaction, the concentrations of various blood components change. These changes are nonspecific indicators of inflammation, and only a few of them have general clinical application. The two most commonly used tests for nonspecific inflammatory disorders are C-reactive protein (CRP) and erythrocyte sedimentation rate.

### C-reactive protein test

This beta globulin is produced by the liver and excreted into the bloodstream during the acute phase of inflammation. It promotes phagocytosis of bacteria by polymorphonuclear neutrophils. To detect CRP, antiserum is used in several immunoassays—radioimmunoassay, capillary precipitation, gel diffusion, and latex agglutination. Normal serum is negative for CRP. A positive reaction for CRP strongly suggests active inflammation but is nonspecific for any single disorder.

### Erythrocyte sedimentation rate

This test measures the distance RBCs fall in a specially marked tube within 1 hour. As sample RBCs descend in the tube, they displace plasma upward, which retards the downward progress of other settling blood elements. Factors affecting the sedimentation rate include RBC volume, surface area, density, aggregation, and surface charge. Normally, RBCs fall from 0 to 10 mm/hour in males and from 0 to 20 mm/hour in females. Accelerated rates occur in infection, rheumatoid arthritis, rheumatic fever, hemolytic anemia, thyroid disease, some malignancies, and autoimmune disorders.

### Patient teaching is the key

Although you may not actually perform most immunodiagnostic tests, your nursing responsibilities during the diagnostic workup are significant. Preparing the patient physically, gathering the necessary equipment, and ensuring that appropriate consent forms have been signed are only part of your responsibilities. Preparing the patient emotionally is just as important.

How much you tell the patient depends, of course, on his emotional status, his age, and his ability to comprehend. For example, a patient may fear he's losing too much blood because of the many venipunctures usually required in the immune diagnostic workup. You can ease this fear by explaining that the 30 ml typically drawn is only an ounce. Attending the doctor-patient conferences so you can later explain and reinforce what the doctor has said is one way to help clarify details the patient may not understand. Using special teaching aids, such as colorful charts, diagrams, or informational brochures, is another. And involving family members in patient teaching can help ensure a cooperative patient, especially if he's very young or old and in fear of or unable to comprehend the test procedures. In these ways, your patient teaching may help provide reliable, accurate test results.

**Points to remember**

- Laboratory evaluation of the immune system begins with the complete blood count and differential cell count.
- The specific diagnostic workup may include in vitro techniques, such as immunodiffusion, agglutination, precipitation, immunofluorescence, and radioimmunoassay.
- Normal T- and B-cell counts do not in themselves verify a competent immune system. T and B cells, though present in normal numbers, may not function normally in some immune disorders.
- Hemolytic assay, the most commonly used complement assay, measures the lytic capacity of a plasma sample.
- Invasive procedures, such as bone marrow aspiration and biopsy, percutaneous renal biopsy, and lymph node biopsy, confirm diagnosis.
- Lymphangiography, a radiographic study, aids in the staging of lymphomas, identifies metastatic involvement of lymph nodes, and suggests or evaluates treatment.
- Thorough patient teaching can significantly decrease patient anxiety and help ensure reliable test results.

# 4 MANAGING IMMUNE FUNCTION

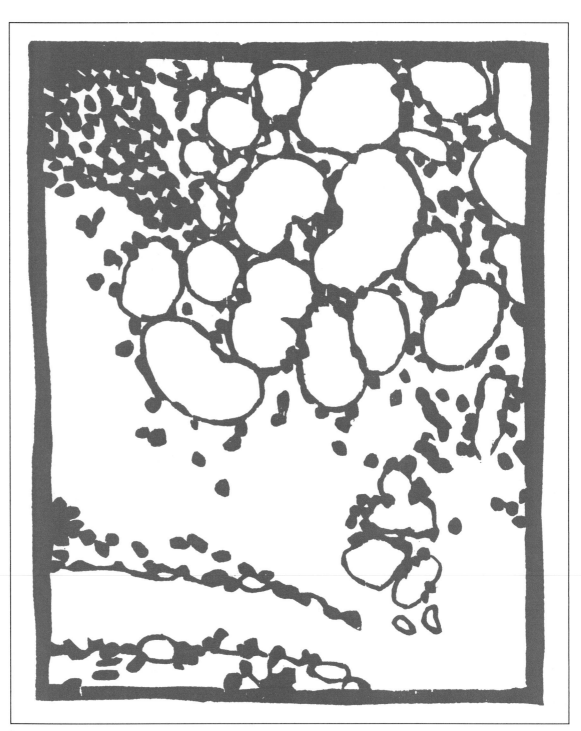

Bone marrow depression

New understanding of immunologic pathophysiology has brought advances in pharmacologic and non-pharmacologic treatment. Such treatment includes new drugs; new uses for some established drugs; and other forms of therapy, such as total nodal irradiation and improved environmental control. These improved approaches to treatment have helped immunodeficient patients recover with fewer complications.

Keeping up with these rapid changes will help you avoid drug errors and prepare you to implement drug therapy tailored to individual needs.

## IMMUNOTHERAPEUTIC AGENTS

Typically, immunotherapeutic agents are prescribed to interrupt a disease's mechanism of action rather than to eliminate its underlying causes. The major groups of immunotherapeutic agents include *anti-inflammatory* agents, *immunosuppressive* agents, *remission-inducing* agents, *antiallergic* agents, and investigational *immunoenhancing* agents.

### Anti-inflammatory agents

These agents act to suppress inflammation by interfering with some portion of the body's inflammatory reaction (such as secretion of histamine, kinins, prostaglandins, and other substances that mediate inflammation). Numerous drugs are available to suppress inflammation. *Nonsteroidal anti-inflammatory drugs (NSAIDs)* and *corticosteroids* are the two main classes of these agents.

**NSAIDs.** These drugs, which also have analgesic properties, include aspirin and newer agents chemically unrelated to aspirin. Although their exact mechanisms of action remain unknown, NSAIDs appear to inhibit prostaglandin synthesis, which may play an important role in suppression of inflammation. (See *Action of prostaglandin inhibitors,* page 52.) These drugs may also be involved in the inhibition of leukocyte activation and migration to inflammation sites and the inhibition of lysosomal enzyme release from phagocytes.

Because prostaglandins help mediate many types of pain, NSAIDs help inhibit joint swelling, pain, morning stiffness, and disease activity; they also improve functional capacity in patients with rheumatoid arthritis.

Among the NSAIDs, aspirin is the drug of choice and the standard to which all other NSAIDs are compared. However, although aspirin has relatively low toxicity, many patients cannot tolerate the gastrointestinal (GI) side effects of the large doses needed to arrest inflammation. For some of these patients and for those whose inflammation doesn't respond to aspirin, other NSAIDs, such as ibuprofen and naproxen, may be tried. Although these drugs share common pharmacologic properties, individual patient responses vary greatly, and trial administration over several weeks may be necessary before the patient achieves clinical benefits. For patients who respond to aspirin but cannot tolerate its side effects, other forms of salicylates, such as sodium salicylate, choline salicylate (Arthropan), choline magnesium trisalicylate (Trilisate), and salsalate (Disalcid) may provide relief and cause fewer GI side effects.

When choosing an NSAID, consider the patient's medical history, his past responses to therapy, and the clinical outcome desired. For example, NSAIDs are used cautiously in peptic ulcer disease or bleeding disorders.

*Consider side effects.* NSAIDs produce many of the same side effects. GI effects are most common and may include epigastric distress; nausea; anorexia; and gastric or intestinal ulceration, which may lead to occult blood loss. NSAIDs may also impair platelet function, causing prolonged bleeding times. Their central nervous system (CNS) effects may include headaches, drowsiness, dizziness, and visual and auditory disturbances. They may also affect renal and hepatic function.

Because of their high incidence of adverse reactions, indomethacin, phenylbutazone, oxyphenbutazone, and meclofenamate sodium should be used only for short periods. Sulindac (Clinoril) may be safer to use in patients with mild to moderate renal impairment.

In caring for patients who are taking NSAIDs, observe for adverse reactions, such as GI disturbances, petechiae, bruises, and melena; monitor blood test results for anemia, decreased platelet count, prolonged prothrombin time, and partial thromboplastin time to detect hematologic disturbances. Report tinnitus, blurred vision, and CNS effects, which are more common with high doses and toxic reactions.

*Watch for therapeutic effects.* Such effects include increased joint mobility and exercise tolerance and decreased pain, edema, and redness. In your patient teaching, stress that NSAIDs treat symptoms of rheumatic disease but do not cure the disease itself. Inform the patient that he may need to try many NSAIDs before finding one that relieves his symptoms

# Action of prostaglandin inhibitors

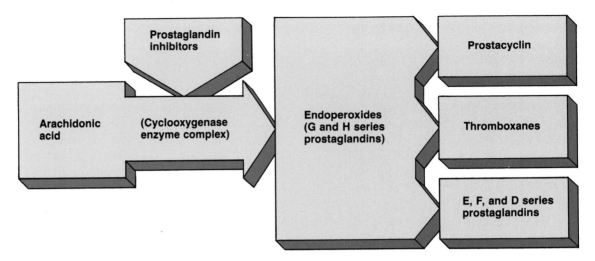

Nonsteroidal anti-inflammatory agents are prostaglandin inhibitors that typically relieve pain and inflammation by blocking an early step in prostaglandin synthesis, an important part of the inflammatory reaction.

Prostaglandins form when cell injury or distortion of cell membranes triggers a chain reaction. First, enzymes produced by phagocytes at the injury site split the phospholipids in the cell membranes, freeing arachidonic acid. This normally dormant fatty acid is then activated by the enzyme cyclooxygenase (prostaglandin synthetase) to create the G and H series prostaglandins called endoperoxides. Next, these endoperoxides convert to thromboxanes and prostacyclin, which respectively promote and prevent platelet aggregation, and to E, F, and D series prostaglandins. These final prostaglandins, particularly the E series, cause inflammation and pain.

Prostaglandin inhibitors check the action of the cyclooxygenase enzyme complex and prevent conversion of arachidonic acid to the endoperoxides or intermediate prostaglandins. Prostaglandin inhibitors mediate but do not arrest the inflammatory response or its consequences. For example, in the patient with rheumatoid arthritis, these drugs may reduce pain, redness, and swelling, but joint destruction continues.

and that maximum effectiveness may require 1 to 2 weeks of therapy. Teach him to recognize side effects and to report them immediately. To avoid GI upset, suggest that he take the drug with food or milk or with a full glass of water. Antacids or special dose formulations such as buffered or enteric-coated aspirin may also be beneficial.

**Corticosteroids.** Produced naturally by the adrenal gland, these hormones are used in synthetic form as potent anti-inflammatory agents in rheumatic diseases, such as rheumatoid arthritis, systemic lupus erythematosus (SLE), and vasculitis. They're effective in every stage of inflammation. Some of the most commonly used corticosteroids include betamethasone acetate, cortisone, dexamethasone, hydrocortisone, and methylprednisolone sodium. These drugs produce such side effects as infection, fluid retention, GI irritation, hypokalemia, hyperglycemia, and development of cushingoid symptoms, which restrict their prolonged use. They may also suppress the hypothalamic-pituitary-adrenal axis after prolonged use or high doses. (See *How the body regulates corticosteroid secretion,* page 55.)

*Administration of corticosteroids can be varied to control or minimize side effects.* Oral preparations should be given with or shortly after meals to decrease GI symptoms. Parenteral forms should be administered according to the manufacturers' instructions. Alternate-day therapy is sometimes used to minimize side effects. In this form of therapy, short-acting steroids such as prednisone are given once every 48 hours, usually at 8 a.m., to mimic the body's normal release of cortisol. Alternate-day therapy has proven beneficial in some patients with rheumatoid arthritis, acute rheumatic fever, nephritis, SLE, vasculitis, and some chronic dermatoses. In other patients, however, symptoms recur on nontreatment days.

*Watch for therapeutic effects.* Such effects include improved range of motion, decreased joint pain and edema, and ability to perform activities of daily living. Monitor blood pressure and electrolyte status, and note adverse reactions, such as CNS effects (ranging from depression to euphoria), osteoporosis or pathologic fractures (particularly in postmenopausal women and immobilized patients), myopathy, and delayed growth in children. Also check for GI distress (nausea, vomiting, peptic ulcer, increased appetite, and obesity), increased susceptibility to infection, delayed wound healing, menstrual irregularities, and hirsutism. Be alert for adverse reactions to long-term corticosteroid therapy, especially adrenocortical insufficiency marked by fainting, weakness, anorexia, nausea, vomiting, hypotension, and shock. Most adverse reactions result from excessive doses of corticosteroids and cause redistribution of fat and a cushingoid appearance (moon face, buffalo hump, and truncal obesity). These effects may change the patient's self-image and impair his psychological well-being.

Because corticosteroids are gluconeogenic, you need to assess blood and urine glucose levels frequently in diabetic patients. Such patients may require increased doses of insulin or oral hypoglycemic agents. Concurrent use of diuretics may lead to excessive potassium depletion, and concomitant use of NSAIDs may increase ulcerogenic effects. Antihistamines, barbiturates, chloral hydrate, phenytoin, and rifampin may impair steroid effectiveness.

*Teach special precautions.* Warn the patient not to discontinue steroid therapy without his doctor's approval because of the risk of potentially life-threatening adrenal insufficiency. Tell him that if he can't take the drug orally (for example, if he's experiencing nausea or vomiting), he must receive it parenterally. When corticosteroids are to be discontinued, tell him the dosage must be tapered gradually, over several weeks to months, to ensure the return of normal pituitary-adrenal function.

Warn the patient that infections, extremes in temperature, surgical procedures, or other stressful events may require increased doses of corticosteroids. Suggest that he reduce exposure to infections by avoiding large crowds and practicing good hygiene. Advise him to wear a special bracelet to alert medical personnel of his need for additional corticosteroids in emergencies.

Instruct him to weigh himself weekly to detect possible fluid retention. If he experiences this side effect, suggest dietary changes, particularly limiting salt intake. Tell the hyperglycemic patient to closely monitor his condition and to report unusual responses to any medication. Finally, stress the importance of regular medical supervision, and advise the patient to report such reactions as sore throat, fever, weekly weight gain of 5 lb (2.3 kg) or more, ankle swelling (edema), depression, and mood changes.

## Immunosuppressive agents

Pharmacologic suppression of immune responses may be necessary to control disease activity in autoimmune disorders such as rheumatoid arthritis and glomerulonephritis and to combat organ transplant rejection. Many anticancer agents have been used successfully for this purpose. In addition, new drugs (such as cyclosporine) have been developed specifically to suppress the immune response. Immunosuppressive drugs are usually most effective when administered during the induction phase of the cell-mediated response; once the immune response has progressed to the effector phase, these agents become less effective. As a result, it's common practice to induce immunosuppression as soon as possible in autoimmune diseases and before organ transplantation.

**Therapeutic uses.** The *anticancer agents azathioprine* (Imuran), *cyclophosphamide* (Cytoxan), *chlorambucil,* and *methotrexate* effectively suppress both humoral and cell-mediated immune responses. However, many factors influence their immunosuppressive effects. For example, primary immune responses are more easily suppressed than secondary responses. Azathioprine and its active metabolite 6-mercaptopurine kill proliferating cells, which accounts for many serious side effects, especially bone marrow suppression. Cyclophosphamide effectively suppresses B lymphocytes (thus inhibiting antibody formation) but has little value in preventing rejection. And chlorambucil and methotrexate seem less potent than cyclophosphamide.

*Specific immunosuppressive agents* include *cyclosporine, antilymphocyte globulin (ALG),* and *monoclonal antibodies.* Cyclosporine (Sandimmune), a new immunosuppressive agent, is used with corticosteroids to prevent rejection and to combat chronic rejection in patients treated with other immunosuppressants. Its mechanisms of action are unknown, but it may inhibit the production of T-lymphocyte growth factor (interleukin 2). This effect seems more specific for helper T lymphocytes, causing their numbers to diminish during therapy. Cyclosporine, which is not cytotoxic and does not suppress bone marrow, has successfully increased graft survival in kidney, liver, bone marrow, and heart transplants.

ALG, prepared by immunizing horses with human thymus cells, has been developed to prevent and treat organ transplant rejection and aplastic anemia. A purified preparation of ALG antibodies, *lymphocyte immune globulin (LIG)* is used to deplete T lymphocytes in a patient's blood to suppress his cell-mediated immunity. Although LIG is immunosuppressive, its clinical benefit is controversial.

Monoclonal antibodies are being used successfully to prevent organ transplant rejection. They are specific for antigens on T lymphocytes and cause lymphopenia (decreased lymphocytes) and immunosuppression. Their use, however, is largely experimental.

**Side effects.** The most serious side effect of immunosuppressive therapy is bone marrow suppression, which produces leukopenia (a decreased white blood cell [WBC] count), thrombocytopenia (a decreased platelet count), and anemia (decreased hemoglobin, hematocrit, and red blood cell counts) and predisposes the patient to infection. To determine bone marrow suppression, monitor the complete blood count (CBC) and platelet count. Observe the patient with leukopenia for signs of infection, such as sore throat, mouth sores or ulcerations, fever, chills, dysuria, and malaise. To prevent infection, practice aseptic technique, promote adequate oral hygiene, encourage a nutritious diet, and take meticulous care with any indwelling (Foley) and urinary catheters.

Observe the patient for bruises and signs of bleeding. Check urine and stools for blood. In the patient with thrombocytopenia, avoid I.M. injections. Severe leukopenia or thrombocytopenia may require dosage adjustment or discontinuation of therapy.

If ordered, administer antiemetics for GI symptoms such as nausea, vomiting, abdominal cramps, or diarrhea. Watch for alterations in nutritional status. Warn the patient that these drugs commonly induce alopecia, nausea, and vomiting. Remember also that menstrual irregularities have been associated with the use of cytotoxic drugs, and hypertension and cholestasis have been associated with the use of cyclosporine.

**Precautions.** Immunosuppressive drugs must be used cautiously in patients with renal or hepatic diseases. Monitor blood values—blood urea nitrogen, creatinine, serum glutamic-oxaloacetic transaminase, serum glutamic-pyruvic transaminase, and alkaline phosphatase levels. Report changes in urinary output or signs of jaundice. To avoid hemorrhagic cystitis, which occurs in 5% to 10% of patients receiving cyclophosphamide, push at least 2 to 3 liters of fluids per day, unless contraindicated. Encourage the patient to urinate frequently.

In patients receiving cyclophosphamide, anticoagulants may increase bleeding tendencies, and concurrent use of allopurinol may require decreased dosages of azathioprine and 6-mercaptopurine. (Concurrent use of allopurinol may also require decreased dosages of cyclophosphamide.)

Before administering ALG, ask the patient if he's ever had a reaction to horse serum. Adverse reactions associated with ALG include fever, chills, rash, pain at the injection site, and in some cases, anaphylaxis. To reduce or prevent these reactions, diphenhydramine hydrochloride (Benadryl) may be administered before or during ALG therapy.

**Administration and teaching.** Advise the patient of the correct dosage and scheduling of immunosuppressive agents, and teach him to watch for adverse reactions. Promote good oral and personal hygiene, and encourage him to avoid exposure to infections. Be sure he can identify early signs of infection. Teach him to observe for signs of bleeding, especially if he's on anticoagulant therapy. To prevent internal bleeding, tell him to avoid aspirin and aspirin-containing preparations. Encourage him to use an electric razor to decrease the risk of external bleeding.

Counsel the patient to avoid pregnancy, if possible, because of the teratogenic effects of these drugs. If the patient experiences alopecia, suggest the use of wigs or scarves. Advise the patient who's taking methotrexate to avoid prolonged exposure to sunlight or sunlamps to prevent a photosensitivity reaction.

## Remission-inducing agents

Three classes of agents induce full or partial remission of severe, progressive rheumatoid arthritis: gold compounds, antimalarial agents, and penicillamine. But because of their extremely toxic effects, these agents are reserved for patients who have not responded adequately to NSAIDs and other treatment.

**Gold compounds.** These drugs, including aurothioglucose (Solganal) and gold sodium thiomalate (Myochrysine), are effective against rheumatoid arthritis. They must be administered I.M. at weekly to monthly inter-

## How the body regulates corticosteroid secretion

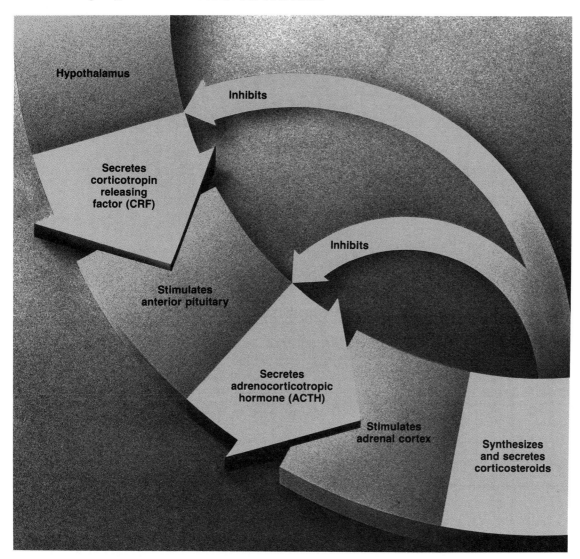

**Hypothalamus**

Inhibits

**Secretes corticotropin releasing factor (CRF)**

Inhibits

**Stimulates anterior pituitary**

**Secretes adrenocorticotropic hormone (ACTH)**

**Stimulates adrenal cortex**

**Synthesizes and secretes corticosteroids**

When blood corticosteroid levels are low, the hypothalamus secretes corticotropin releasing factor (CRF), which stimulates the anterior pituitary gland to release adrenocorticotropic hormone (ACTH). This, in turn, stimulates the adrenal cortex to secrete corticosteroids as needed. If the blood contains an adequate or elevated concentration of corticosteroids (as when synthetic corticosteroids are administered), a negative feedback mechanism inhibits the hypothalamus from secreting CRF, which would otherwise trigger the sequence of ACTH secretion.

vals. Auranofin (Ridaura), a new oral form of gold, seems as effective as parenteral gold salts and may produce fewer serious side effects. Although their mechanisms of action are unknown, gold compounds have been shown to suppress many immunologic functions, including antibody synthesis, lymphocyte activation, and phagocytosis.

*Precautions and side effects.* When administering gold compounds, watch for common side effects, including dermatitis; stomatitis; proteinuria; and bone marrow suppression, which results in low WBC and platelet counts. Tell the patient to report immediately any skin rash, which may progress to fatal exfoliative dermatitis if drug therapy continues. And advise him that beneficial effects may not appear for 8 weeks or longer. If he's receiving aurothioglucose, an oil suspension of gold, be sure to warm it and shake it thoroughly

before injection. Observe the patient for anaphylactic reactions for 30 minutes after I.M. injections.

**Antimalarial agents.** The antimalarials chloroquine hydrochloride and hydroxychloroquine sulfate (Plaquenil) have been used to suppress lymphocyte activation and chemotaxis (cell migration) in rheumatoid arthritis and SLE. However, chloroquine has been abandoned in recent years because it causes ocular toxicity.

*Precautions and side effects.* The patient who's receiving antimalarial drugs should have periodic CBCs and liver function tests. Because these drugs have been associated with blindness, baseline and periodic ophthalmologic exams are also necessary. Advise the patient to report blurred vision or light sensitivity. And watch for CNS effects, including headaches, dizziness, and neuromyopathy.

**Penicillamine.** Traditionally used for treating heavy metal poisoning, penicillamine (Cuprimine) has more recently been used to treat rheumatoid arthritis. It suppresses T- and B-lymphocyte activity and decreases antibody responses, but the mechanism of its antirheumatic action remains unknown.

*Precautions and side effects.* Advise the patient receiving penicillamine that onset of beneficial effects may take 6 weeks to 6 months. Because thrombocytopenia may occur, watch for signs of bleeding. Notify the doctor if the platelet count goes below 100,000/mm³. Also report any signs of rash. Loss of taste sensation is common but reversible, whether or not the drug is discontinued.

### Antiallergic agents

When exposed to specific allergens, sensitized mast cells release vasoactive or bronchospastic mediators, such as histamine and slow-reacting substance of anaphylaxis, which is also known as leukotrienes C, D, and E. These mediators are responsible for allergic symptoms such as urticaria, asthma, rhinitis, and atopic dermatitis. Many of these symptoms can be inhibited or counteracted with antihistamines, bronchodilators, decongestants, xanthine derivatives, glucocorticoids, cromolyn sodium, and other drugs.

**Antihistamines.** These agents block histamine receptors on various tissues, preventing histamine released by mast cells from interacting with the histamine receptors on adjacent tissue cells. They also have varying degrees of anticholinergic, sedative, antiemetic, and local anesthetic effects. They're particularly useful for treating allergic rhinitis, vasomotor rhinitis, allergic conjunctivitis, urticaria, and allergic reactions to blood products. Because receptor sites can be blocked before histamine is released from mast cells, antihistamines produce better therapeutic results when administered regularly rather than sporadically. (See *Chemical classes of antihistamines.*)

*Precautions and side effects.* Antihistamines are contraindicated in narrow angle glaucoma, acute asthmatic attack, urinary retention, and prostatic hypertrophy. They are generally well tolerated but may produce drowsiness and dry mouth. Drowsiness, sedation, and hypotension are more likely in elderly patients. Warn the patient about these side effects, and tell him to avoid alcohol and other CNS depressants. To alleviate dry mouth, give the patient sugarless gum, hard candy, or ice chips. To avoid GI upset, administer antihistamines with food or milk.

**Bronchodilators.** These drugs mimic beta-adrenergic stimulation by acting upon β-2 receptors in bronchial tissue, dilating the lung's airways to relieve reversible bronchospasm in asthma, bronchitis, and emphysema. Some bronchodilators also stimulate β-1 receptors in the heart, which may produce life-threatening side effects. Inhalant forms of sympathomimetic bronchodilators act rapidly when administered via metered-dose inhaler, nebulizer, or intermittent positive-pressure breathing. Oral preparations are often used when rapid response is unnecessary or when the patient has difficulty using an inhaler. However, oral forms require larger doses and their systemic distribution produces more side effects. Parenteral bronchodilators are usually reserved for emergency treatment of status asthmaticus.

*Precautions and side effects.* Increased blood pressure and tachycardia commonly accompany use of bronchodilators, so you need to monitor patients closely. Also watch for CNS stimulation (particularly in elderly patients), including hallucinations, convulsions, anxiety, nervousness, insomnia, and (with oral β-2 sympathomimetics) tremor. Use all sympathomimetic bronchodilators cautiously in patients with coronary artery disease, cardiac dysrhythmias, and hypertension. If the patient has difficulty using an inhaler, teach him how to use it correctly. (See *Using a metered-dose nebulizer,* page 58.) Warn him not to exceed his prescribed dosage since bronchodilators lose effectiveness with overuse.

**Decongestants.** These agents stimulate alpha-adrenergic receptors of vascular smooth muscle to constrict dilated blood vessels within the nasal mucosa. They are often combined with antihistamines to treat allergic rhinitis accompanied by nasal obstruction. Commonly used decongestants include ephedrine, pseudoephedrine, phenylpropanolamine, and phenylephrine. Although both oral and topical nasal decongestants are effective, topical preparations may produce fewer systemic side effects.

*Precautions and side effects.* Nasal decongestants are vasoconstricting agents and may elevate blood pressure. Use them cautiously in patients with coronary artery disease, hypertension, and diabetes mellitus. Monitor for dysrhythmias, elevations in blood pressure, nervousness, insomnia, headache, and dizziness. Stress that overuse of topical nasal

## Chemical classes of antihistamines

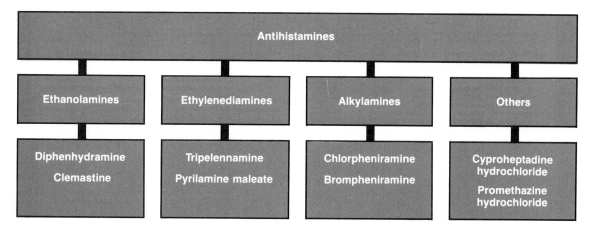

decongestants leads to rebound phenomenon, exaggerating nasal symptoms.

**Xanthine derivatives.** Chemically related to caffeine, these drugs have been used as potent bronchodilators, providing relief of acute asthmatic symptoms. The most popular xanthine derivative is theophylline, which dilates bronchioles by relaxing smooth muscle. Although its mechanism of action is unknown, it may be related to inhibition of phosphodiesterase, the enzyme that degrades cyclic adenosine monophosphate in smooth muscle.

Theophylline is available in oral and rectal forms. Aminophylline, a form of theophylline, is administered I.V. and ensures rapid delivery for acute symptoms. Plain, uncoated tablets or liquids may be satisfactory in treating nonacute symptoms. A sustained-release form is preferred for chronic symptoms. Oral xanthine derivatives include theophylline, aminophylline, oxtriphylline (Choledyl) and dyphylline (Lufyllin). Generally, rectal forms are less dependable and variably absorbed.

The dosage needed to maintain therapeutic levels of theophylline varies according to the patient's age, smoking history, and medications. For example, children and smokers need higher doses to ensure adequate blood levels. To achieve optimal bronchodilation, serum levels should be maintained within therapeutic range (10 to 20 mcg/ml). Higher levels may be toxic. Sustained-release forms emit theophylline slowly over 12 or 24 hours to maintain a relatively constant serum level. Immediate-release forms produce wide variations in serum levels.

*Administration and teaching.* An infusion pump ensures consistent administration of aminophylline and avoids the transient hypotension associated with rapid I.V. administration. (I.M. injection of aminophylline is painful and should be avoided.) Oral sustained-release forms are specially coated to release medication over long periods: tell the patient to swallow them whole without chewing or crushing them. However, if the patient has difficulty swallowing them, the contents of sustained-release capsules may be mixed with food, such as applesauce.

If the patient complains of nausea or queasiness when theophylline treatment begins, check to ensure that levels are within therapeutic range. GI complaints may be an early sign of toxicity.

*Side effects.* Theophylline may worsen pre-existing dysrhythmia, so you need to watch for tachycardia, premature ventricular contractions, ventricular fibrillation, and, rarely, cardiovascular collapse. Check the patient's heart rate before each dose of medication. (Cardiac side effects usually do not occur with therapeutic levels of theophylline.) Grand mal seizures may occur, particularly when serum levels exceed 50 mcg/ml.

Since xanthine derivatives are related to caffeine, they may produce diuresis, CNS stimulation, and increased gastric acid secretion. Watch for signs of CNS stimulation, including irritability, restlessness, dizziness, nervousness, headache, insomnia, and convulsions. Sympathomimetic agents may cause CNS stimulation and increase theophylline's side effects.

**Glucocorticoids.** This class of corticosteroids is most effective for treating symptoms of allergic disorders. In asthma, glucocorticoids enhance the action of catecholamines, increase the number of beta-adrenergic receptors for catecholamines, and suppress late-phase allergic inflammatory reactions. Systemic and nonsystemic (topical inhaled) glucocorticoids are useful in adjuvant therapy

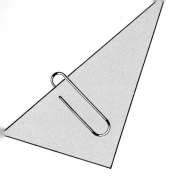

# Using a metered-dose nebulizer

*Dear* _____

You will be taking the drug your doctor has prescribed as an aerosol. To get the most benefit from your treatment, follow these instructions carefully.
• Insert the drug container into the short end of the plastic mouthpiece so that the container nozzle engages in the small hole (illustration 1).
• Then, holding the apparatus upside down, place the mouthpiece well into your mouth, closing your lips tightly over it (illustration 2).
• Exhale through your nose as completely as possible.
• Then, inhale deeply through your mouth, while pressing the container firmly into the mouthpiece to release the medication (illustration 3).
• After you've released the medication, hold your breath for 10 seconds.
• Remove the inhaler, and exhale (illustration 4).

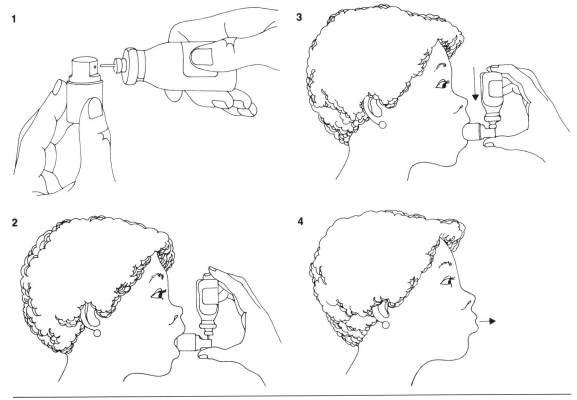

for severe asthma; intranasal forms are highly effective in allergic rhinitis; and topical preparations relieve many skin disorders.

Parenteral (I.V.) glucocorticoids, usually administered in high doses, help alleviate status asthmaticus. Oral glucocorticoids help control symptoms of allergic diseases; if possible, they should be administered in alternate-day therapy to avoid suppression of the hypothalamic-pituitary-adrenal axis. (However, only those steroids with a short half-life—prednisone, prednisolone, and methylprednisolone—are suitable for alternate-day therapy.)

Topical inhaled glucocorticoids include dexamethasone (Decadron) and beclomethasone dipropionate (Beclovent). Beclomethasone, the preferred agent, has fewer side effects and is indicated for long-term therapy. Unlike dexamethasone, beclomethasone that's absorbed through the lungs into systemic circulation is metabolized to an inactive form. Thus, use of beclomethasone avoids the side effects of systemic corticosteroids.

In many asthmatic patients, either oral or inhaled forms of glucocorticoids may be effective; however, inhaled forms should not be used to treat *acute* asthmatic attacks because they may not deliver an adequate dose to the lung tissue.

The effect of topical glucocorticoids in allergic skin disorders (such as atopic dermatitis and contact dermatitis) depends upon percutaneous absorption. Of these agents, the fluorinated corticosteroids (such as fluocinolone acetonide) are the most potent.

*Administration and side effects.* When an inhaled glucocorticoid is prescribed with a sympathomimetic agent, administer the sympathomimetic several minutes before the glucocorticoid. The sympathomimetic opens airways, allowing the glucocorticoid to penetrate deep into the respiratory tract. Allow at least 1 minute between inhalations when multiple inhalations are indicated.

The most serious side effects of aerosol glucocorticoids are oral and pharyngeal *Candida* infections, hoarseness, and cough. To avoid these, instruct the patient to gargle with water and to rinse his mouth after each use. Also instruct him not to exceed his prescribed dose because high doses may cause adrenal suppression.

Lightly apply ointments and creams containing glucocorticoids, and cover the site with an occlusive dressing to increase absorption. Topical glucocorticoids may cause local skin reactions, so watch for signs of irritation, including dryness, infection, and skin atrophy. Excessive or prolonged use of topical corticosteroids can produce systemic side effects, especially when these agents are applied to broken skin, over a large area, or with an occlusive dressing.

**Miscellaneous drugs.** Cromolyn sodium is useful for treating asthma. It prevents mediator release from mast cells and may reduce bronchial hyperreactivity in some asthmatic patients. However, it's poorly absorbed from the GI tract and must be inhaled directly into the lungs through a Spinhaler.

The anticholinergic agent atropine and similar compounds have been used to block cholinergic receptors, relieving bronchoconstriction and mucous gland secretions in some asthmatic patients.

*Precautions and side effects.* When cromolyn sodium is prescribed in capsule form, instruct the patient not to swallow the capsule. Teach him how to use the drug with the Spinhaler. Advise him that beneficial effects of this drug may take 2 to 4 weeks to appear.

Because cromolyn sodium is not systemically absorbed, most of its side effects occur in the respiratory tract. Watch for broncho-

spasm, cough, nasal congestion, pharyngeal irritation, and wheezing. Cromolyn sodium is contraindicated in acute asthmatic attacks.

Atropine is not used extensively because it commonly produces such side effects as flushed skin; dry mouth, nose, and skin; blurred vision; bradycardia; tachycardia with palpitations; and headache. Ipratropium (Atrovent), an atropine-like drug currently being investigated, appears to be better tolerated than atropine.

**Experimental immunoenhancing agents**

Experimental immunotherapy focuses on drugs currently being used to treat nonimmune diseases, such as the peptic ulcer drug cimetidine, as well as purely experimental agents such as Interferon (a group of proteins released by cells after antigen stimulation).

**Levamisole.** This drug has been shown to enhance and restore blunted cell-mediated immune responses by stimulating both helper and suppressor T lymphocytes. It's useful in some patients with severe, progressive rheumatic diseases. Its mechanism of action is unknown, but levamisole structurally resembles the thymic hormones thymin and thymopoietin. Because levamisole is long-acting, it's administered only once weekly.

The most serious side effect of levamisole therapy is neutropenia, which increases susceptibility to infection. When administering levamisole, monitor the patient's blood count periodically, and watch for signs of infection, such as fever and chills. Also watch for adverse reactions, such as nausea, insomnia, and alterations in taste and smell.

**Interferons.** A group of heterogeneous proteins produced by several cell types in the body, interferons have antiviral and antineoplastic effects under laboratory conditions. Although their mechanisms of action remain unknown, interferons inhibit viral replication and tumor cell growth and enhance natural killer-lymphocyte activity and phagocytosis. Clinical trials of Interferon in neoplastic and infectious diseases have suggested tumor regression, increased survival, and effective treatment of viral infections in immunocompromised patients. These investigations have benefited from new technology that produces large quantities of Interferon through genetic manipulation of bacteria.

Fever, a common side effect of Interferon administration, usually peaks at the start of treatment and subsides with continued therapy. Other side effects include pain at the

## Understanding transfer factor

Transfer factor, a leukocyte extract, confers sensitivity to a specific antigen on an immunodeficient recipient. To prepare transfer factor, leukocytes from an immunologically positive donor (one with positive skin tests) are freeze-thawed, enzymatically treated, and dialyzed. When the leukocyte extract is injected into an immunologically negative recipient (one with negative skin tests), his lymphocytes become sensitized and confer cell-mediated immunity. For example, immunity to *Mycobacterium tuberculosis* can be transferred by this method, which results in a tuberculin-positive skin test reaction.

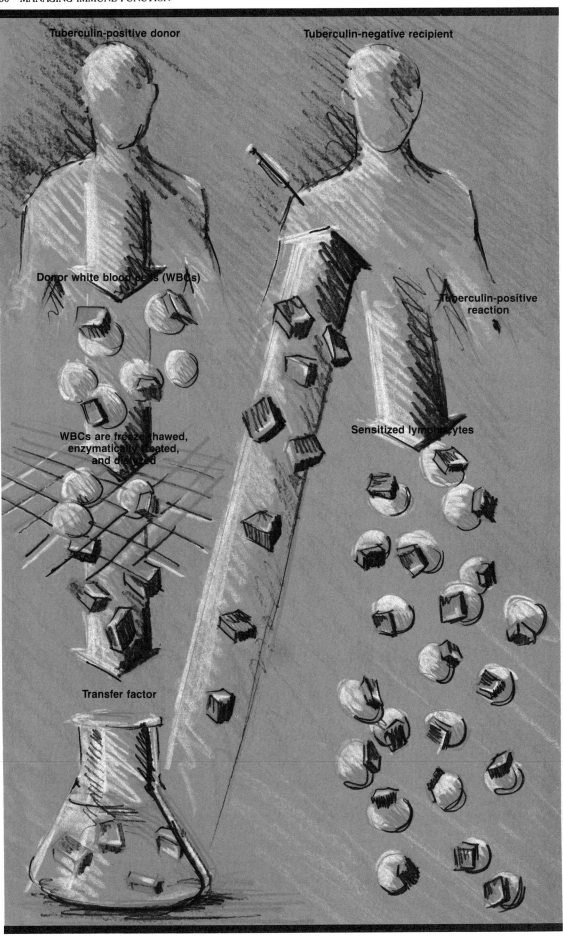

Tuberculin-positive donor

Tuberculin-negative recipient

Donor white blood cells (WBCs)

Tuberculin-positive reaction

WBCs are freeze-thawed, enzymatically treated, and dialyzed

Sensitized lymphocytes

Transfer factor

injection site, shivering, and fatigue.

**Thymic hormones.** The thymus gland produces many hormones essential to the development and maturation of T lymphocytes. Thymic hormones isolated and used in clinical trials include thymin, thymosin, and facteur thymique serique. These agents are being tested for their ability to restore cell-mediated immunity in patients with acquired and congenital T-lymphocyte defects and in those with autoimmune diseases. In some patients, allergic reactions have been reported after injection of these hormones.

**Cimetidine.** This peptic ulcer drug has successfully restored cell-mediated immunity in some patients. Although the mechanism of action is not understood, it may be related to cimetidine's ability to block $H_2$ histamine receptors on suppressor T lymphocytes. Cimetidine has been shown to induce cell-mediated immunity in patients with chronic mucocutaneous candidiasis. Cimetidine has also restored delayed cutaneous hypersensitivity in patients with negative reactions to common skin test antigens, such as mumps and *Candida*. Potential side effects of cimetidine use include headache; constipation; dizziness; fatigue; gynecomastia; azoospermia; and mental confusion, particularly in the elderly.

**Transfer factor.** Also known as dialyzable leukocyte extract, transfer factor has been used successfully to treat recurrent infections in immunodeficient patients. It has also improved the survival rate in some patients with malignant disease. Transfer factor confers specific immunity from the donor. It does not affect antibody production. (See *Understanding transfer factor.*)

**Bacille Calmette-Guérin (BCG).** A strain of *Mycobacterium bovis*, BCG nonspecifically helps stimulate T lymphocytes and natural killer lymphocytes. Its mechanism of action remains unknown. This agent is usually administered by scarification. In this technique, a special device must be used to make 20 scratches—each 2″ (5 cm) long—on a 2″ × 2″ area. (Each scratch must be deep enough to produce some bleeding.) Although BCG may be administered by intradermal injection, it usually produces severe local reactions. It may also be injected directly into lesions; however, this method increases side effects, such as fever, chills, and granulomatous hepatitis. BCG has been used with varying success as an adjuvant to cancer chemotherapy.

***Corynebacterium parvum.*** *C. parvum* is a gram-positive bacterium that, when heat-killed, can be used to enhance immune responses. Although *C. parvum* has been reported to cause tumor remission, its severe side effects, including high fever, headache, and hypertension, will probably limit its usefulness.

## IMMUNOBIOLOGIC AGENTS
The concept of immunization has been recognized for centuries, and modern immunization has reduced the incidence and morbidity of many diseases and has even eradicated smallpox.

New vaccines are being developed to overcome the problem of increased pathogenic resistance to standard antibiotics. Immunizations against gonorrhea, dental caries, and certain tumors are now being tried, with promising results.

**Major types.** The following definitions can help you understand the action and clinical uses of immunobiologic agents.

A *vaccine* is a suspension of attenuated live or killed microorganisms or of antigenic determinants of organisms administered to induce immunity and prevent infectious disease.

A *toxoid* contains exotoxins (heat-labile, proteinaceous toxins formed by bacteria and secreted outside the bacterial cell). These substances are chemically changed to make them nontoxic, but they retain the ability to stimulate antitoxin (antibody formation). Immunization with a toxoid induces production of antibodies and memory lymphocytes, which give lasting protection against the toxin.

An *immune serum globulin* provides passive immunity against infectious diseases or suppresses antibody formation, as in Rh incompatibility. These globulins are obtained from hyperimmunized human or animal donors, or from pooled plasma. These products are then purified and standardized. Immune serums are effective only for prophylaxis.

A *specific immune globulin* is a special preparation obtained from selected donors who possess a high concentration of antibodies against a specific illness. For example, hepatitis B immune globulin is obtained from patients who have recovered from hepatitis B.

An *antitoxin* is a solution of antibodies from animals (usually horses) that have been immunized with a specific toxin. Antitoxins bind to and neutralize bacterial toxins, but they must be administered early in the course of the infection and in adequate doses.

## Common vaccines for inducing active immunity

| Disease | Agents | Use |
|---------|--------|-----|
| Diphtheria | Toxoid | Infancy and childhood; three I.M. injections during the first year and at age 4 to 6; > 90% effective |
| Pertussis | Heat-killed *Bordetella pertussis* (DPT) | |
| Tetanus | Toxoid | |
| Poliomyelitis | Live, attenuated poliovirus; three types | Three doses of trivalent vaccine given orally during first year; boosters at ages 1½ and age 4 to 6; > 95% effective |
| Rubeola (measles) | Live, attenuated virus | At age 1; 95% effective |
| Rubella (German measles) | Live, attenuated virus | After age 1 and at puberty; > 95% effective |
| Mumps | Live, attenuated virus | After age 1; 95% effective |
| Influenza | Formalin-ethylene oxide, inactivated; multiple types | Used primarily in elderly patients with chronic lung and heart disease; 60% to 75% effective |
| Smallpox | Live vaccinia virus | No longer recommended for United States residents; > 90% effective |
| Rabies | Virus grown in duck embryos or human diploid cells; inactivated with beta-propiolactone | Used under special conditions; 80% effective |
| Yellow fever | Live, attenuated virus | Only for travel in epidemic areas |
| Cholera | Phenol-killed *Vibrio cholerae* | For travel to certain areas of the world |
| Typhoid | Acetone-killed *Salmonella typhosa* | For travel to certain areas of the world |
| Plague | Heat-killed *Yersinia pestis* | For travel to certain areas of the world |

## Immunization

Immunization induces or augments resistance to disease. *Active immunization* involves natural exposure to an infecting organism or use of vaccines and toxoids. *Passive immunization* involves administration of preformed antibodies to a nonimmunized person.

**Active immunization.** Following exposure to an immunizing substance, the body produces antibodies specific for the substance. Upon first exposure to a vaccine, a latent period of 1 to 2 weeks must pass before antibody production begins. Typically, a patient's IgM is the first immunoglobulin synthesized after initial antigenic exposure. A second exposure elicits a faster response in antibody production, with formation of IgG immunoglobulin. These subsequent responses to antigens are typically referred to as secondary, or anamnestic, responses. The ability to produce a secondary response may persist for many years after initial exposure to the immunizing substance but eventually declines. This decline is the reason for booster immunizations.

(See *Common vaccines for inducing active immunity.*)

Although immunization may be achieved with live or dead vaccines or toxoids, live vaccines pose a slight risk of disease, even in immunocompetent persons. Active immunizations rarely cause serious complications, but they may produce fever, malaise, and soreness at the injection site. Some reactions are specific for certain agents and induce symptoms of the natural disease, such as the arthralgia that occurs after rubella vaccination. However, these reactions are less frequent and less severe than in the natural disease.

Allergic reactions may follow exposure to the egg protein commonly found in viral vaccines. For this reason, patients with severe allergy to egg products should receive a vaccine whose culture was grown in an alternate medium.

Administration of live vaccines is contraindicated in pregnant patients because of potential teratogenic effects, in patients receiving corticosteroids or immunosuppressive drugs,

## Sera commonly used for passive immunization

| Disease | Serum source and preparation | Valuable | Adverse reactions |
|---------|------------------------------|----------|-------------------|
| Tetanus | Human, hyperimmune | Yes | Local pain, swelling, tenderness |
| Diphtheria | Equine◊, purified; | Yes | Serum sickness |
| | Immune human serum globulin | Yes | Local pain, swelling, tenderness |
| Hepatitis A | Immune human serum globulin | Yes | Local pain, swelling, tenderness |
| Hepatitis B | Human, hyperimmune | Probably | Local pain, swelling, tenderness |
| Non-A, non-B hepatitis | Immune human serum globulin | Unknown | Local pain, swelling, tenderness |
| Rubeola | Immune human serum globulin | Yes | Local pain, swelling, tenderness |
| Varicella zoster | Human, hyperimmune† | Yes | Local pain, swelling, tenderness |
| Rabies | Human, hyperimmune | Yes | Local pain, swelling, tenderness |
| | Equine◊ | Yes | Serum sickness |
| Poliomyelitis | Immune human serum globulin | Yes | Local pain, swelling, tenderness |
| Smallpox | Human, hyperimmune | Yes | Local pain, swelling, tenderness |
| Mumps | Human, hyperimmune | Doubtful | Local pain, swelling, tenderness |
| Rubella | Immune human serum globulin | Doubtful | Local pain, swelling, tenderness |
| Clostridial myonecrosis (gas gangrene) | Equine◊, polyvalent | Doubtful | Serum sickness |
| Botulism | Equine◊, polyvalent | Yes | Serum sickness |

◊Purified and concentrated horse serum      †Obtainable from Centers for Disease Control, Atlanta

and in those with immunodeficiencies.

A person who has received live oral polio vaccine may cause inadequately immunized persons who are exposed to his viral excretions to develop poliomyelitis. Therefore, parents whose vaccination histories indicate inadequate immunization should be immunized with inactivated polio vaccine before a child's immunization.

**Passive immunization.** Immune serum globulins and maternal antibodies, which cross the placental barrier, are examples of passive immunizing substances. The effect of passive immunization is immediate but transient; it's most useful after exposure to toxins or microorganisms in persons who cannot produce antibodies or who risk developing disease before active immunization can stimulate antibody production.

Antibodies for passive immunization may be obtained from humans or animals; animal serum, however, can be immunogenic and cause allergic reactions and life-threatening anaphylaxis in patients who have previously been exposed to an animal serum. (See *Sera commonly used for passive immunization.*) Therefore, do not administer animal antiserum without obtaining a history of exposure or allergic reaction to any product from the specific animal source used to prepare the antitoxin. Have epinephrine readily available when administering such antiserums.

Animal serum may also produce serum sickness reactions, including arthritis, pruritus, fever, rashes, and lymphadenopathy, which may occur within hours or weeks after immunization. Adverse reactions to human serum globulin injections are rare and usually confined to the injection site.

### OTHER IMMUNOTHERAPIES
When immune disorders fail to respond to conventional therapy, they may respond to immunotherapeutic techniques. For example, in a bone marrow transplant, the patient may require total nodal irradiation to suppress immune response and prevent graft rejection. *(continued on page 66)*

# How apheresis works

Therapeutic apheresis allows the selective removal of unwanted components (plasma or cellular elements) from the blood of a patient suffering from an autoimmune disease (such as rheumatoid arthritis or systemic lupus erythematosus).

In this procedure, whole blood is channeled via a venous access line to a blood cell separator (see drawing), then centrifuged to separate the blood components. Acid citrate dextrose (ACD) is added to the system as an anticoagulant throughout the procedure.

As whole blood passes through the system, it is separated into component-rich plasma and red blood cells (RBCs). RBCs are returned to the donor, the unwanted immune component is removed from the plasma and retained in the system, and the component-poor plasma is then returned to the donor. The system is primed with saline solution and flushed with additional saline solution after the procedure.

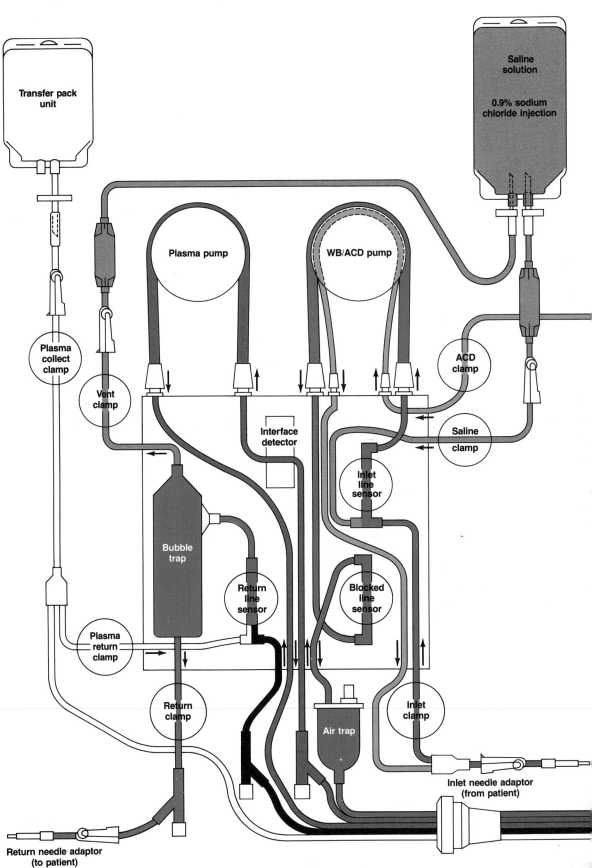

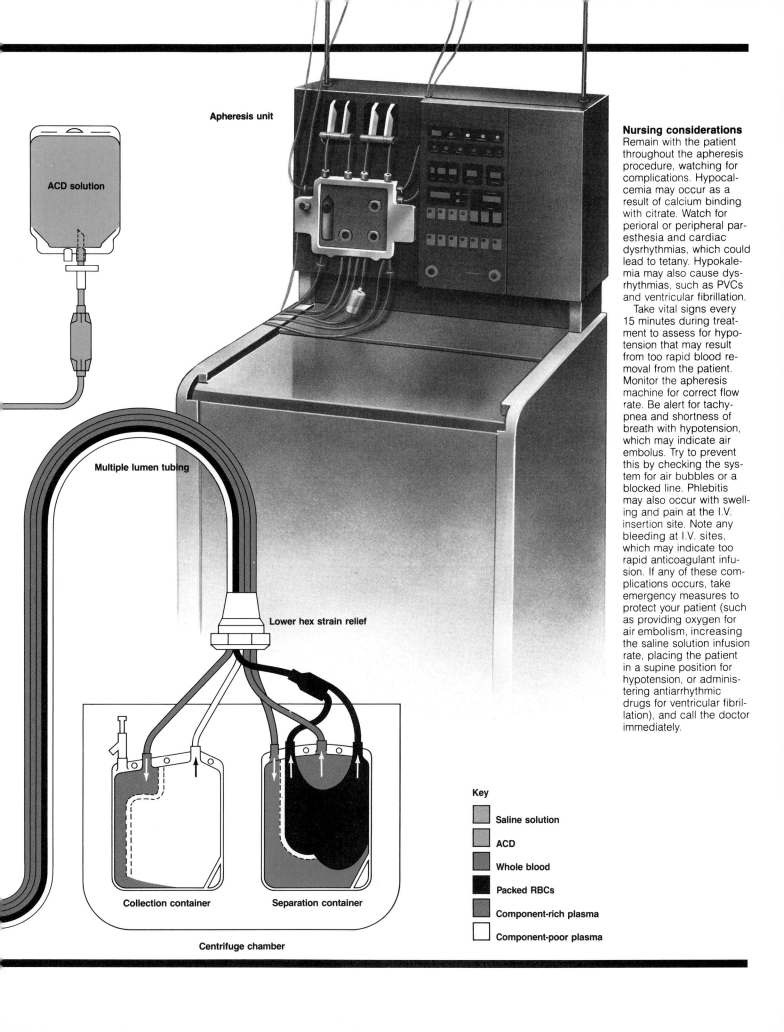

**ACD solution**

**Apheresis unit**

**Multiple lumen tubing**

**Lower hex strain relief**

**Collection container**

**Separation container**

**Centrifuge chamber**

**Key**

- Saline solution
- ACD
- Whole blood
- Packed RBCs
- Component-rich plasma
- Component-poor plasma

**Nursing considerations**
Remain with the patient throughout the apheresis procedure, watching for complications. Hypocalcemia may occur as a result of calcium binding with citrate. Watch for perioral or peripheral paresthesia and cardiac dysrhythmias, which could lead to tetany. Hypokalemia may also cause dysrhythmias, such as PVCs and ventricular fibrillation.

Take vital signs every 15 minutes during treatment to assess for hypotension that may result from too rapid blood removal from the patient. Monitor the apheresis machine for correct flow rate. Be alert for tachypnea and shortness of breath with hypotension, which may indicate air embolus. Try to prevent this by checking the system for air bubbles or a blocked line. Phlebitis may also occur with swelling and pain at the I.V. insertion site. Note any bleeding at I.V. sites, which may indicate too rapid anticoagulant infusion. If any of these complications occurs, take emergency measures to protect your patient (such as providing oxygen for air embolism, increasing the saline solution infusion rate, placing the patient in a supine position for hypotension, or administering antiarrhythmic drugs for ventricular fibrillation), and call the doctor immediately.

## Reducing the risk of infection: The laminar airflow room

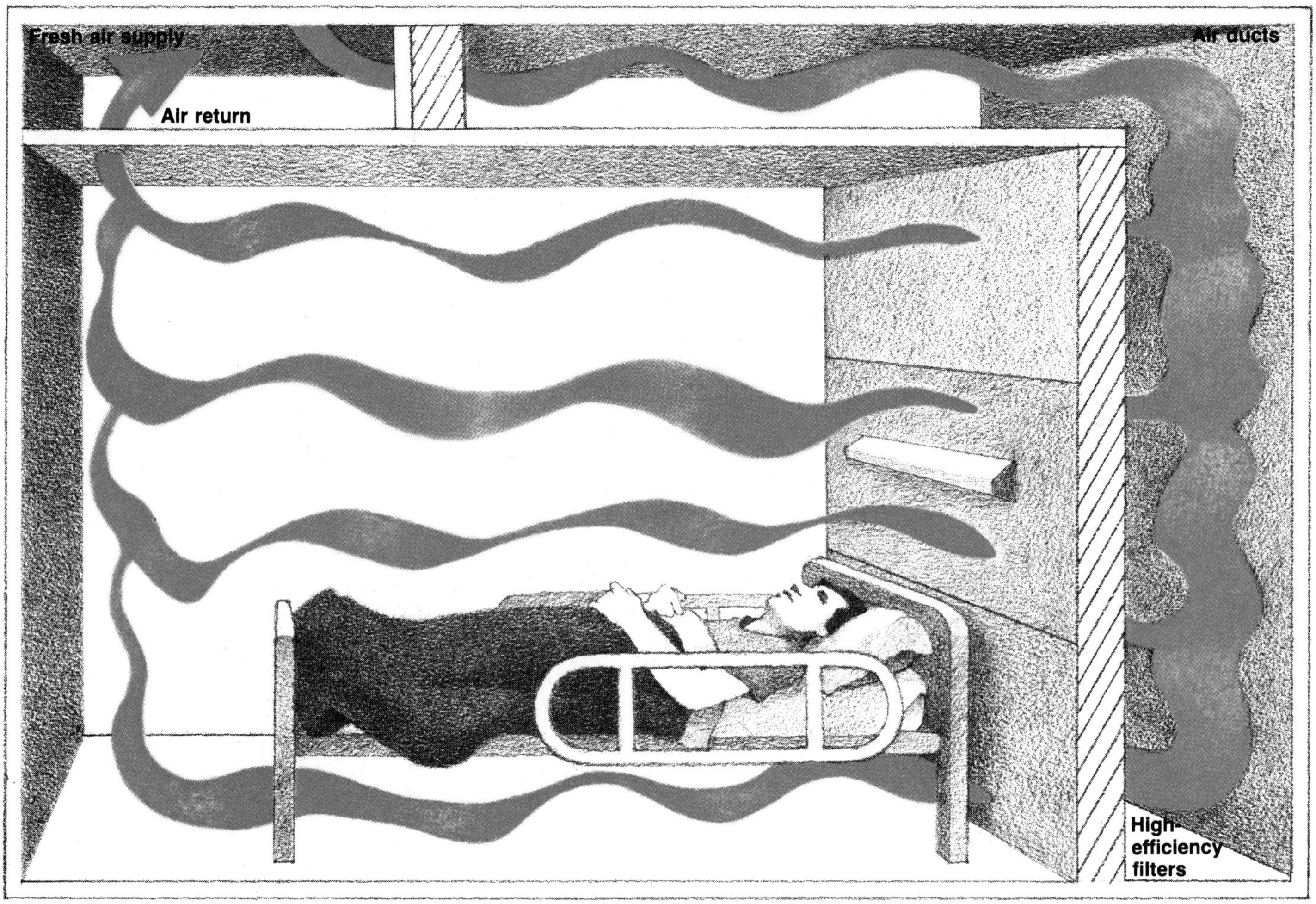

Fresh air supply

Air ducts

Air return

High-efficiency filters

The laminar airflow room provides a germ-free environment for patients at high risk—for example, those experiencing disease relapse or those receiving nonhistocompatible transplants. This room contains a high-efficiency air filter in one wall or in the ceiling. Filtered air flows across the room with a laminar distribution, providing several hundred air exchanges per hour. To further minimize the chance of infection, the room and its furnishings may be cleaned with germicidal cleansers, and the patient's food and clothing may be sterilized.

And afterward, he may require meticulous environmental control, in addition to careful monitoring, to prevent life-threatening infections.

### Bone marrow transplant

Bone marrow is transplanted primarily to reconstitute hematologic and immunologic function in patients who have not responded to conventional immunotherapy. It is the treatment of choice in aplastic anemia and immunodeficiency.

Four major types of bone marrow transplantation are *syngeneic, human-leukocyte-antigen– (HLA–) matched allogeneic, HLA-mismatched allogeneic,* and *autologous.* In syngeneic transplants, the recipient and donor are identical twins—a perfect match. In HLA-matched allogeneic transplants, the donor and recipient are compatible—usually siblings. A new technique, the HLA-mismatched allogeneic transplant, allows transplantation between an incompatible donor and recipient. In this procedure, harmful, mature T lympho-

cytes are removed from donor marrow by agglutination with soybean lectin. In autologous transplants, the patient's own marrow is frozen and stored for reinfusion after chemotherapy or radiotherapy.

**Preparation.** To ensure a successful transplant and prevent graft-versus-host disease (GVHD), the recipient and donor are matched for compatibility. Before transplantation, the recipient must undergo intensive immunosuppression to remove malignant cells, to prepare bone marrow spaces for engraftment, and to help prevent graft rejection. Typically, the recipient receives total body irradiation or total nodal irradiation in addition to immunosuppressive chemotherapy with cyclophosphamide or ALG.

Cultures of the patient's skin, throat, mouth, stool, and vagina are taken and stored to recontaminate the patient with normal bacterial flora before discharge. Other cultures are taken to determine negative bacterial and fungal growth.

To eliminate bacteria, the patient bathes in

chlorhexidine twice a day and uses sterile clothing and sheets. To sterilize the GI tract, antibiotics (cefamandole nafate, gentamicin, and nystatin) are given. Women receive clotrimazole intravaginally.

Despite meticulous care in transplant technique, GVHD may occur when newly grafted immunocompetent cells recognize foreign antigens in the recipient's body. Its characteristic symptom is a maculopapular rash; it may also produce diarrhea, hepatosplenomegaly, jaundice, cardiac irregularity, CNS irritation, and pulmonary infiltrates. In patients with this condition, corticosteroids or immunosuppressive agents increase the risk of fatal infection. Most immunodeficient patients who develop GVHD die from this complication or its accompanying infections.

Several controlled environments are currently being used for transplant patients. These include room isolation and, to decrease the risk of major infections or septicemia, laminar airflow in a clean or sterile environment. (See *Reducing the risk of infection: The laminar airflow room.*)

**Precautions.** The first 2 to 4 weeks after bone marrow transplant are the most critical. During this time, the patient lacks functional marrow—a direct result of the massive immunosuppressive chemotherapy and total body irradiation he has undergone. Posttransplant complications include bleeding, infection, stomatitis, and GVHD, as well as psychological effects related to isolation and the disease itself.

Watch for signs of infection, fever, chills, cough, and dysuria, and report these immediately. The doctor may order blood and urine studies and a chest X-ray. He may also prescribe antibiotics. Because the patient's platelet count is low, watch for signs of bleeding, such as petechiae, ecchymoses, and hematuria. Monitor the WBC count, and if possible, avoid invasive procedures such as rectal temperatures and injections. Promote meticulous oral care to help prevent stomatitis. Perform routine oral assessment, observing for white plaques, ulcerations, and redness. As ordered, administer immunosuppressant chemotherapy, watching closely for signs of GVHD. Its cardinal sign—a red, maculopapular rash—appears 7 to 14 days after the transplant, usually beginning on the face, palms, and soles, and later spreading to the trunk.

**Apheresis**
In this procedure, certain elements of the patient's blood are removed and the remainder is retransfused. For example, plasmapheresis (removal of all plasma) and leukapheresis (removal of cellular elements) have been used for SLE, multiple sclerosis, rheumatoid arthritis, myasthenia gravis, Goodpasture's syndrome, and thrombotic thrombocytopenic purpura. (See *How apheresis works,* pages 64 and 65.)

**Precautions.** Throughout the procedure, watch the patient for such complications as phlebitis, hypotension, and electrolyte imbalance. Monitor the cell-separator return tube for clotted or hemolyzed blood and air emboli. Check patency of tubes and connections, and watch the pump speed for correct flow.

After apheresis, observe the transfusion sites for bleeding and hematoma formation. Monitor the patient for signs of electrolyte imbalance, particularly hypokalemia. Observe for cardiac dysrhythmias, leg cramps, and mental confusion. Because minor blood loss occurs with apheresis, watch for signs of hypovolemia, such as orthostatic hypotension. Also watch for signs of infection, particularly in the immunosuppressed patient.

## Total nodal irradiation
Irradiation of major lymph node areas effectively induces immunosuppression and may help prevent graft rejection. This procedure typically induces a prolonged period of lymphopenia and has been used experimentally to treat autoimmune disorders such as rheumatoid arthritis and SLE. Such use needs continued investigation to evaluate its clinical benefit.

**Side effects.** Side effects of total nodal irradiation are related to the site chosen for treatment and to radiation dosage levels. The skin surrounding the treatment site typically becomes dry and erythematous; scaling, edema, and hair loss may also occur. The patient may also experience GI disturbances. Sterility is common.

## To stay current, stay informed
Understanding advances in immunotherapy poses a continuing challenge. Understanding immunotherapeutic drugs and other forms of immunotherapy enables you to care most effectively for patients with immune disorders. Such knowledge enables you to set realistic care goals and to develop appropriate nursing interventions. It also enables you to help the patient understand, accept, and manage his disease.

**Points to remember**

- Drugs that control the inflammatory process are classified as nonsteroidal anti-inflammatory drugs and corticosteroids.
- Pharmacologic suppression of the immune response may be required in severe rheumatoid arthritis, glomerulonephritis, and bone marrow and organ transplantation.
- Bone marrow is typically transplanted to reconstitute hematologic and immunologic function in patients with immunodeficiencies, acute leukemia, or severe aplastic anemia.
- Experimental immunoenhancing agents include levamisole, Interferon, thymic hormones, and transfer factor.
- Active immunization (by natural exposure or administration of vaccines or toxoids) causes production of specific antibodies.

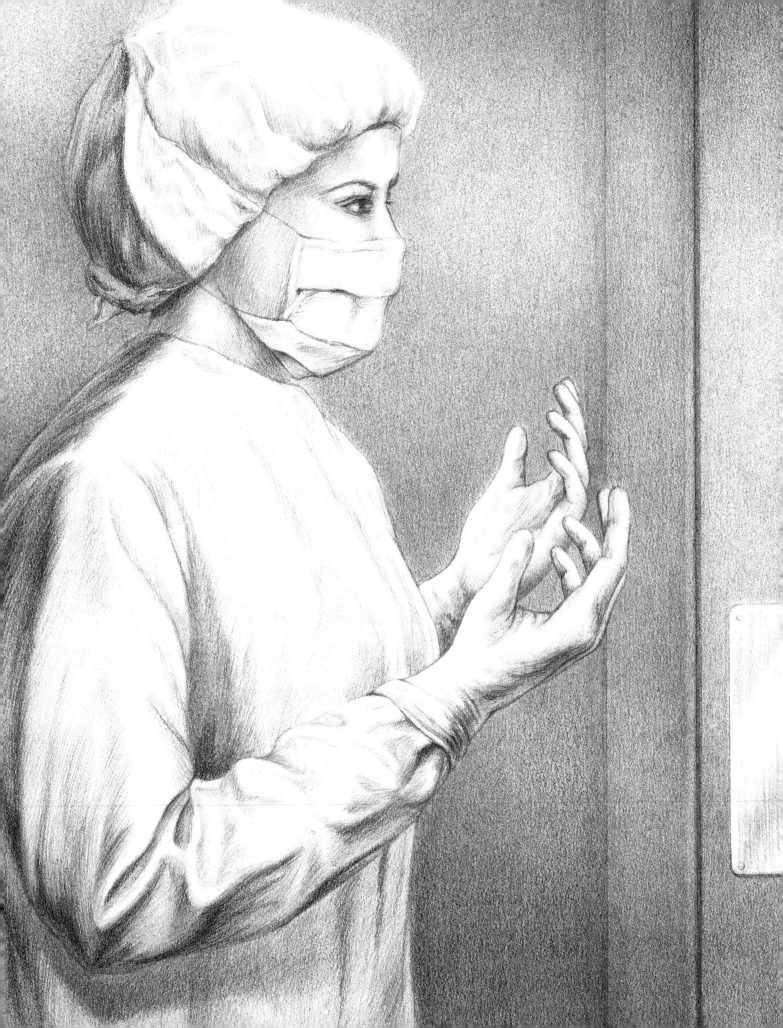

# DISORDERS OF
# THE IMMUNE
# SYSTEM

# 5 OVERCOMING IMMUNODEFICIENCIES

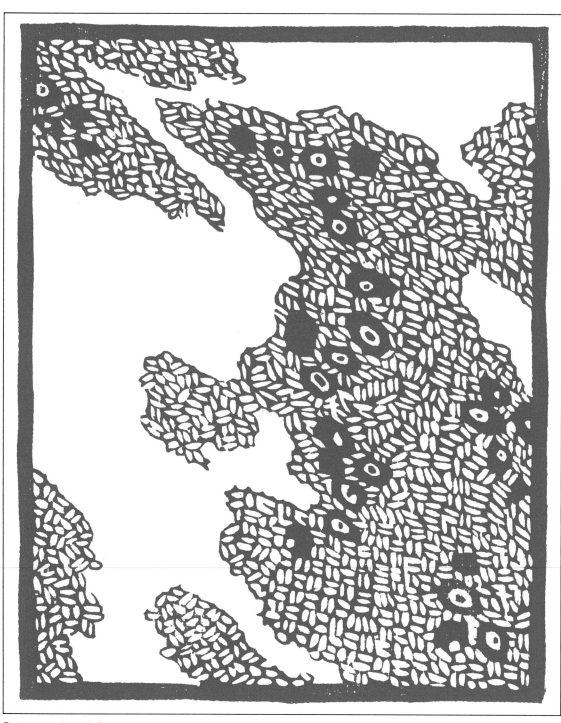

*Pneumocystis carinii*

The normal immune system protects the body from potentially harmful environmental and internal substances. When this complex system fails or functions inadequately, these substances can overwhelm the body; thus, the immunodeficient patient falls prey even to ordinarily nonpathogenic agents.

Caring for an immunodeficient patient poses a challenge at every turn. You need keen assessment skills to detect multiple and often subtle symptoms of immunodeficiencies. You need to know basic immune mechanisms to understand how dysfunction can affect this patient (see Chapter 1). You must be able to identify and counsel high-risk groups and to offer support, teaching, and advice to those with chronic immunodeficiencies. Finally, you need to be aware of recent advances in identifying, treating, and preventing immunodeficiencies to ensure you're providing this patient with the best care possible.

## Many forms

Acquired immunodeficiency syndrome (AIDS) has brought public attention to one of many types of immunodeficiencies. These disorders may be primary—either congenital or acquired—and may result in other problems, such as infection or malignancy; or they may be secondary to another disease or to aggressive treatment for a disease.

**Primary congenital immunodeficiency.** Some individuals are born lacking a specific substance or function essential to normal immune function. Their primary congenital immunodeficiency has been genetically transmitted, either as an X-linked trait (as in Bruton's hypogammaglobulinemia or Wiskott-Aldrich syndrome), or as an autosomal recessive trait (as in Swiss-type severe combined immunodeficiency [SCID] or immunodeficiency with ataxia-telangiectasia). Generally, such deficiency shows itself early in life; but in B-cell deficiencies, the infant is usually protected by his mother's IgG, which crosses the placenta and circulates in sufficient quantities for about 6 months. Thus, an infant with hypogammaglobulinemia, a defect in humoral immunity, will begin to have recurrent infections at about age 6 months. An infant who also has defects in cell-mediated immunity will show symptoms even earlier. (See *Primary congenital immunodeficiencies,* page 72.)

**Primary acquired immunodeficiency.** Others are born with normally functioning immunity but, for unknown reasons, develop immuno-deficiencies during their lifetime.

**Secondary immunodeficiency.** Still others develop immunodeficiency secondary to a known disease or injury or as a consequence of immunosuppressive therapy.

## Immunodeficiency: Why and who?

Immunodeficiency has varied causes, some of them age-related. An infant begins to produce IgM in utero and receives short-term passive immunity in the form of IgG across the placenta from the maternal circulation. During the early years, he receives probably the greatest antigenic stimulation of his life and is continuously differentiating self from nonself. When he reaches age 6 or 7, his immune system is completely mature. Until that time, he's more susceptible to infections.

The immune system—and immunocompetence—changes with age. Beginning at about midlife, both humoral and cell-mediated responses decline, either because of a progressive breakdown of the immune system or through some unknown mechanism of genetic control. Aging promotes susceptibility to injury and infection and increases vulnerability to autoimmune diseases and malignancies. This growing vulnerability to disease stems mainly from declining numbers and diminishing function of T lymphocytes (T cells), which may prove to be an intrinsic part of aging.

Other factors, such as environment and lifestyle, also appear to affect immunocompetence. Exposure to powerful drugs, noxious chemicals, thermal injury, and radiation can suppress immune function by destroying lymphocytes or inhibiting their maturation and function. Malnutrition can also reduce T-cell response.

Stress, when coupled with ineffective coping, can also induce temporary or prolonged immunosuppression. Stress profoundly inhibits the body's immune response through its associated rise in endogenous corticosteroids and catecholamines. This immunosuppression involves decreased chemotaxis and migration of neutrophils and monocytes as well as sequestration of T cells and, possibly, increased function of suppressor T cells.

## Incidence varies

Primary congenital immunodeficiency is considered rare. Isolated IgA deficiency, however, is more common, affecting roughly 1 out of 600 individuals in the United States. SCID, the most severe of all congenital immunodeficiencies, affects 1:100,000 to 1:500,000. AIDS has

# Primary congenital immunodeficiencies

| Disorder | Clinical findings | Pathologic findings |
|---|---|---|
| **Humoral** | | |
| Bruton's hypogamma-globulinemia | Recurrent pyogenic infections, especially pneumonia, sinusitis, otitis, furunculosis, meningitis, sepsis, panhy-pogammaglobulinemia, arthritis of the large joints | Absence of plasma cells; decreased B cells; pre–B cells fail to secrete immunoglobulin (decreased IgA, IgG, IgM) |
| Transient hypogamma-globulinemia of infancy | Recurrent respiratory tract infections beginning 5 to 6 months after birth, with recovery in 1 to 2 years | Uncertain cause; decreased IgG; low or normal IgA and IgM |
| Selective IgA deficiency | Bacterial infections of respiratory, gastrointestinal, and genitourinary tracts; diarrhea; malabsorption; frequently associated with autoimmune disease | IgA synthesis but not secretion; possible high-circulating anti-IgA antibody |
| Common variable immune deficiency (may be acquired) | Recurrent pyogenic infections (similar to Bruton's); malabsorption; diarrhea; giardiasis; autoimmune disease; lymphoreticular malignancy | Normal B-cell count; low immunoglobulin levels suggesting diminished synthesis or secretion |
| **Cell-mediated** | | |
| DiGeorge's syndrome | Thymic hypoplasia, hypocalcemia, parathyroid hypoplasia, otitis, tuberculosis, *Candida albicans,* abnormal facies, congenital cardiac anomalies, chronic diarrhea, failure to thrive, esophageal atresia | Thymic and parathyroid hypoplasia; deficient T cells; often increased B cells |
| Chronic mucocutaneous candidiasis | Chronic, resistant *C. albicans* infections of skin, nails, and mucous membranes; rarely life-threatening; possibly some endocrine abnormalities | Normal T-cell count, but failure of lymphokine production in the clone responsive to candida antigen |
| **Combined** | | |
| Severe combined immunodeficiency | Multiple, severe infections (bacterial, fungal, and viral); graft-versus-host disease; diarrhea; extreme wasting | Decreased T and B cells; little or no antibody |
| Immunodeficiency with ataxia-telangiectasia | Progressive cerebellar ataxia; multiple telangiectasia of skin and ocular mucosa; recurrent sinopulmonary infections; endocrine abnormalities; lymphomas | Possible decreased T cells; impaired T-cell function; decreased IgA and IgE in some patients |
| Wiskott-Aldrich syndrome | Thrombocytopenia with hemorrhagic tendency; eczema; recurrent infection; lymphoreticular malignancy | Possible hypercatabolism of immunoglobulin; decreased IgM and IgG; increased IgA and IgE; decreased T cells |
| **Phagocytic** | | |
| Chronic granulomatous disease | Marked lymphadenopathy with draining lymph nodes; hepatosplenomegaly; recurrent pneumonias; abscesses; dermatitis; conjunctivitis; osteomyelitis usually with unusual organisms of low virulence | Abnormal neutrophil function; impaired intracellular killing by the phagocyte because of enzyme deficiency (NADH or NADPH oxidase) |
| Jobs/Hyper IgE | Recurrent "cold" abscesses of skin, lymph nodes, and subcutaneous tissue; eczema; otitis media | Abnormal chemotaxis; increased eosinophils and IgE; abnormal antibody synthesis |
| "Lazy leukocyte" syndrome | Recurrent bacterial infections | Defective chemotaxis; decreased migration of peripheral neutrophils |
| Chédiak-Higashi syndrome | Recurrent cutaneous bacterial infections; hepatosplenomegaly; partial albinism; progressive central nervous system abnormality; lymphoreticular malignancy | Depressed neutrophil response to normal chemotactic stimuli; delayed neutrophil killing time |
| **Complement** | | |
| C1r | Autoimmune disease; infections; glomerulonephritis | Impaired ability to clear immune complexes |
| C3 | Multiple serious pyogenic infections, especially of skin and lungs; autoimmune disease | Impaired ability to opsonize bacteria; inability to activate C5 through C9 |
| C5 | Recurrent bacterial infections; diarrhea; seborrhea; autoimmune disease | Impaired chemotaxis and cytolysis |
| Hereditary angioedema | Episodic edema of throat, abdomen, face | Decreased C1 esterase inhibitor |

struck with increasing frequency since it was first recognized in 1979. (See *Acquired immunodeficiency syndrome [AIDS]: Incidence,* page 74, and *What you should know about AIDS,* pages 80 and 81).

Secondary immunodeficiency, from other diseases or aggressive treatments, is the most common immunodeficiency. When it results from the use of drugs that hamper inflammation and the immune response, it's also the most common cause of nosocomial infections.

## PATHOPHYSIOLOGY

Immunodeficiency implies inadequate numbers or function of any of the immune system's components. So immune disorders are classified according to the deficient structural component as humoral (B-cell) immunodeficiency, cell-mediated (T-cell) immunodeficiency, combined B- and T-cell immunodeficiency, phagocytic dysfunction, and complement deficiency.

### Humoral (B-cell) immunodeficiency

These disorders reflect decreased levels of any or all of the immunoglobulin classes. Abnormally low levels of all immunoglobulins (gamma globulins) is called hypogammaglobulinemia. Sometimes this condition is mistakenly called agammaglobulinemia, or absence of gamma globulin; actually, however, a small amount of immunoglobulin is usually present. Conversely, a deficiency in one or more, but not all, immunoglobulin classes is called dysgammaglobulinemia, as in selective IgA deficiency.

The patient with hypogammaglobulinemia can't respond adequately to antigenic stimulation, specifically to high-grade encapsulated bacteria and some viruses. Consequently, he's especially vulnerable to infection from such pyogenic organisms as streptococcus, staphylococcus, *Pseudomonas, Hemophilus influenzae,* and various pneumococci. The resulting infections, especially pneumonia, sinusitis, osteomyelitis, dermatitis, and septicemia, tend to be recurrent and severe. The patient with hypogammaglobulinemia doesn't show the same vulnerability to fungal and most viral infections since the latter infections are controlled by cell-mediated immunity.

Since plasma cells normally produce antibodies, antibody deficiency may result from defects at any step of the sequence in which plasma cells form from activated B cells.

### Cell-mediated (T-cell) immunodeficiency

These disorders involve inadequate or dysfunctional T cells. T-cell deficiency usually causes abnormal B-cell function because of a lack of helper T cells ($T_4$), but serum immunoglobulins may be normal or even elevated. The patient with cell-mediated immunodeficiency has little immunity against fungal and most viral infections and is highly susceptible to low-grade or opportunistic infections from organisms such as *Candida albicans* and *Pneumocystis carinii.* He may suffer severe and even fatal reactions to normally mild childhood diseases, such as chicken pox, and to vaccination with live virus or bacille Calmette-Guérin. Also, since he can't respond adequately to tumor antigens, he suffers exaggerated risk of malignancy.

The T-cell–deficient patient can't produce an adequate delayed hypersensitivity skin reaction; this is known as anergy. The main reason seems to be active suppression, but other conditions besides congenital T-cell deficiency can cause anergy. These include inadequate production of lymphokines, which promotes T-cell proliferation and differentiation into effector T cells; inadequate response by monocytes to lymphokines released after antigen exposure; and use of drugs such as corticosteroids that inhibit the inflammatory response.

Cell-mediated immunodeficiency also promotes susceptibility to graft-versus-host disease (GVHD) if the patient receives a transplant or transfused lymphocytes. In this form of immunodeficiency, the patient's cells can't avoid attack by the donor's immunocompetent cells (see Chapter 9).

The causes and nature of T-cell deficiencies vary. For example, DiGeorge's syndrome stems from abnormal embryonic development—an absent or hypoplastic thymus gland. (See *How immunodeficiencies develop,* page 77.) In AIDS, deficiency is in one subset of T lymphocytes, the $T_4$ subset, which results in an abnormal or reversed $T_4$:$T_8$ ratio.

### Combined T- and B-cell immunodeficiency

This most severe immunodeficiency reflects profound defects in both T- and B-cell immunity, as in SCID. In these disorders, all or many adaptive immune mechanisms are congenitally underdeveloped or absent, perhaps from failure of the bone marrow stem cell to produce T and B cells, from lack of certain essential enzymes, or from an unidentified genetic mutation.

A patient lacking T- and B-cell immunity falls prey to nearly every kind of infection.

# Acquired immunodeficiency syndrome (AIDS): Incidence

## Age

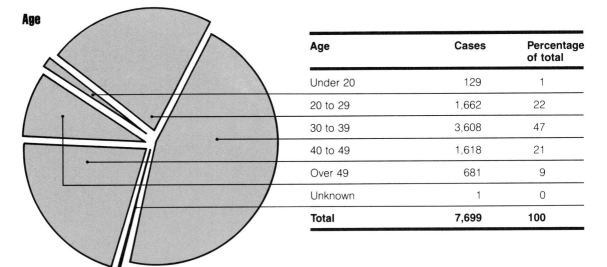

| Age | Cases | Percentage of total |
| --- | --- | --- |
| Under 20 | 129 | 1 |
| 20 to 29 | 1,662 | 22 |
| 30 to 39 | 3,608 | 47 |
| 40 to 49 | 1,618 | 21 |
| Over 49 | 681 | 9 |
| Unknown | 1 | 0 |
| **Total** | **7,699** | **100** |

## Race/ethnicity

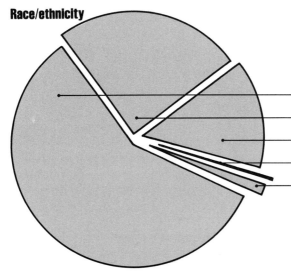

| Race/ethnicity | Cases | Percentage of total |
| --- | --- | --- |
| White | 4,486 | 59 |
| Black | 1,948 | 25 |
| Hispanic | 1,129 | 15 |
| Other | 31 | <1 |
| Unknown | 105 | 1 |
| **Total** | **7,699** | **100** |

## High-risk groups

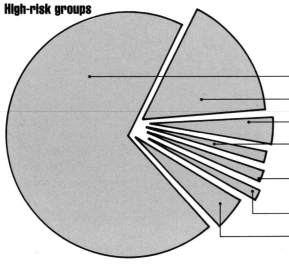

| High-risk groups | Cases | Percentage of total |
| --- | --- | --- |
| Homosexual or bisexual | 5,541 | 72 |
| I.V. drug user | 1,317 | 17 |
| Haitian | 263 | 3 |
| Hemophiliac | 53 | 1 |
| Transfusion with blood/ blood products | 102 | 1 |
| Child whose parent has AIDS or is at increased risk for AIDS | 64 | 1 |
| Other | 359 | 5 |
| **Total** | **7,699** | **100** |

Unless his condition is diagnosed and treated early and aggressively, he's likely to die from overwhelming infection during his first year of life. He may also be susceptible to GVHD in response to circulating maternal T cells. He should never receive live, attenuated viral immunization, as he may develop fatal vaccinia or poliomyelitis.

**Phagocytic dysfunction**
These disorders—both primary and secondary—result from deficient numbers or function of neutrophils or macrophages, the two major phagocytic cells.

Primary phagocytic disorders generally reflect abnormal metabolism, abnormal chemotaxis, or a killing (phagocytosis) defect. For example, in the patient with defective chemotaxis, either a lack of chemotactic substance or a poor neutrophil response to the chemotactic substance so reduces the number of neutrophils attracted to the damaged area that they are too few to phagocytize the antigen. In chronic granulomatous disease, neutrophils and monocytes can ingest bacteria. However, they lack the specific enzyme to kill and digest these bacteria, such as *Staphylococcus aureus,* and the patient typically suffers from chronic suppurative infections.

Many associated or secondary phagocytic defects may occur. These conditions are usually from a reduced number of neutrophils (neutropenia) because of suppressed bone marrow function, as in aplastic anemia, various malignancies, and immunosuppressive therapy.

The patient with phagocytic dysfunction is susceptible to a wide range of bacterial and fungal infections, from mild, recurrent skin infections to severe and fatal systemic infections. However, he tends to resist viral or protozoal infections.

**Complement deficiency**
These disorders reflect absence or deficiency of complement components that aid phagocytosis by acting as chemotaxins or opsonins. This inhibits the normal complement cascade so that the membrane attack component (C5 to C9) can't destroy the immune complex and antigen (see *The complement cascade,* page 20). Thus, a patient with a complement abnormality can't combat bacteria by complement fixation and has many severe infections. But some complement deficiencies also contribute to autoimmune disorders because of a decreased ability to clear immune complexes.

Complement deficiency may also stem from deficiency of an inhibitor. For example, in hereditary angioedema, complement is activated but the normal control for shutting it off—the C1 esterase inhibitor—is missing, so that tissue destruction and cell lysis continue unabated until the antigen or the available complement has been consumed. A patient with this disorder has repeated episodes of edema in the skin, GI tract, and respiratory tract. Laryngeal angioedema may prove fatal.

**Other secondary factors**
Probably most of the immunodeficient patients you'll care for have acquired the deficiency secondary to other conditions, such as malnutrition, disease, stress and injury, or iatrogenic factors. (See *Disorders with associated secondary immunodeficiency.*)

**Malnutrition.** For example, malnutrition hinders lymphocyte production, particularly reducing T-cell number and function. It may be the most common contemporary cause of immunodeficiency. The malnourished patient suffers anergy, susceptibility to multiple infections, and poor wound healing.

**Disease.** Similarly, malignant tumors can suppress the production and function of lymphocytes and neutrophils. Lymphomas and leukemias produce direct immunodeficiency by causing abnormal production or function of immature or pathologic immune components.

**Stress and injury.** Severe or chronic stress, especially associated with ineffective coping, can result in temporary or long-standing immunosuppression, with atrophy of the lymphoid organs, lymphopenia, and decreased resistance to infection and disease.

Trauma, especially involving burns or hemorrhage, results in massive protein and tissue loss as well as in damage to skin and other first-line defenses. Loss of blood, tissue, and cellular components leaves the trauma victim with a low neutrophil count and low immunoglobulin levels. Reserves quickly deplete, and replacement can't keep up with demand.

**Iatrogenic factors.** Many drugs and specific treatments can cause immunosuppression. Sometimes immunosuppression is desired, as in organ transplant or in treating certain autoimmune and hyperinflammatory processes. Other times, it's an undesirable complication, as in cancer chemotherapy or treatment with certain antimicrobials, and it may require modification of treatment.

How do drugs induce immunosuppression? Cyclophosphamide, azathioprine, methotrexate,

## Disorders with associated secondary immunodeficiency

**Humoral disorders**
Multiple myeloma
Nephrotic syndrome
Protein-losing
  enteropathy
Prematurity
Sickle cell disease

**Cell-mediated disorders**
Tuberculosis
Hodgkin's lymphoma
Nonlymphoid
  malignancies
Malnutrition
Acute viral infections
Autoimmune diseases
  (systemic lupus
  erythematosus,
  rheumatoid arthritis)

**Combined humoral and cell-mediated disorders**
Acute and chronic
  leukemias (more T-
  than B-cell
  dysfunction)
Crohn's disease
Burns
Rubella

**Phagocytic disorders**
Chronic infections
Diabetes mellitus
Hodgkin's lymphoma
Aplastic anemia
Malnutrition

**Complement disorders**
Nonlymphoid
  malignancies
Systemic lupus
  erythematosus
Alcoholic cirrhosis
Malnutrition
Prematurity

and other cytotoxic agents may decrease T-cell number and function, primary humoral (antibody) response, and neutrophil and monocyte counts. Corticosteroids cause deficient immunoglobulin synthesis; inadequate phagocytic migration; decreased lysosomal enzyme release, with decreased killing at the inflammation site; reduced T-cell effectiveness; and poor wound healing.

A newer drug, cyclosporine, acts by inhibiting synthesis of $T_4$ cells, causing deficient cell-mediated immunity. In renal and other organ transplants, it's currently the preferred drug to prevent graft rejection.

Antibiotics and other antimicrobials are known to alter the normal bacterial balance in the pharynx and GI tract, sometimes producing resistant microbes. Prolonged antibiotic therapy may allow proliferation of *Candida* and gram-negative bacilli, such as *Pseudomonas, Klebsiella,* and *Proteus,* risking superinfection by resistant organisms.

X-rays cause immunosuppression because lymphocytes are X-ray–sensitive. Therefore, radiation induces profound lymphopenia in the lymphoid organs and general circulation and suppresses T-cell function.

In many patients, secondary immunodeficiencies have multiple causes. For example, in a patient with malignancy, immunodeficiency may result from the tumor and its treatment as well as from the accompanying stress and malnutrition.

## MEDICAL MANAGEMENT
First and foremost, good medical management requires a comprehensive history of the patient's present and previous illnesses and infections as well as a careful family history.

### Diagnostic tests: Confirming the characteristics
When the history and a detailed physical examination suggest one of the immunodeficiency disorders, specific tests can help establish a differential diagnosis.

**Tests for humoral immunodeficiency.** A history of recurrent bacterial pneumonia, sepsis, meningitis, and other bacterial infections characterizes a humoral immunodeficiency. *Quantitative immunoglobulin serum levels* by radioimmunoassay or immune electrophoresis confirm or rule out this condition in about 90% of patients. Normal levels of the three major immunoglobulins (IgG, IgM, and IgA) probably rule out a serious defect in humoral immunity, although infrequently an IgG or IgA subclass may be missing. However, a significant decrease in one or more immunoglobulins probably indicates humoral immunodeficiency.

The *Schick test* evaluates IgG function. A delayed hypersensitivity reaction 3 to 4 days after intradermal injection with diphtheria toxin in a patient previously immunized with DPT vaccine indicates the lack of circulating antibody. An *isohemagglutinin titer* evaluates IgM function; low or absent titers indicate the lack of antibody.

A *total lymphocyte count* may be part of a preliminary screen for immunodeficiencies, but it helps little in diagnosing humoral deficiency because B cells constitute 20% or less of total lymphocytes. Tests are now available to isolate and count B cells; although reduced numbers of B cells indicate humoral deficiency, many humoral deficiencies involve function, not numbers.

If other diagnostic tests point to humoral immunodeficiency, in vitro tests can determine lymphocyte function by measuring *B-cell response* to a polysaccharide mitogen, such as pokeweed. A low or absent response indicates a depressed or defective humoral immune system. Pokeweed also stimulates T cells, though to a lesser degree.

**Tests for cell-mediated immunodeficiency.** A history of recurrent or severe fungal, viral, or other opportunistic infections characterizes cell-mediated immunodeficiency. A *complete blood count and differential* may aid diagnosis because low total lymphocytes can usually be attributed to low T-cell number.

The patient with cell-mediated immunodeficiency is generally anergic, and an important test, the *hypersensitivity skin test,* shows his inability to react to a battery of common skin antigens. Another test, *dinitrochlorobenzene (DNCB) sensitization,* is used occasionally to establish or rule out cutaneous anergy. It detects the failure of the cell-mediated immune system to respond to a new antigen.

A *T-cell count* can quantify T cells themselves as well as T-cell subpopulations by fluorescent activated cell sorter (FACS) analysis. This method separates cells by type using monoclonal antibodies. A patient with DiGeorge's syndrome has few T cells, whereas a patient with AIDS shows a low number of $T_4$ cells.

**Tests for combined T- and B-cell immunodeficiency.** A history of early, repeated, and severe infections of various kinds characterizes combined T- and B-cell immunodeficiency.

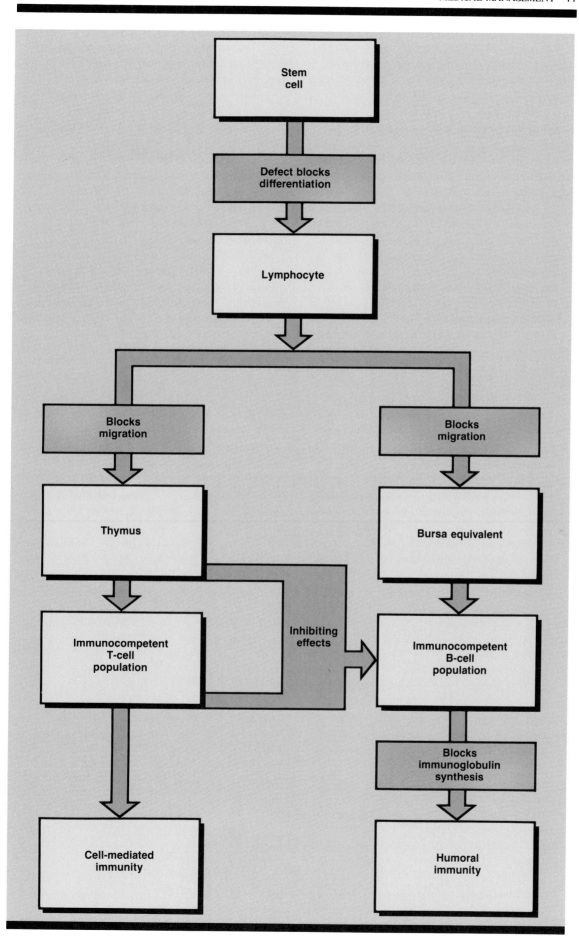

## How immunodeficiencies develop

T- and B-cell immunodeficiencies originate in various developmental defects that interrupt cell maturation.

Combined humoral and cell-mediated immunodeficiencies are caused by defects that impair stem cell differentiation into B and T lymphocytes. They may be congenital (X-linked) or acquired and of unknown cause.

Blocked migration of B lymphocytes to the bursa equivalent and blocked antibody synthesis result in hypogammaglobulinemia.

Blocked migration of T lymphocytes to or from the thymus may impair both cell-mediated and humoral immunity.

Laboratory studies of T- and B-cell number and function show abnormal results with marked reduction in the lymphocyte count, low immunoglobulin levels, lack of lymphocyte response to mitogens, and anergy.

**Tests for phagocytic dysfunction.** A history of infections with various unusual and normally nonpathogenic organisms characterizes phagocytic disorders. *A white blood cell count with differential* may show neutropenia if the patient has a deficient number of neutrophils. *The Rebuck skin window technique, nitroblue tetrazolium (NBT) test, intracellular killing curve (neutrophil microbicidal assay),* and *neutrophil chemotaxis and migration tests* may be done to evaluate a qualitative neutrophil defect in which numbers are normal or even elevated.

For example, a patient with a chronic granulomatous disease (CGD) shows no nitroblue tetrazolium dye reduction. This test is based on the increased metabolic activity of normal granulocytes after phagocytosis. Defective granulocytes in CGD are unable to generate superoxide and hydrogen peroxide and thus can't reduce NBT. The patient's killing curves for organisms to which he's susceptible show little or no killing in 2 hours.

Diagnosing specific bacteria and other microorganisms such as fungi, viruses, and parasites may require other tests, such as *blood cultures, liver and open lung biopsies,* and *aspiration of draining lymph nodes.*

**Tests for complement deficiency.** Low $CH_{50}$ *(total hemolytic complement) levels* characterize complement deficiency. *Assays of specific components* may be necessary to identify the deficient protein. A patient with hereditary angioedema has a characteristic history and hereditary pattern with low levels of C1 esterase inhibitor, C2, or C4.

**Tests for secondary immunodeficiency.** Frequent infections also characterize secondary immunodeficiency. Diagnosis may rely on tests for quantity and function of T and B cells, neutrophils, immunoglobulins, phagocytes, and complement.

## Treatment: Prompt and aggressive

In the immunocompromised patient, any infection may be life-threatening. Treatment aims to detect infection promptly, combat it aggressively, and, when possible, replace deficient substances.

**In humoral immunodeficiency.** A patient with humoral immunodeficiency usually needs episodic and appropriate antibiotics, some-times in combination, to treat life-threatening infections; and he needs antibody replacement with immune globulin or plasma transfusions. Immune globulin is usually given I.M. but it may be given I.V. if the patient fails to respond to I.M. administration or if he needs large amounts of antibody. (See *Gamimune: Tips for safe administration.*)

Immune globulin should not be given to patients with selective IgA deficiency or transient hypogammaglobulinemia of infancy. Some patients with IgA deficiency have suffered severe anaphylactoid reactions to immune globulin, and high anti-IgA antibody levels were found in their circulation. Presently, deficient IgA cannot be safely replaced. A patient with transient hypogammaglobulinemia of infancy should not receive immune globulin primarily because it may depress his own endogenous IgG production.

Plasma transfusions may be used to replace all classes of immunoglobulins but not without the associated risk of transmitting hepatitis or AIDS. To lessen this risk, a patient should receive plasma from the same reliable donor whenever possible.

**In cell-mediated immunodeficiency.** The patient with cell-mediated immunodeficiency needs immunologic reconstitution or enhancement by bone marrow or fetal thymus transplant along with treatment of his infections, which may be more severe than those in patients with immunoglobulin deficiency.

Fetal thymus transplants have proven successful in DiGeorge's syndrome but have proven less beneficial in other T-cell disorders. A fetal thymus—of less than 14 weeks' gestation, to minimize GVHD—should be transplanted as soon as possible after diagnosis.

No method of immunologic enhancement or reconstitution has thus far proven effective in AIDS.

Agents such as transfer factor and thymosin may be given to augment or enhance T-cell function. Thymosin, alone and in combination with transfer factor, bone marrow transplants, or other therapies, has been used with variable success in Wiskott-Aldrich syndrome, immunodeficiency with ataxia-telangiectasia, and other cell-mediated immunodeficiencies.

Antiviral and antifungal agents may be used to combat infections. Amphotericin B administered I.V. effectively controls systemic fungal infections; however, this drug should not be used repeatedly, since a large, cumulative dose (and sometimes even a small dose) risks nephrotoxicity. Another antifungal drug, ketoconazole (Nizoral), is also proving effective. Acyclovir I.V. is now being used to control some systemic viral infection.

**In combined T- and B-cell immunodeficiency.** A patient with combined immunodeficiency needs careful surveillance and aggressive treatment for any infection. Protective isolation, ranging from careful cleanliness to plastic bubbles with laminar airflow, may be necessary. Immune globulin should be administered; live, attenuated viral vaccine should be avoided; and blood products should be irradiated with 3,000 to 6,000 rads before administration to prevent GVHD from potentially viable lymphocytes.

For the patient with SCID, bone marrow transplant offers the best hope because it supplies normal lymphoid precursors that may correct the immunodeficiency. The development of lectin-separated bone marrow transplant, which allows non-HLA identical transplants, has dramatically improved the prognosis in SCID; however, the procedure carries risks, the greatest of which is GVHD.

Other forms of therapy, including fetal liver and thymus transplant, have had some success. Enzyme replacement therapy offers an alternative in adenosine deaminase (ADA)–deficient SCID when no histocompatible donor can be found for bone marrow transplant; it consists of giving the patient 15 ml/kg of glycerol-frozen, irradiated, packed normal erythrocytes every 2 to 4 weeks.

**In phagocytic disorders.** The patient with a phagocytic disorder may need surgical removal or drainage of abscesses. He should receive broad-spectrum or combination antibiotic therapy even before culture results are available. Therapy usually must be prolonged for maximum effectiveness despite the risk of encouraging resistant organisms. The patient with widespread fungal infections may need administration of I.V. amphotericin B. The patient with neutrophil dysfunction who fails treatment or who has a potentially fatal infection may need granulocyte transfusions. Also, sometimes transfusions help localize infection.

**In complement disorders.** The patient with a complement deficiency can receive replacement complement components through whole blood or fresh plasma transfusions. However, since complement component infusion frequently results in increased activation and increased immune complex disease, treatment for complement deficiency is usually symptomatic. In patients with hereditary angioede-

ma, fibrinolytic agents or anabolic steroids such as danazol have effectively reduced the frequency of attacks.

**In secondary immunodeficiency.** Such a patient may benefit from immune serum globulin or from reconstituting or enhancing immune mechanisms. Although iatrogenic immunosuppression is often the desired effect of certain drugs and therapies, close and continuous patient monitoring for signs of infection is crucial. If the patient's immune profile drops below his minimum parameters, immunosuppressive therapy may be stopped or altered.

## NURSING MANAGEMENT

Because immunodeficiency manifests itself in so many forms and in so many body systems, your assessment—including a thorough history and an exacting physical examination—becomes increasingly important.

### Nursing history: The best clues

Begin by seeking pertinent biographic data, including the patient's age. Remember that the very young and the elderly are at increased risk for immunodeficiency. However, primary congenital immunodeficiency rarely surfaces before age 3 months because the newborn infant is still protected by maternal antibody.

Ask about occupational exposure to chemicals and radiation because these may suppress the immune system.

Note psychosocial factors. A history of stress coupled with ineffective coping may depress the immune system. Homosexuality with a history of many sexual partners constitutes a high-risk factor for AIDS.

**Ask about the chief complaint.** Commonly, it's related to infection. Respiratory infections occur most frequently, so ask about coughing and shortness of breath. Fever, the prime sign of infection, may be the chief complaint; its pattern may be significant. Intermittent fever, falling to or below normal each day and then rising again, occurs in bacteremia. Marked temperature swings, usually with chills and sweating, occur in local infections such as acute osteomyelitis, empyema, and intraabdominal abscess. Relapsing fever, febrile episodes alternating with 1 or more days of normal temperature, occurs in chronic meningococcemia. Patients receiving immunosuppression may have a blunted febrile response.

Pain may be related to an infection. Ask the patient to define and locate any pain and *(continued on page 82)*

(continued on page 82)

# What you should know about AIDS

AIDS refers to a disease characterized by weakened or diminished cell-mediated immunity. Typically, the AIDS patient has a low helper-T-cell number, which results in an abnormal $T_4$:$T_8$ ratio. As his cell-mediated immunity weakens, the patient becomes vulnerable to infectious organisms such as *Pneumocystis carinii,* which causes potentially fatal pneumonia because of progressive alveolar occlusion. He's also at high risk for infections from yeast, cytomegalovirus, herpesvirus, and toxoplasmosis. And he's more susceptible to particular malignancies, such as lymphoma of the brain and Kaposi's sarcoma. (See *Incidence and mortality in AIDS.*)

**No definitive findings**
The Centers for Disease Control defines AIDS as the presence of an opportunistic infection or Kaposi's sarcoma in someone with no known cause of immunodeficiency. Onset of AIDS is usually insidious, with no definitive signs or symptoms, although fever, loss of appetite and weight, extreme fatigue, and lymphadenopathy have been reported. Other manifestations of weakened immunity include white patches of candidiasis in the mouth, throat (thrush), or esophagus; lesions around the mouth and anus from herpes simplex types I and II; and, in Kaposi's sarcoma, flat, asymptomatic lesions on the skin and mucous membranes. As these lesions age, they turn from pink to red to plum, as red blood cells extravasate into the surrounding stroma and coalesce into plaques. If death occurs, it's generally caused by infection or by tumors of vital organs.

**Treatment usually supportive**
To date, AIDS has no cure. Its

## Incidence and mortality in AIDS*

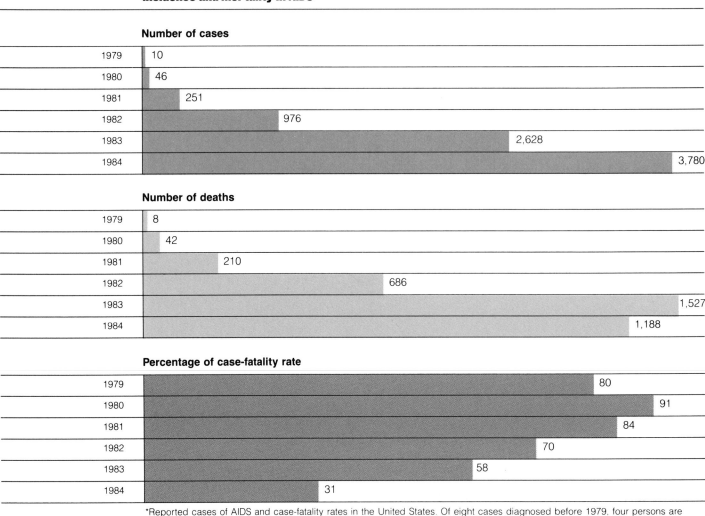

**Number of cases**

| Year | Cases |
|------|-------|
| 1979 | 10 |
| 1980 | 46 |
| 1981 | 251 |
| 1982 | 976 |
| 1983 | 2,628 |
| 1984 | 3,780 |

**Number of deaths**

| Year | Deaths |
|------|--------|
| 1979 | 8 |
| 1980 | 42 |
| 1981 | 210 |
| 1982 | 686 |
| 1983 | 1,527 |
| 1984 | 1,188 |

**Percentage of case-fatality rate**

| Year | Percentage |
|------|------------|
| 1979 | 80 |
| 1980 | 91 |
| 1981 | 84 |
| 1982 | 70 |
| 1983 | 58 |
| 1984 | 31 |

*Reported cases of AIDS and case-fatality rates in the United States. Of eight cases diagnosed before 1979, four persons are known to have died.

treatment is largely supportive and may include drug and radiation therapy.

Supportive measures in AIDS aim to reduce the risk of infection, to treat existing infections and malignancies, to maintain adequate nutrition, and to provide emotional and psychological support.

Drug treatment for infections in AIDS varies. The drug of choice for *P. carinii* pneumonia is an oral or I.V. preparation of trimethoprim and sulfamethoxazole (Bactrim or Septra). If treatment fails or if toxicity occurs, pentamidine (Pentam-300) may be substituted; however, this drug may cause side effects, such as azotemia, liver dysfunction, tachycardia, hypotension, hypoglycemia, and skin rashes. Even with successful treatment, pneumonia recurs in about 20% of patients.

Radiation therapy and antineoplastic drugs may be used to treat Kaposi's sarcoma. But aggressive treatment increases the likelihood of infection, and, when treatment is stopped, often the disease returns.

Interferon has proven no more successful than chemotherapy alone.

To reduce the risk of contracting AIDS, the U.S. Public Health Service recommends avoiding sexual contact with persons known to have or suspected of having AIDS. It also advises that members of high-risk groups refrain from donating blood.

To help the public better understand AIDS, a toll-free number has been established to provide information on recent developments in the struggle against AIDS. The number is 800-342-AIDS. Persons in Hawaii and Alaska may call this number collect: 202-245-6867. Persons in Washington, D.C., may call 646-8182.

**Finally, some good news**
Recently, the probable cause of AIDS was identified as a variant of a known cancer virus, human T-cell lymphotrophic virus, or HTLV-III. Mass production of this virus has led to the development of a new blood test to identify persons having antibodies to the AIDS virus. This test is expected to be available soon. And because this test will identify most carriers of the AIDS virus, the risk of transmitting AIDS through blood transfusions can be greatly reduced. Scientists hope to have an AIDS vaccine available within the next 3 years.

## Opportunistic diseases in AIDS*

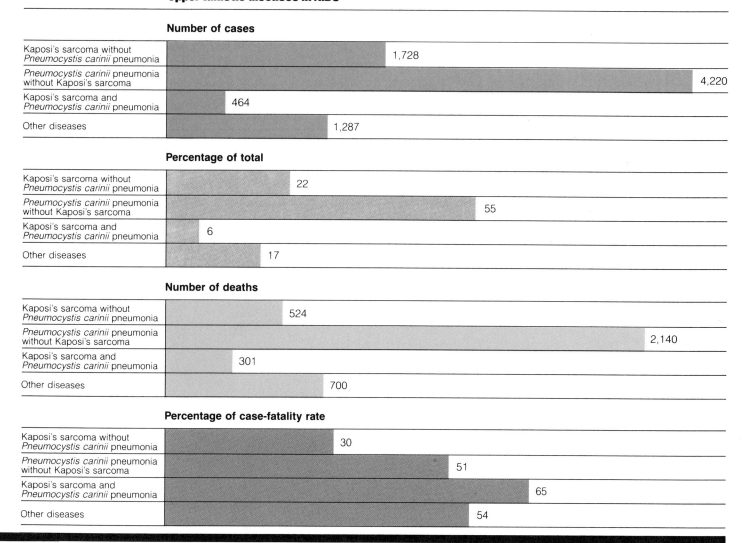

**Number of cases**

| | |
|---|---|
| Kaposi's sarcoma without *Pneumocystis carinii* pneumonia | 1,728 |
| *Pneumocystis carinii* pneumonia without Kaposi's sarcoma | 4,220 |
| Kaposi's sarcoma and *Pneumocystis carinii* pneumonia | 464 |
| Other diseases | 1,287 |

**Percentage of total**

| | |
|---|---|
| Kaposi's sarcoma without *Pneumocystis carinii* pneumonia | 22 |
| *Pneumocystis carinii* pneumonia without Kaposi's sarcoma | 55 |
| Kaposi's sarcoma and *Pneumocystis carinii* pneumonia | 6 |
| Other diseases | 17 |

**Number of deaths**

| | |
|---|---|
| Kaposi's sarcoma without *Pneumocystis carinii* pneumonia | 524 |
| *Pneumocystis carinii* pneumonia without Kaposi's sarcoma | 2,140 |
| Kaposi's sarcoma and *Pneumocystis carinii* pneumonia | 301 |
| Other diseases | 700 |

**Percentage of case-fatality rate**

| | |
|---|---|
| Kaposi's sarcoma without *Pneumocystis carinii* pneumonia | 30 |
| *Pneumocystis carinii* pneumonia without Kaposi's sarcoma | 51 |
| Kaposi's sarcoma and *Pneumocystis carinii* pneumonia | 65 |
| Other diseases | 54 |

to describe how it interferes with daily activities. If the patient is a child, ask his parents to describe any behavior reflecting pain, such as crying and pulling on the ears, which is related to otitis media.

The chief complaint may also be related to malignancy, such as the skin eruptions characteristic of Kaposi's sarcoma and frequently seen in the patient with AIDS.

**Explore present and past illnesses.** Record all information related to the present illness. Ask about onset, duration, course, and severity. Ask about accompanying symptoms, which may help to determine the nature of the infection. For example, the typical clinical course of a fungal infection is usually chronic with vague, seldom intense signs and symptoms that include fever, chills, night sweats, anorexia, weight loss, malaise, and depression. Signs and symptoms of viral infection are usually nonspecific, including persistent fever, headaches, myalgias, fatigue, enlarged lymph nodes, GI disturbances, and sometimes skin lesions such as measles or herpes zoster. Pyogenic bacterial infections may produce pus-laden secretions that drain from skin lesions or appear in sputum.

Ask especially about prior acute and chronic infections. Those that were chronic and tended to recur, those in which the infecting agent was unusual, those in which the infection did not completely clear between episodes, and those in which response to treatment was incomplete should arouse your suspicion of immunodeficiency.

However, remember that, in children, not the number but the type of infection is the important factor and also that congenital immunodeficiency occurs only rarely. Even as many as 9 or 10 episodes of respiratory infections per year may occur in the healthy child. However, infections such as meningitis, pneumonia, osteomyelitis, or bloodstream infections occurring more than once should prompt you to investigate for immune dysfunction. Other conditions, such as persistent thrush of the mouth, chronic skin infections, continued diarrhea, and failure to thrive should also prompt your suspicion of immunodeficiency; the type of infection sometimes offers a clue to the type of immune defect.

Ask about previous immunizations and the patient's reaction to them to evaluate the type and severity of the immune defect. Usually, the patient with severe immunodeficiency will report previous severe reactions to live, attenuated virus. This data also helps in planning which antigens to use in the skin tests.

Ask if the patient has arthritis, leukemia, diabetes, nephrotic syndrome, or any other condition that might be related to secondary immunodeficiency. Ask about previous hospitalizations, blood transfusions, and specific treatments, including radiation therapy and any drugs prescribed in the past and present. These facts may help explain the patient's current immunosuppressive findings. Ask about previous surgery; the patient who has undergone splenectomy or tonsillectomy is more susceptible to infection. Ask about allergies, and find out how they are manifested.

Ask about congenital anomalies, as these may accompany congenital immunodeficiency disorders. For instance, the patient with DiGeorge's syndrome may have various cardiac and parathyroid anomalies.

Check for familial patterns of infection, malignancy, or autoimmunity. Remember, most of the primary immunodeficiencies have been transmitted genetically; even though the patient's parents, who transmitted the gene of immunodeficiency, may not have the disease themselves, the patient's siblings, cousins, or other family members may have some sort of immunodeficiency problem or may have died from an unknown cause.

Conclude your history taking with a complete systems review. Neurologic, endocrine, or bleeding abnormalities or signs of autoimmunity may help in diagnosing such complex immunodeficiencies as hypogammaglobulinemia, Wiskott-Aldrich syndrome, ataxiatelangiectasia, and DiGeorge's syndrome.

Note respiratory symptoms, which are often related to infection or its aftermath. Ask about GI problems, especially chronic diarrhea. Ask about skin problems; rashes in mucous membranes of the mouth, throat, and vagina typically accompany candida infections. Skin rashes also occur in other diseases, such as herpes.

**Physical assessment: Infection anywhere**
Data gathered during the physical examination may confirm the diagnosis. You'll be hunting the often elusive signs of infection in every body system. But remember that swelling, erythema, tenderness, and other signs of inflammation and infection may not appear in the immunodeficient patient because of diminished responsivity. So, in your assessment you need to be especially diligent to detect such easily missed signs as tenderness in the perianal area without edema or erythema,

mild inflammation of the pharynx, or subtle rales, all of which may signal infection.

Start by taking the patient's vital signs. Check for fever, tachycardia, and, if the infection is severe, hypotension.

**Examine the skin.** Look for draining lesions or other evidence of current infection and scars from past infections. Look for eczema and dermatitis, which may appear in Bruton's hypogammaglobulinemia or Wiskott-Aldrich syndrome but may also appear in enzyme and nutritional deficiencies. Look for purpura; its presence may be the result of an immune reaction to a bacterium that damaged the vascular endothelium. And watch for palpable, nonpainful, and purplish lesions, which may signal Kaposi's sarcoma, a malignancy associated with AIDS.

**Palpate the skin and organs.** Note skin temperature and turgor. Palpate the abdomen, noting the size and condition of the liver and spleen. Also palpate the lymph nodes, noting any enlargement. Liver, spleen, or lymph node enlargement suggests possible malignancy or acute or chronic infection.

**Assess respiration.** Check for altered respiratory rate and depth or for signs of distress, such as nasal flaring. Auscultate the chest, noting adventitious or diminished breath sounds. Inspect the larynx for inflammation.

**Evaluate neurologic status.** Assess coordination, gait, and cerebellar function. Neurologic abnormalities are common in ataxia-telangiectasia. Also look for signs of decreased level of consciousness, including restlessness and confusion, which frequently accompany serious infection.

## Nursing diagnoses: Planning care

With your assessment data complete, now look to your nursing diagnoses and plan your interventions to protect your immunodeficient patient against infection and other complications. Your diagnoses, no doubt, will include the following typical nursing diagnoses for the immunosuppressed patient.

**Potential for infection related to immune system deficiency.** Your goal is to keep the patient from developing an infection and to prevent the spread of an existing infection. *To avoid infection in the patient,* check him frequently for signs and symptoms of infection. Inspect susceptible areas daily, such as the skin, mouth, pharynx, axilla, perineum, and rectal area. Auscultate the lungs for abnormal breath sounds that may occur with respiratory infections. Monitor vital signs frequently.

Examine secretions and excretions for changes in color or consistency. Monitor white cell and neutrophil counts daily for changes.

Watch especially for fever, and take necessary measures to control it. Remember, however, that such control impairs a valuable indicator of the infection's course. If the fever is extremely high or prolonged, debilitating, discomforting, or affecting central nervous system function, administer acetaminophen or aspirin for antipyresis.

Ask about signs of inflammation, increased fatigue, burning on urination, or sore throat. If you suspect infection at any site, report it immediately and obtain a culture as ordered.

If necessary, isolate the patient for his protection. Protective isolation may range from a gown, mask, and gloves for anyone entering the room to complete sterile isolation in life islands or laminar airflow units. Carry out any prescribed infection-prevention measures, such as granulocyte transfusions.

Give special attention to cleanliness and asepsis; wash your hands immediately before and after contact with the patient and after contact with any contaminated or potentially infectious material. Be sure to instruct the patient's family about the need for thorough hand washing and the patient about the need for good personal hygiene. Ensure scrupulous mouth care to prevent stomatitis.

Keep skin and mucous membranes intact. If the patient is confined to bed, give meticulous skin care and turn him every 2 hours.

Try to avoid manipulative and invasive procedures because the immunodeficient patient is susceptible to local or systemic infections. Such procedures include dental manipulation, bronchoscopy, liver biopsy, I.V. pyelography, and barium enemas. Avoid the use of urinary or intravenous catheters and respiratory equipment when possible. Before any necessary invasive procedure, prepare the patient carefully and change any dressing or tubing according to institutional policy.

Keep the patient's room and immediate environment free of dirt, dust, and excess equipment. Control the temperature, humidity, and airflow as much as possible.

Remember that every person and item entering the room is potentially dangerous to the patient. You may want to exclude flowers, plants, and other sources of bacteria or fungi. Monitor visitors and staff to prevent exposure to infection and to maintain a calm environment. Ensure adequate rest, since chronic fatigue increases susceptibility to infection.

# Precautions for care of an AIDS patient

Although AIDS is not thought to be transmitted by casual contact with persons who've contracted it or persons in high-risk groups, health-care workers need to observe special precautions when caring for an AIDS patient. The Centers for Disease Control suggests the following:

• If the AIDS patient cannot maintain good hygiene—for example, if he has profuse diarrhea or fecal incontinence or if he exhibits altered behavior secondary to central nervous system infections—provide him with a private room.

• Avoid accidentally wounding yourself with sharp instruments contaminated with potentially infectious materials.

• Avoid contacting open skin lesions with material from the AIDS patient.

• Wear gloves and a gown when handling blood specimens, blood-soiled articles, body fluids, excretions, and secretions, as well as surfaces and materials exposed to them.

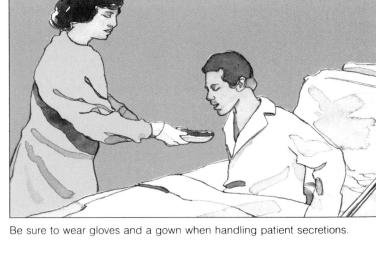

Be sure to wear gloves and a gown when handling patient secretions.

• Wash your hands thoroughly and immediately if they become contaminated. Also wash your hands after removing gowns and gloves and before leaving the patient's room.

• Label blood and other specimen containers prominently with a special warning, such as "AIDS Precaution." If the outside of the specimen container is visibly contaminated with blood, clean it with a disinfectant, such as a 1:10 solution of 5.25% sodium hypochlorite (household bleach) and water. Examine the container carefully for leaks or cracks. Place blood specimens in an impervious second container for transport. Clean blood and other spills promptly with the same disinfectant.

• Put soiled articles in an impervious bag and clearly label it.

Or put such items in a colored plastic bag designed for infectious waste disposal. Incinerate or dispose of contaminated items as your institution directs; reprocess reuseable items accordingly.

• Sterilize lensed instruments after use.

• Use disposable needles, when possible. Also, use only needle-locking syringes or one-piece needle-syringe units to aspirate fluids from the patient, so that collected fluid can be safely discharged through the needle. If you use reuseable syringes, decontaminate them before reprocessing.

• Avoid needle puncture by discarding used needles in a puncture-resistant container. Do not bend needles or reinsert them into their original sheaths.

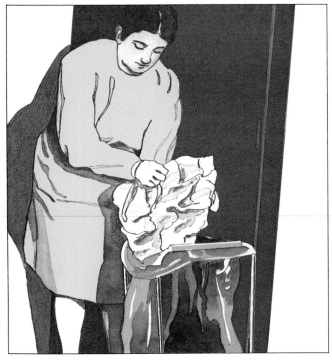

Dispose of soiled linens by double-bagging.

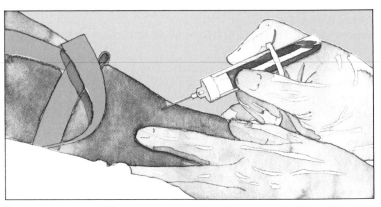

Avoid sticking yourself with contaminated needles when obtaining blood.

Try to minimize environmental stress as much as possible.

Encourage the patient to eat a well-balanced diet that's high in proteins, which is needed for immunoglobulin production. If needed, add vitamin supplements, as ordered, to prevent debilitation. Give adequate hydration to keep respiratory secretions thin and to promote adequate flushing of the urinary tract, thus inhibiting bacterial proliferation.

*To prevent the spread of an existing infection,* provide the patient with tissues and a waste receptacle, and instruct him to cover his nose and mouth and to turn away from others when he must cough. Advise frequent hand washing by both the patient and staff. If possible, place the patient in a private room during the acute phase of infection. Use respiratory or other isolation procedures, as required. (See *Precautions for care of an AIDS patient.*)

Consider your interventions successful if the patient remains infection-free or receives early treatment for infection and if staff and visitors don't contract an existing infection.

**Ineffective coping related to diagnosis, prognosis, treatment, or inadequate support systems.** To promote effective coping behavior, first assess the factors that may be contributing to the patient's poor coping ability. These may include inadequate problem solving, inadequate support systems, and sudden or progressive deterioration in health. Assess the patient's present and past coping patterns. Listen to him attentively, and carefully observe his nonverbal behavior, such as eye contact and body positioning. Facilitate insights, encourage verbalization, and support the patient's strengths. Stay alert for signs portending suicide, especially in a patient with a poor prognosis. Look for clues, such as a history of attempted or threatened suicide; personality or behavioral changes; sexual dysfunction, loss of appetite, or sleep disturbances; giving away personal possessions; or sudden euphoria. If you detect any of these, report your suspicions and implement suicide precautions. Refer the patient for counseling, as appropriate.

Help the patient develop appropriate coping techniques by exploring and promoting previous effective coping efforts. Discuss possible alternatives to his problems. Above all, be nonjudgmental. Let the patient know that you care about his situation and are willing to listen. Encourage him to share his feelings with friends and family members, and, if necessary, help him to establish good emotional support systems.

Teach the patient relaxation techniques if he needs them. Help him to find or renew outlets that promote fulfillment and self-esteem, such as crafts, reading, or artwork. Encourage good grooming and assist him with it, if necessary, to improve his appearance.

Bend the rules sometimes, if necessary. Your depressed and critically ill patient may need to talk to a special friend even though policy allows only family visitors. If the special friend helps the patient, let him visit.

Consider your interventions successful if the patient shows a positive change in behavior, achieves an ability to make decisions, reduces his anger, and shows less depression.

**Potential alterations in health maintenance related to chronic immunodeficiency.** Your goal is to teach the patient and his family how the patient can maintain good health and how to recognize and manage infection or other complications.

Encourage the patient to live a normal life, but advise him to avoid potentially harmful situations and activities such as shopping in a crowded mall.

Teach the patient and his family early signs of bacterial, fungal, and viral infection and to report these signs to his doctor immediately. Also, teach the patient how to administer medications he will need at home and what side effects to watch for. Often, you need to teach the patient special hygiene techniques and how to apply his own dressings. Finally, help the patient plan his daily activities around treatments.

Consider your interventions successful if the patient maintains a healthy life-style, complies with necessary precautions, and observes his treatment regimen.

### The guardian role

As you know, the patient with immunodeficiency faces an uncertain future. While he's in your care, you can help protect him from his faulty immune system. To do so, you must assess him continuously to guard against the infections that constantly threaten him; and you must be ready for rapid emergency intervention. But when your patient leaves your care, he must be prepared to assume the guardian role for himself and be able to cope with fear and uncertainty. Whether he takes effective charge of his life or lets his disorder defeat him may rest on your skill, your teaching, and your caring.

**Points to remember**

- Although congenital immunodeficiencies occur only rarely, secondary immunodeficiencies occur commonly and increase susceptibility to nosocomial infections.
- Immunodeficiency renders the patient susceptible to infections, malignancies, and disease, even from normally innocuous substances.
- Lectin-separated bone marrow transplants and enzyme replacement make treatment possible and more effective for SCID patients.
- Preventing infection is the main goal of nursing care for the immunodeficient patient.

# 6 DEALING WITH ALLERGY

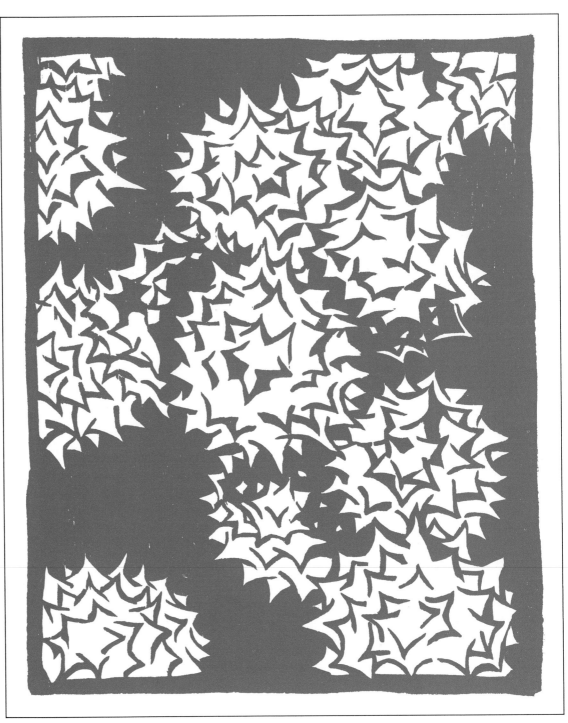

Ragweed pollen

Considering the statistics (about one in every four Americans has a serious allergy), you shouldn't be surprised that allergy is the immune disorder you see most often. Why are many people allergic to milk, pollen, poison ivy, and other substances that do little or no harm to others? The answer lies in an inappropriate and excessive response of the immune system—called a hypersensitivity response. This response may be bothersome, as in hay fever, or life-threatening, as in systemic anaphylaxis following a bee sting.

Understanding allergic reactions and the various antigens, or allergens, that can trigger them enables you to assess patients for early signs and symptoms of hypersensitivity and to act promptly to prevent or minimize allergic reactions. This chapter gives you a firm basis for dealing effectively with allergic disorders.

### Routes of allergen entry

Before discussing pathophysiology, let's first review how allergens enter the body. Food allergens, such as eggs and wheat, enter via the gastrointestinal (GI) tract and are called *ingestants.* Typically, allergic reactions to food allergens first appear in infancy. Airborne allergens enter via the respiratory tract and are called *inhalants.* Indoor inhalants include house dust; plant and animal products used for stuffing furniture and toys, such as feathers; animal danders (exfoliated epithelial cells); and molds. Chief among outdoor inhalants is pollen. Topical allergens, such as cosmetics and plant toxins derived from poison ivy or poison oak, are called *contactants.* Such allergens as saliva and venom from insect stings enter the body via *injection.* Drug allergens may enter via ingestion, injection, or topical application. Typically, allergic reactions to penicillin and other drugs are most common in adults.

### PATHOPHYSIOLOGY

Allergic disorders have been appropriately described as "immunity gone wrong," because they involve normal immune mechanisms with a hair-trigger sensitivity to substances that are not intrinsically harmful. One theory proposes that this heightened responsiveness stems from unexplained dysfunction of the regulatory action of helper and suppressor T cells.

Of the four types of hypersensitivity (see *Gell and Coombs classification of hypersensitivity reactions,* pages 22 and 23), most allergies express either a Type I or Type IV reaction.

### Type I hypersensitivity reaction

Also known as immediate or anaphylactic hypersensitivity, this reaction develops within minutes after exposure to an antigen. However, continued release of chemical mediators may cause a delayed or persistent reaction for up to 24 hours. It's mediated almost exclusively by IgE antibodies, also called reagins.

The Type I reaction requires previous sensitization or exposure to the specific antigen, resulting in the production of specific IgE antibodies by plasma cells. This antibody production takes place in the lymph nodes (primarily in tonsillar tissue, Peyer's patches, and the lamina propria of the GI tract) and is enhanced by helper T cells. IgE antibodies then bind to membrane receptors on mast cells (found throughout connective tissue) and basophils, setting the stage for a Type I reaction.

On reexposure, the antigen binds to adjacent IgE antibodies or cross-linked IgE receptors, activating a series of cellular reactions that trigger degranulation—the release of powerful chemical mediators. This process is strongly influenced by the interaction of cyclic nucleotides: cyclic $3':5'$-adenosine monophosphate (cAMP) and cyclic $3':5'$-guanosine monophosphate (cGMP).

Chemical mediators are classified as primary mediators (preformed), found in specific granules in mast cells and basophils, or as secondary mediators (inactive precursors or newly synthesized substances), formed or released in response to primary mediators. Through their effects on target organs, such as the skin, lungs, and GI tract, these mediators are responsible for the clinical features of Type I reactions (see *Chemical mediators and their actions,* page 90).

Typically, such clinical features reflect the route of allergen entry, but they may vary with the amount of allergen, the amount of mediator released, and the sensitivity of the target organ.

The Type I reaction operates in local and systemic anaphylaxis. Some examples of local anaphylaxis include extrinsic bronchial asthma (see *Asthma: Immediate hypersensitivity,* page 89), allergic rhinitis (such as hay fever), and allergic conjunctivitis. Systemic anaphylaxis, a more severe, generalized IgE-mediated reaction, occurs with certain drugs, food allergies, and most insect stings. It can result in widespread urticaria, pruritus, angioedema, laryngeal edema, asthma, hypotension, and, at times, coma and death. Anaphylactoid reactions to radiocontrast dye or to such drugs as codeine and dextran preparations clinically resemble anaphylaxis but are not mediated by IgE.

### Type IV hypersensitivity reaction

Also known as delayed or cellular hypersensitivity, this reaction occurs 24 to 72 hours after exposure to an allergen. It's mediated by sensitized T cells and macrophages.

The events that follow intradermal injection of tuberculin antigen or purified protein derivative exemplify the Type IV reaction. Sensitized T cells react with the antigen at or near its site of injection. Release of soluble mediators (lymphokines) attracts, activates, and retains macrophages at this site. By releasing lysozymes, macrophages are mainly responsible for tissue damage. Edema and fibrin deposition cause the induration characteristic of a positive tuberculin reaction.

Contact dermatitis, another Type IV reaction, results from cutaneous exposure to allergens, including cosmetics, adhesive tape, topical drugs, drug additives (like lanolin), and plant toxins derived from poison ivy or poison oak. Initial exposure causes sensitization; reexposure triggers a hypersensitivity reaction involving low-weight molecules (haptens) that bind with proteins (carriers) and are processed by Langerhans' cells in the skin, which causes intense itching, erythema, and papulovesicular lesions.

### MEDICAL MANAGEMENT

Whether allergic disorders present dramatically (as in anaphylaxis) or insidiously (as in contact dermatitis), a thorough medical history and physical examination provide clues that pinpoint allergy as the cause of symptoms. Remember that symptoms may be influenced by nonimmunologic factors, such as infection, fatigue, and emotional stress. Diagnostic tests confirm allergy and help identify the offending allergen(s).

### Diagnostic tests

Tests commonly ordered to evaluate allergy include:

**Routine laboratory tests.** The *white blood cell (WBC) differential count* typically reveals eosinophilia in allergy.

*Stool examination* helps exclude parasitic infection, one of several disorders associated with marked eosinophilia or unexplained urticaria. *Smear and stain of nasal secretions* may show dramatically increased levels of eosinophils, suggesting allergic rhinitis. *Gram stain, culture,* and *cytologic examination of sputum* may help distinguish atopic asthma from infectious or neoplastic disorders.

**Radiologic tests.** Although a chest X-ray is of minimal value in diagnosing asthma or evaluating the severity of an acute attack, this test helps rule out other disorders, such as bronchopulmonary aspergillosis and bronchiectasis. X-rays can also identify chronic changes, such as increased anterior-posterior diameter and widened intercostal spaces.

**Pulmonary function tests.** These tests determine the severity of an acute asthmatic attack; rule out asthmatic complications, such as pneumothorax; and evaluate the patient's response to therapy. During an acute asthmatic attack, spirometry may reveal abnormal ventilatory capacity and abnormal lung volume. Pulmonary function tests also are used to aid differential diagnosis of obstructive lung disease.

**IgE-mediated (Type I) hypersensitivity tests.** Considered sensitive and reliable, *skin testing* confirms sensitivity to a specific allergen. It's performed using prick, scratch, or intradermal methods. Intradermal testing is most sensitive, but least specific, and carries the greatest risk of anaphylaxis.

Skin testing involves topical or intradermal placement of minute doses of a specific allergen, followed by observation of the site for at least 15 minutes. Appearance of the classic wheal (hive) and flare (erythema) accompanied by intense itching confirms IgE-mediated hypersensitivity. Wheal formation with projections (pseudopodia) signals a definitive positive reaction, which commonly occurs in hay fever and animal dander rhinitis. A positive reaction strongly suggests allergy to inhalants, such as pollens, dander, and dust, but is less reliable in food allergy.

*Radioimmunoassay tests* measure serum IgE levels. As screening tests for allergy, they should be interpreted in light of skin test results. One type, the *radioimmunosorbent test,* measures total serum IgE levels; however, its two variations—*paper radioimmunosorbent test* and *double immune assay*—are more sensitive. Elevated serum IgE levels suggest allergy, but normal or even decreased serum IgE levels may occur in IgE-mediated hypersensitivity.

# Asthma: Immediate hypersensitivity

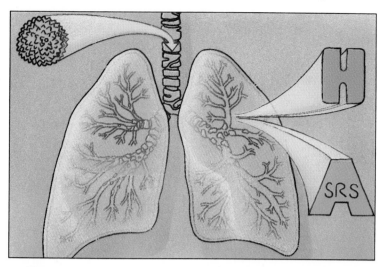

Asthma, a syndrome marked by episodes of dyspnea, bronchoconstriction, abnormal mucus production, and wheezing, exemplifies the Type I, or immediate hypersensitivity, reaction.

When the patient inhales an allergenic substance (upper left), sensitized IgE antibodies trigger mast cell degranulation in the lung interstitium, releasing histamine and slow-reacting substance of anaphylaxis (SRS-A), or leukotrienes (right).

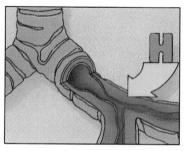
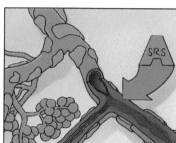

At left, histamine then attaches to receptor sites in the larger bronchi, causing irritation, inflammation, and edema.

At right, SRS-A attaches to receptor sites in the smaller bronchi, causing edema and attracting prostaglandins, which enhance the effects of histamine in the lungs.

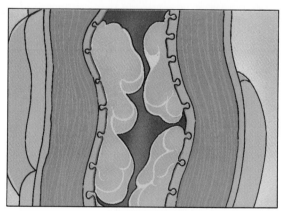
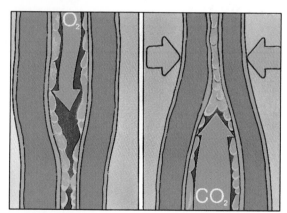

With the help of prostaglandins, histamine also stimulates excessive mucous secretion, further narrowing the bronchial lumen (above left).

When the patient inhales, the narrowed bronchial lumen can still expand slightly, allowing air to reach the alveoli. However, when the patient exhales, increased intrathoracic pressure closes the bronchial lumen completely (above center). Air can enter but cannot exit (above right).

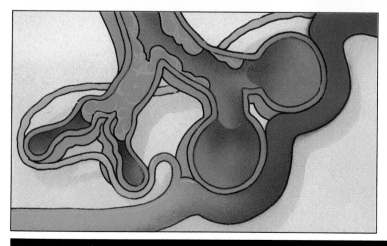

Mucus then fills the lung bases, inhibiting alveolar ventilation (left). Shunting of blood to other alveoli fails to compensate for this, and respiratory acidosis follows.

## Chemical mediators and their actions

| Mediator | Action |
|---|---|
| **Primary mediators** | |
| Histamine (preformed in mast cells) | • Increases vascular permeability<br>• Increases respiratory mucous secretions<br>• Causes smooth-muscle contraction, pruritus, small blood vessel dilation, and pulmonary vagal stimulation |
| Eosinophil chemotactic factor of anaphylaxis (ECF-A) (preformed in mast cells) | • Is chemotactic for eosinophils |
| Platelet activating factor (PAF) (synthesized by neutrophils, mast cells, and macrophages) | • Triggers platelet aggregation with release of histamine and serotonin<br>• Causes bronchoconstriction and vasodilation |
| Neutrophil chemotactic factor of anaphylaxis (NCF-A) (preformed in mast cells) | • Is chemotactic for neutrophils |
| Prostaglandins (chemically derived from arachidonic acid)<br>    D and F series<br>    E series | <br><br>• Cause bronchoconstriction and vasodilation<br>• Cause bronchodilation and vasodilation |
| Basophil kallikrein of anaphylaxis (preformed in mast cells) | • Liberates bradykinin, which causes bronchoconstriction; vasodilation; decreased blood pressure; increased vascular permeability; increased mucous secretion; and nerve stimulation, which produces pain and burning |
| **Secondary mediators** | |
| Bradykinin (derived from precursor kininogen) | • Causes smooth-muscle contraction<br>• Increases vascular permeability<br>• Induces pain |
| Serotonin (preformed in platelets) | • Increases vascular permeability |
| Slow-reacting substance of anaphylaxis (SRS-A), or leukotrienes C, D, and E (chemically derived from arachidonic acid; synthesis triggered by mast cell degranulation) | • Causes smooth-muscle contraction<br>• Increases vascular permeability |

The most commonly used IgE test is the *radioallergosorbent test (RAST)*, which measures a specific IgE antibody against a specific allergen; for example, the number of IgE molecules for ragweed pollen. RAST correlates well with skin testing, is safe, and doesn't vary in response to drugs or existing dermatoses like atopic eczema. However, it's not as reliable or sensitive as skin testing, and it's more expensive.

Another IgE test, the *basophil histamine release test,* measures the amount of histamine released from IgE antibody–bound basophils in response to a specific antigen added to the blood. This in vitro test correlates well with skin testing and helps evaluate suspected food allergy. However, it's currently used more commonly as a research tool because it's expensive.

**Provocative tests.** These tests, called challenges, simulate allergen contact in the environment and may rival skin testing for diagnostic value. However, because inhalation, topical application, or ingestion of allergens is not without risk if reactivity is high, provocative tests require close supervision and are preferably performed in a hospital.

*Food challenges* use double- or single-blind placebo control to evaluate suspected food allergy. In these tests, the patient ingests the suspected food in progressively larger amounts until he exceeds the amount that had allegedly evoked an allergic reaction. If overt symptoms of erythema, urticaria, itching, vomiting, or diarrhea develop, the test is considered positive. Other symptoms, such as fatigue, depression, and restlessness, aren't conclusive.

Another provocative test, *patch testing,* is used to evaluate suspected contact dermatitis. Because the Type IV hypersensitivity reaction operates in contact dermatitis, the clinical response is observed 24 to 48 hours after exposure to the allergen. Patch testing is contraindicated in patients with extensive dermatitis to avoid aggravating this condition.

**Other dietary tests.** The *elimination diet*, a tedious 1- to 2-week course of dietary manipulation, identifies food allergens by eliminating them one by one from the diet. Improvement or alleviation of symptoms when specific foods are restricted implies that such foods or the additives they contain (particularly sulfites) are allergens. Another diagnostic test, the *dietary diary* involves carefully recording intake and any associated symptoms. Typically, symptoms develop within 48 hours after ingesting an allergen.

## Treatment aims to bar allergic reaction
Because allergy typically follows a chronic course, treatment is often prolonged and may incorporate one or more of the following approaches: avoidance therapy, symptomatic therapy, or immunotherapy.

**Avoidance therapy.** As its name implies, avoidance therapy involves removing the offending allergen from the patient's environment. For example, avoidance of dust or pet dander may resolve allergic rhinitis, whereas avoidance of poison oak or poison ivy may prevent contact dermatitis. However, patients usually are allergic not to one but to several allergens. So therapy must aim to minimize contact with as many offending allergens as possible.

Avoidance therapy may help in allergy to airborne allergens, such as pollen, mold spores, and house dust, and allergy to certain foods and drugs. Occasionally, dietary restrictions apply in childhood asthma because some foods trigger asthmatic attacks.

**Symptomatic therapy.** This form of therapy focuses on several drugs that prevent or minimize the effects of chemical mediators released upon reexposure to a specific allergen (see *How drugs affect degranulation*, page 92). Among other drugs, antihistamines play a role in symptomatic therapy. These drugs help minimize sneezing, rhinorrhea, and associated itching in allergic rhinitis, but they're less effective for nasal congestion and eye symptoms. Antihistamines also help treat food and drug allergies and contact dermatitis. However, the side effects of drowsiness and dry mouth may limit their use.

Oral sympathomimetic amines (decongestants) help relieve allergic symptoms by mimicking the effects of epinephrine and nor-

epinephrine. Alpha-adrenergic sympathomimetics reduce nasal congestion by causing vasoconstriction. Combinations of sympathomimetics and antihistamines—for example, Ornade, Dimetapp, and Naldecon—offer decongestant effects with stimulatory effects to decrease drowsiness. Such drug combinations should be used cautiously in patients with hypertension, angina pectoris, or hyperthyroidism. Nose drops and nasal sprays containing alpha-adrenergic sympathomimetics temporarily relieve nasal congestion. However, prolonged use of these drugs (more than 3 or 4 days) usually exacerbates nasal obstruction by causing rebound congestion (rhinitis medicamentosa).

Beta-adrenergic sympathomimetics (isoproterenol) and theophyllines help treat extrinsic asthma by relaxing smooth muscle, causing bronchodilation. These drugs may also interfere with mast cell degranulation by increasing cellular cAMP.

Sympathomimetics alone or in combination with anticholinergics help relieve symptoms of food allergy.

Adrenocorticosteroids are useful in various allergic disorders because of their immunosuppressive and anti-inflammatory effects. Oral corticosteroids may benefit allergic rhinitis when other drugs are ineffective, for example, at the height of the pollen season. Topical corticosteroids, such as dexamethasone nasal spray (Turbinaire), are especially useful in treating rhinitis medicamentosa. Beclomethasone dipropionate and flunisolide, new steroidal aerosols for treating allergic rhinitis, have fewer adverse effects than dexamethasone. Currently, beclomethasone via inhalation is the corticosteroid of choice for asthma. Topical corticosteroids, antipruritics, and bland topical applications are useful in treating contact dermatitis.

Cromolyn sodium, a topical drug recently approved by the Food and Drug Administration for allergic rhinitis and conjunctivitis, may prevent the release of chemical mediators, such as histamine and slow-reacting substance of anaphylaxis, from mast cells. However, it can't relieve an acute asthmatic attack in progress.

**Immunotherapy.** This therapy begins with accurate identification of the specific IgE antibody for an allergen. It then involves serial subcutaneous injections of the allergen's immunogenic extract in progressively larger doses to establish a maximal tolerated dose. This dose raises the threshold for symptoms

# How drugs affect degranulation

Degranulation, the release of powerful chemical mediators from the secretory granules of mast cells and basophils, is a key step in the allergic reaction. Several drugs can inhibit or greatly reduce the effects of degranulation.

Cromolyn sodium is thought to inhibit the entry of calcium ions into mast cells, which initiates degranulation. This drug also prevents release of the mediators histamine and slow-reacting substance of anaphylaxis (SRS-A) from mast cells. Corticosteroid hormones and drugs that increase cyclic 3':5'-adenosine monophosphate (cAMP) inhibit the migration of granules to the cell membrane. However, if granules fuse with the cell membrane and discharge their chemical mediators, antihistamines and other drugs can neutralize or counteract their effects. Isoproterenol can ease reduced airway diameter caused by smooth-muscle contraction and can inhibit release of histamine and SRS-A. Decongestants can break up thick, tenacious secretions caused by increased mucous secretion.

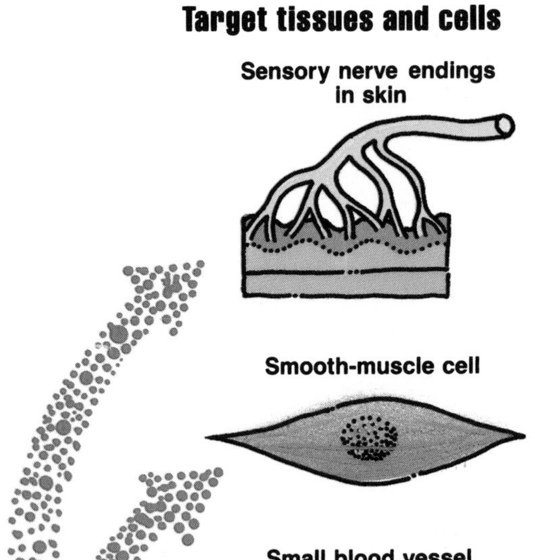

## Target tissues and cells

Sensory nerve endings in skin

Smooth-muscle cell

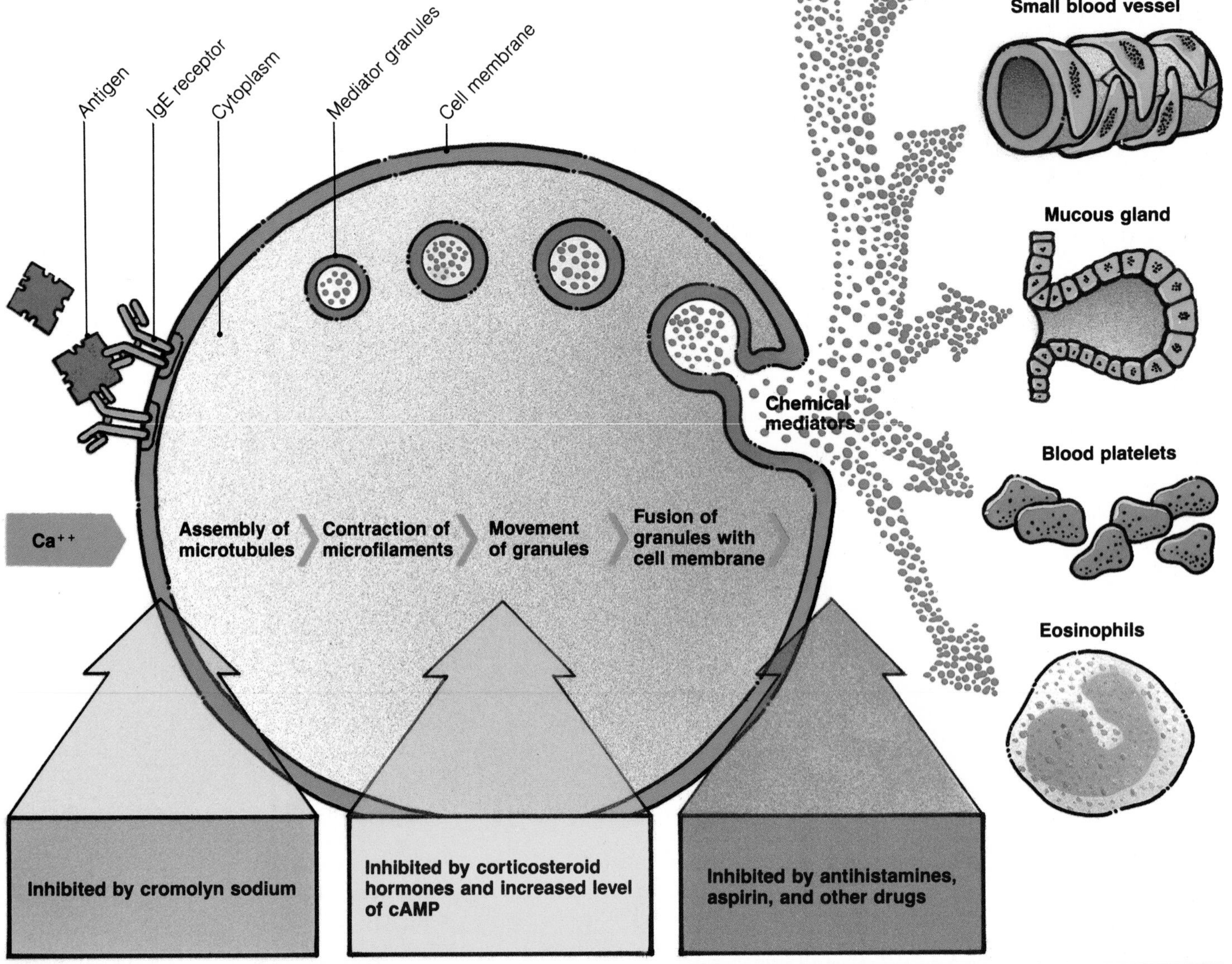

Small blood vessel

Mucous gland

Blood platelets

Eosinophils

Antigen

IgE receptor

Cytoplasm

Mediator granules

Cell membrane

Chemical mediators

Ca++

Assembly of microtubules

Contraction of microfilaments

Movement of granules

Fusion of granules with cell membrane

Inhibited by cromolyn sodium

Inhibited by corticosteroid hormones and increased level of cAMP

Inhibited by antihistamines, aspirin, and other drugs

resulting from exposure to the allergen, although the precise mechanism needs further investigation. The dose may trigger the development of new IgG antibodies called blocking antibodies and may increase suppressor T-cell function.

Immunotherapy is useful in allergic rhinitis associated with ragweed, in hypersensitivity to insect venom, and in asthma. However, compliance with therapy is challenging because it's prolonged and requires numerous injections.

## NURSING MANAGEMENT

Because allergy appears in many forms with varying severity, it's certain to challenge your nursing skills. You must be able to adapt your nursing care to each patient's needs, whether his allergy is merely bothersome or potentially life-threatening. A detailed nursing history provides the basis for an effective care plan.

### Comprehensive history first

Begin by gathering biographic information. Then, to obtain a comprehensive history, be sure to ask about:

**Symptoms.** Have the patient describe his chief complaint. Nasal stuffiness and a cold that won't go away are common complaints in allergy. Next, explore other symptoms that may point to an allergic disorder, including urticaria, itching, sneezing, rhinitis, eye irritation, poor hearing, wheezing, dyspnea, cough, abdominal pain, nausea, and diarrhea. In fact, a complex set of symptoms often occurs in allergy. For example, if the patient's chief complaint is rhinitis, the presence of conjunctivitis or nasal pruritus usually confirms allergic rhinitis. Conversely, rhinitis without conjunctivitis or pruritus is probably not related to allergy.

Are symptoms continuous or intermittent? In allergic disorders, symptoms are usually intermittent or sporadic. Note when and where the patient has had symptoms. Pinpoint specific dates or times of the year, if possible. Seasonal variations in allergic disorders may correlate with pollen eruption. Are particular places, such as the basement, attic, field, factory, warehouse, or home, associated with exacerbation of symptoms?

**Diet.** Have the patient describe his diet. Does he associate adverse effects with specific foods? Differentiate allergic signs, like rash and swelling, from indigestion.

**Home, school, and work environment.** Does the patient have any pets? Note the type of furnishings in his home, such as draperies, carpeting, bed mattress, and pillows. What type of heating is in his home? Find out if he's exposed to inhalants (such as industrial fumes) or contactants (such as nickel) at work. Does he associate a particular agent with his allergy? Ask about recent exposure to possible allergens—plants, insects, and certain foods—and to primary irritants—cigarette smoke, paint, perfumes, or pollutants.

**Childhood and infectious diseases.** Has the patient had common childhood diseases, such as measles, mumps, and chicken pox? How often does he have bacterial or viral infections?

**Previous hospitalizations.** Has the patient ever been hospitalized for an allergic disorder? If so, for how long? What was the course of treatment? Did he undergo any tests using radiocontrast dye? If so, did he experience an allergic reaction? Did the patient's symptoms worsen shortly after discharge? This may pinpoint allergens in the home.

**Allergic and immunologic history.** Does the patient have a known sensitivity to pollens, certain foods, danders, or drugs? Ask about dermatitis, urticaria, angioedema, eczema, hay fever, vasomotor rhinitis, asthma, migraine, and seasonal conjunctivitis. Learn the results of previous skin tests. Also ask about desensitization, vaccinations, and immunizations. Has immunotherapy ever been tried?

**Medication history.** What over-the-counter or prescription drugs is the patient currently taking? What is his response to them? Also note drugs prescribed in the past and the patient's response. If he mentions a drug allergy, be sure to differentiate between adverse effects and hypersensitivity. Seek medical documentation of hypersensitivity.

**Family history.** Do any family members have allergic disorders? The tendency toward allergic disorders is probably hereditary, although the exact mechanism of transmission is unclear.

**Psychosocial history.** To determine how the patient copes with his allergic disorder, ask about relationships with family, friends, and co-workers. Identify life-style changes associated with allergy symptoms. Also assess his knowledge level and readiness to learn.

### Next, the physical examination

Begin by taking the patient's vital signs and his height and weight. Fever may indicate secondary infection, such as sinusitis or pneu-

## Common agents that trigger anaphylaxis or anaphylactoid reactions

**Local anesthetics**
Lidocaine
Procaine

**Antibiotics**
Aminoglycosides
Amphotericin B
Cephalosporins
Nitrofurantoin
Penicillins
Sulfonamides
Tetracyclines

**Dextran**
Iron dextran

**Diagnostic agents**
Radiocontrast dyes

**Other drugs**
Barbiturates
Diazepam
Phenytoin
Protamine

**Enzymes**
Chymopapain
Chymotrypsin
Penicillinase
Trypsin

**Food additives**
Bisulfites

**Foods**
Beans
Chocolate
Cottonseed oil
Eggs
Fruits
Grains
Nuts
Seafood (shellfish)

**Hormones**
Adrenocorticotropic
  hormone
Estradiol
Insulin
Parathyroid hormone
Vasopressin

**Pollens**
Grass
Ragweed

**Proteins**
Horse and rabbit serum

**Venoms**
Fire ant
Hymenoptera
Snake

monia. Weight loss and delayed growth are possible in some children with chronic asthma or in those treated with corticosteroids or dietary restrictions.

Then, systematically examine the patient, watching for symptoms that suggest allergy.

**Skin.** Observe the skin for rashes, eruptions, scaling, dryness, and pigmentation changes. Note the location, distribution, and appearance of any abnormalities. Flexural lichenification (thickening and hardening) is common in adults with atopic dermatitis, whereas facial and extensor lichenification appears in infants. Erythema, edema, and papulovesicular lesions typically accompany allergic contact dermatitis. Ask about itching. Urticaria usually points to food or drug allergy.

**Lymph nodes.** Assess for lymph node enlargement, tenderness, or pain, which may result from adjacent throat or ear infection or from severe allergic contact dermatitis.

**Eyes.** Observe for inflammation, excessive tearing, swollen lids, and itching. Some children have dark circles under the eyes called allergic shiners. Contact dermatitis due to cosmetics may produce the same signs.

**Ears.** Inspect the external ears for lesions. Contact dermatitis, usually associated with earrings containing nickel, silver, or chrome, is most common in adults. Atopic eczema occurs more frequently in children, but its lesions also appear elsewhere on the body. Such lesions may be erythematous, papular, or vesicular. Examine the middle ear for fluid and bubbles, which indicate middle-ear effusion (serous otitis media). Also ask about a stopped-up or popping sensation in the ear and about poor hearing.

**Nose.** Assess the inferior turbinates for swelling; paleness; and thin, clear secretions; and the adjacent mucosa for erythema. In children, look for a horizontal nasal crease due to constant rubbing. Note thick, viscid, purulent, and possibly blood-tinged nasal discharge, which signals secondary infection.

**Throat.** Ask about sore throat and palatal itch, which are common in allergy, and look for signs of infection.

**Mouth.** Assess for swelling and soreness of lips, tongue, and buccal mucosa.

**Respiratory system.** Observe for chest deformity. Ask about shortness of breath, wheezing, dyspnea, cough, and sputum production. Also check for other respiratory infections. Auscultate for wheezes during forced expiration. Recognize that wheezing is typically absent or minimal with severe bronchocon-

striction and warns of impending respiratory failure. Note the use of accessory muscles and intercostal retraction, which may accompany an acute asthmatic attack. In pregnant patients with asthma, expect normal vital capacity but decreased residual volume and functional residual capacity, possibly due to elevation of the diaphragm by the enlarging uterus.

**Cardiovascular system.** Assess for palpitations, tachycardia, and irregular rhythm, which may signal an acute asthmatic attack. Such symptoms reflect severe hypoxemia, carbon dioxide retention, and increased work of breathing. Be alert for cyanosis, tachypnea, and pulsus paradoxus.

**GI system.** Ask about changes in appetite or weight, nausea vomiting, diarrhea, and flatulence. Such symptoms may reflect food allergy or other GI disorders, such as intestinal viral or bacterial infection.

**Reproductive system (female).** Note existing pregnancy. Allergic rhinitis may worsen during pregnancy, then moderate soon after delivery. Mild asthma occasionally improves during pregnancy.

### Shape nursing diagnoses

Using data collected from the nursing history and physical examination, identify the patient's actual or potential problems that you're qualified to treat. The following nursing diagnoses will probably be part of your care plan.

**Knowledge deficit related to disease.** Your goals are to help the patient understand allergy and its signs and symptoms and to prevent or minimize systemic anaphylaxis and local allergic reactions. Begin by assessing the patient's ability and readiness to learn. Include the parents if the patient is a child. Provide written educational material to reinforce your teaching.

Clearly define allergy to eliminate any misconceptions. Explain that allergy represents an inappropriate, excessive reaction to usually harmless substances. Inform the patient that allergies develop only with exposure to various substances.

Not surprisingly, food allergy is the first concern in infancy. Have parents immediately report signs and symptoms of food allergy, such as unusual appetite or crying immediately after eating. Instruct them to avoid suspected food allergens but to be sure to provide comparable nutritional substitutes, such as milk substitutes. Warn them to be alert for other allergies once a food allergy

## EMERGENCY MANAGEMENT

# Anaphylaxis

**Angioedema**

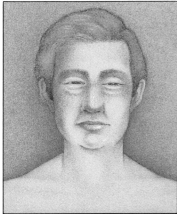

**Urticaria with itching**

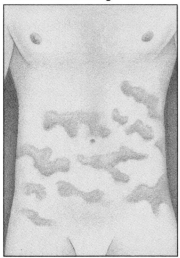

Anaphylaxis, an extreme hypersensitivity response, is usually mediated by IgE antibodies and occurs within a few seconds to hours after antigen exposure. As a nurse, you'll probably see drug-induced anaphylaxis most often. Early recognition can be lifesaving. Typically, the patient reports feeling a sense of doom immediately before anaphylaxis.

Most dramatic signs and symptoms of anaphylaxis affect the cutaneous, circulatory, and respiratory systems.

Urticaria, angioedema, pruritus, and erythema may be the early warning signs of anaphylaxis. In most instances, these cutaneous signs are self-limiting and resolve in 48 hours.

Circulatory collapse follows hypotension, shock, and cardiac dysrhythmias caused by reduced cardiac perfusion and oxygenation.

Respiratory failure may involve the upper airway or the bronchi. Edema of the larynx and epiglottis causes hoarseness, stridor, dyspnea, and hypersecretion of mucus.

Other signs and symptoms of anaphylaxis include nausea, vomiting, diarrhea, and urinary urgency and incontinence.

When you recognize an anaphylactic reaction, here's what you should do:
• Remove the offending antigen, if possible.
• Maintain a patent airway. Be prepared to assist the doctor with insertion of an oropharyngeal airway or endotracheal tube or a tracheotomy and to administer oxygen.
• Administer aqueous epinephrine, as ordered. Repeat dose if anaphylaxis is not immediately reversed.
• Administer antihistamines such as diphenhydramine for urticaria and angioedema, as ordered.
• Start an I.V. infusion to administer fluids and additional drugs.
• Monitor the patient for circulatory shock. Provide fluid therapy, as ordered, to restore circulation and blood pressure.
• Monitor the patient's blood pressure, central venous pressure, and urinary output. If volume repletion and I.V. epinephrine do not reverse vascular collapse, other pressor agents, such as norepinephrine, may be needed.
• If cardiac arrest occurs, perform cardiopulmonary resuscitation, and administer specific drug therapy, as ordered.
• Provide mechanical ventilation for respiratory arrest.

Administer other drugs as ordered, such as subcutaneous

**Bronchospasm**

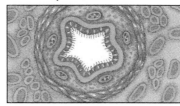

**Laryngeal edema**

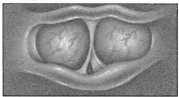

**Hypotension**

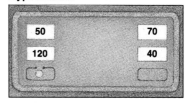

**Cardiac dysrhythmias**

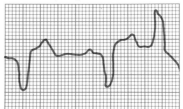

**GI and genitourinary cramps**

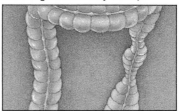

epinephrine (longer acting), corticosteroids to prevent protracted laryngeal edema, and aminophylline for bronchospasm. Avoid rapid infusion, which may precipitate or aggravate hypotension.

Give the patient written information on how to avoid exposure to potentially threatening allergens. Stress that avoidance is the most effective treatment for anaphylaxis. Also suggest desensitization to prevent future reactions to known allergens.

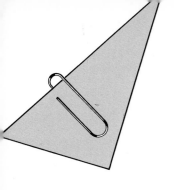

**PATIENT-TEACHING AID**

# Using an anaphylaxis kit

*Dear* _____

1. Contact your doctor, if possible; then proceed with the emergency kit.
2. For a reaction to an insect sting, remove the stinger if it's still there. Be careful not to push, pinch, squeeze, or imbed the stinger farther into the skin. If you were stung on an arm or leg, apply a tourniquet between the sting and your body. To tighten, pull the end of one string. Release the tourniquet every 10 minutes by pulling the metal ring. If you were stung on the body, neck, or face, apply ice to the area.
3. If time allows, use an alcohol swab to cleanse a 4" (10-cm) area on your arm or thigh (above the tourniquet).
4. Prepare a prefilled syringe. First, remove the needle cover. Then, expel air from the syringe

by holding it with the needle pointing up and carefully pushing the plunger.
5. Inject epinephrine. Insert the whole needle straight down into the cleansed skin area. Then, pull back on the plunger. If blood enters the syringe, the needle is in a blood vessel. Withdraw the needle, and reinsert in another site. For adults and children over age 12, push the plunger until it stops (0.3 ml). Do not force it farther. Remove the needle, and replace the needle cover. A second injection of 0.3 ml remains in the syringe. For children age 12 or younger, the epinephrine 1:1,000 syringe has graduations of 0.1 ml for measurement of doses less than 0.3 ml; for ages 6 to 12, 0.2 ml; for ages 2 to 6, 0.15 ml; and for infants to

age 2, 0.05 to 0.1 ml.
6. Chew and swallow chlorpheniramine tablets. Adults and children over age 12 should take four tablets; children age 12 or younger, two tablets.
7. For local reactions, apply cold compresses to ease pain and reduce swelling.
8. Keep warm; avoid exertion.
9. Prepare the prefilled syringe for a second injection. Turn the rectangular plunger one quarter turn to the right to line up with the rectangular slot in the syringe. Do not depress the plunger until you're ready for a second injection.
10. Second injection: If erythema, itching, swelling, and other symptoms don't subside in 10 minutes, repeat steps 4, 5, and 6.
11. See your doctor as soon as possible.

appears.

Tell the patient or his parents that signs and symptoms vary with the type of allergen and the amount of exposure and may involve many body systems. Emphasize the signs and symptoms requiring immediate attention, such as an intractable asthmatic attack.

Explain diagnostic tests used to confirm allergy and to identify the offending allergen(s). Then discuss treatment realistically, including avoidance of the allergen, drugs prescribed for symptomatic relief, and immunotherapy.

*Insect stings.* Avoid using scented soaps and perfumes and wearing bright colors, which attract insects, especially bees. Wear shoes whenever outdoors. Avoid flower beds, orchards with ripe fruit, and garbage pails. Keep car windows closed. Have an experienced exterminator destroy bee hives and hornet or wasp nests.

*Food.* Watch for allergens disguised in other foods, for example, nuts in cookies. Read all food labels carefully. Avoid inhaling cooking odors of known food allergens, since these may also precipitate a reaction.

*Dust.* Eliminate dust-collecting items, such as wool blankets, rugs, chenille bedspreads,

flannel pajamas, and venetian blinds. Place bookcases or boxes containing old books in a distant room or storage area. Dust daily, using a damp or oiled cloth and mop; thoroughly clean weekly. Keep the allergic child away from the room being cleaned. Instruct the allergic adult to wear a mask to filter dust particles during cleaning.

Close off forced-air heating ducts in the patient's bedroom, within limits necessary to maintain a comfortable temperature. Obtain an electrostatic precipitator and central heating and air conditioning, if affordable. Or use a nonelectronic precipitator (HEPA room or central filter). Use an air conditioner, room air filters, or both; and clean these devices often.

Encase feather pillows, mattresses, and boxsprings in impermeable plastic covers. (New Dacron or rubber pillows don't require encasing; old ones do because they may harbor molds.) Remove upholstered furniture, carpeting, bed pads, and stuffed animals and toys from the patient's bedroom.

*Mold.* Avoid damp, unfinished basements and attics; barns; moldy hay; and straw. Limit house plants, as their soil harbors molds. Clean humidifiers and vaporizers with Clorox or vinegar solutions to control mold growth.

*Pollen.* Stay indoors as much as possible during peak pollen seasons. Keep windows closed, since most pollens are from trees, weeds, and grasses and are dispersed by the wind. Listen for pollen count reports on the local radio, and use them as a guide for outdoor activities.

Explain the purpose, dosage, schedule, and adverse effects of prescribed drugs. Also teach the patient how to use an inhaler properly. Inform him that immunotherapy takes several months to show positive results. Stress the importance of his cooperation and the need for continued medical follow-up.

To prevent or minimize systemic anaphylaxis and local allergic reactions, first teach the patient early signs of hypersensitivity, such as pruritus, erythema, urticaria, and edema. Have him report such signs immediately to prevent more severe laryngeal edema and shock. Emphasize that prompt treatment may be lifesaving.

Explain how to use an emergency kit to prevent anaphylaxis (see *Using an anaphylaxis kit*). Have the patient keep the kit stocked and with him—not in the refrigerator—when he's outdoors. Teach him and his family how to administer the injection.

Advise the patient to wear Medic Alert jewelry or to carry a card that describes his allergy in his wallet.

To minimize anaphylaxis from an insect sting, apply ice or a tourniquet proximal to the sting to slow venom absorption. If the stinger is still in place, remove it without squeezing or applying pressure to avoid forcing more venom from the stinger sac. When the acute phase resolves, inform the patient that angioedema may persist for several hours; reassure him, as needed.

Recognize that most drug reactions (about 80%) are predictable and thus preventable. Note that allergy may include all drugs in one family or related substances; for example, sensitivity to penicillin and to dicloxacillin or sensitivity to molds and to antibiotics derived from molds.

Give the patient a hospital identification bracelet that lists known or suspected drug allergies. Also note allergies on the patient's chart, medication and diet Kardexes, and radiology request forms.

Keep emergency equipment nearby, and check its function periodically. Closely monitor the patient receiving drugs with high anaphylactic potential, such as penicillins, synthetic analogues of penicillin, iodides, and aspirin.

Be especially alert when drugs are given by injection, as this administration route is associated with the most severe anaphylaxis.

Before diagnostic studies using radiocontrast dye, premedicate the patient with suspected or known dye allergy with a combination of steroid and antihistamine (prednisone and diphenhydramine), as ordered. Also, closely monitor him during sensitivity testing to penicillin or other drugs, and observe him for 20 to 25 minutes after inoculation.

Have the patient keep a record of any drugs he takes that trigger unusual reactions. Instruct him to clearly describe the reaction, including its severity and how soon after drug administration it occurred.

Closely monitor the patient with known or suspected food allergy during skin testing with food extracts. Have emergency drugs and equipment nearby and be prepared to treat anaphylaxis.

Consider your nursing interventions effective if the patient can define allergy; recognizes signs and symptoms of his disorder; knows about necessary diagnostic tests; understands and adheres to prescribed treatment; knows how to avoid specific allergens; knows the name, purpose, dosage, and adverse effects of prescribed drugs; demonstrates the ability to treat himself to offset anaphylaxis; and confirms plans for ongoing health care.

**Decreased cardiac output related to anaphylaxis.** Of the many possible effects of anaphylaxis, impaired cardiovascular and respiratory function are most life-threatening. To restore cardiac output is therefore a key nursing goal. For your interventions to achieve this goal, see *Emergency management: Anaphylaxis,* page 95.

**Ineffective breathing patterns related to anaphylaxis.** Your nursing goal is to restore optimal respirations to maintain effective gas exchange. For appropriate interventions to achieve this goal, see *Emergency management: Anaphylaxis,* page 95.

### Education plus action
Your role in allergic disorders relies heavily on teaching. For the patient made uncomfortable by an annoying dust or pollen allergy, your tips can make life easier. For the patient with a more serious drug or venom allergy, your tips can be lifesaving. But equally important, your role demands keen assessment to recognize telltale signs and symptoms of anaphylaxis and prompt, appropriate intervention to offset it.

**Points to remember**

- About one in every four Americans has a serious allergy.
- Allergy represents an inappropriate, excessive reaction to substances not intrinsically harmful. Its development probably reflects genetic predisposition, although the mechanism of inheritance is unclear.
- Allergy may be benign yet bothersome, as in allergic rhinitis, or life-threatening, as in acute systemic anaphylaxis.
- Treatment options include avoidance of the allergen(s), drugs for symptomatic relief, and immunotherapy.
- Nursing care focuses on teaching the patient to recognize signs and symptoms of allergy, to know why they develop, to avoid exposure to offending allergen(s), and to know how to administer emergency treatment to offset anaphylaxis.

# 7 MANAGING RHEUMATOID AUTOIMMUNITY

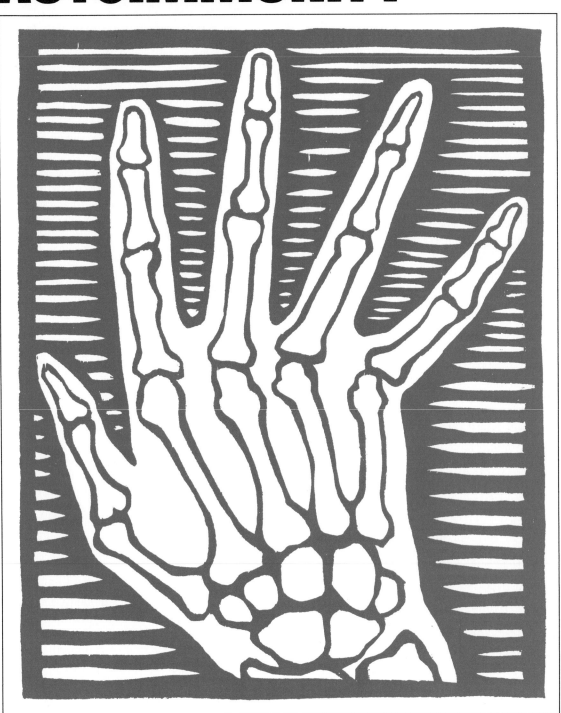

X-ray of rheumatoid arthritis of hand

Systemic autoimmune diseases, also known as rheumatic diseases or collagen-vascular diseases, are marked by an abnormal immune response to self. This leads to a sequence of abnormal tissue reaction and tissue damage that may result in diffuse systemic manifestations. Typical manifestations can vary from minimal localized symptoms to systemic multiorgan involvement with severe impairment of function and life-threatening organ failure.

Some autoimmune disorders are quite common and often have devastating physical, emotional, and financial impact on patients and their families. Managing these disorders is often difficult because of their wide-ranging effects and because they tend to follow an unpredictable course of remission and exacerbation.

### Types of disorders

Systemic autoimmune diseases fall into two categories: diffuse connective tissue diseases and spondyloarthropathies (arthritis associated with spondylitis). (See *Classification of rheumatic diseases,* page 100.) Diffuse connective tissue diseases are more common in females and have a strong potential for multiorgan involvement in addition to arthritis and skin manifestations. Disorders that follow this pattern include rheumatoid arthritis (RA), systemic lupus erythematosus (SLE), scleroderma (also known as progressive systemic sclerosis), and myositis.

Most spondyloarthropathies are more common in males. They share a familial tendency and overlapping clinical features and are now clearly associated with the genetic marker human leukocyte antigen- (HLA-) B27. This group includes ankylosing spondylitis, Reiter's syndrome, psoriatic arthritis, and arthritis associated with chronic inflammatory bowel disease.

The characteristics of many autoimmune disorders overlap: similar autoantibodies (antibodies misdirected against self tissue) are found in many of them, and more than one autoimmune disorder can develop in one person. Autoimmune disorders may also be associated with malignancy or immunodeficiency.

Autoimmune disorders involve disruption of the immunoregulatory mechanism, causing normal cell-mediated and humoral immune responses to turn self-destructive, which results in tissue damage. The immunoregulatory failure appears to result from an immunologic response triggered by an environmental stimulus and promoted by hormonal and viral factors in a genetically susceptible person. (See *SLE: Characteristic immunologic abnormalities,* page 101.)

**Genetic factors.** A familial tendency has long been associated with autoimmune disorders, although no clear inheritance pattern has yet been identified. Family members of patients with autoimmune disease show an abnormally high incidence of serologic markers even when they show no signs of illness.

The complex mechanism of genetic influence on autoimmunity seems related to the HLA histocompatibility complex on chromosome 6. The association between spondyloarthropathy and the presence of the specific antigen HLA-B27 is the most striking. The role of HLA in this and other disorders is still obscure.

**Hormonal factors.** The activity of female sex hormones, rather than a sex-linked genetic factor, seems to explain the higher incidence of many autoimmune disorders in females. Despite this hormonal link, definite hormonal abnormalities haven't been clearly shown. The underlying cause of this link may be abnormal hormone metabolism rather than abnormal hormone production. Pregnancy in autoimmune diseases, especially SLE, has been studied well because onset of the disease is often associated with pregnancy, and patients with SLE may have exacerbations during or shortly after pregnancy.

**Viral factors.** Infection, especially viral infection, may also stimulate the autoimmune response in a genetically susceptible person.

**Stress.** Severe stress or a traumatic event such as an emotional shock, an accident, or illness may be a contributing factor since systemic autoimmune disorders sometimes appear or worsen during stressful periods.

**Environmental factors.** Several other environmental factors have been implicated in the onset of rheumatic diseases. SLE may surface after sunburn or exposure to sunlight. An illness resembling SLE is sometimes associated with certain drugs, such as hydralazine, procainamide, phenytoin, and isoniazid. But such drug-induced SLE is usually mild, resolving when the drug is withdrawn, and rarely has severe systemic complications.

### PATHOPHYSIOLOGY

Several mechanisms may explain the loss of self-tolerance in autoimmune disorders and the antigenicity of self tissue.

## Classification of rheumatic diseases

Systemic autoimmune diseases constitute the first two categories of the rheumatic disease classification system used by the Arthritis Foundation.

**Diffuse connective tissue diseases**
Rheumatoid arthritis
Juvenile arthritis
  Systemic onset
  Polyarticular onset
  Oligoarticular onset
Systemic lupus erythematosus
Progressive systemic sclerosis
Polymyositis/dermatomyositis
Necrotizing vasculitis and other vasculitides
  Polyarteritis nodosa group (includes hepatitis B–associated arteritis and allergic granulomatosis [Churg-Strauss syndrome])
  Hypersensitivity vasculitis (includes Schönlein-Henoch purpura and others)
  Wegener's granulomatosis
  Giant cell arteritis
    Temporal arteritis
    Takayasu's arteritis
  Mucocutaneous lymph node syndrome (Kawasaki disease)
  Behcet's syndrome
Sjögren's syndrome
Overlap syndromes (includes mixed connective tissue disease)
Others (includes polymyalgia rheumatica, panniculitis [Weber-Christian disease], erythema nodosum, relapsing polychondritis, and others)

**Spondyloarthropathies**
Ankylosing spondylitis
Reiter's syndrome
Psoriatic arthritis
Arthritis associated with chronic inflammatory bowel disease

## Changed normal tissue

Normal tissue can be altered by many factors, such as infections, toxins, drugs, and other chemicals. Recognition of this altered tissue as foreign can lead to autoimmune disorders.

## Changed immune components

Autoimmunity may also result from changes in the immune system's cellular components, which maintain normal self-tolerance. These cellular components are found in the lymphoid tissue and the circulation. Cellular components include B cells, which produce antibodies; T cells, which may augment (helper T cells) or diminish (suppressor T cells) the function of other lymphoid cells; macrophages; and mononuclear cells. Cells may change significantly (for example, causing increased B-cell activation and diminished T-cell suppression) after exposure to chemicals, drugs, or infectious organisms.

## Activation of suppressed clones

One function of the suppressor T cell is to prevent activation of T- and B-cell clones that might react to normal self tissue or produce autoantibodies. If this suppressor function is altered or lost, these self-reactive clones can proliferate and destroy normal self tissue.

## Similarity of normal tissue to exogenous antigens

Also known as shared or cross-reactive antigens, exogenous antigens that resemble normal tissue induce the formation of antibodies that may cross-react with structurally similar constituents in normal body tissue.

Any of these four mechanisms could alter the balance of immunoregulatory control. Once this happens, environmental factors may cause further loss of self-tolerance. Then, T and B cells mistake self tissue for nonself, and helper T cells stimulate B cells to produce autoantibodies.

## Autoantibodies

Autoantibodies appear in the serum of many people, even in those without illness. They also appear following tissue damage. In general, they are more likely to appear in older people, perhaps because aging is associated with the gradual breakdown of regulatory control and the decline of whatever factors prevent their synthesis. In fact, at least one type of autoantibody is readily detectable in the serum of more than 50% of people over age 70.

Such autoantibodies may be the source of tissue damage in systemic autoimmune disorders. In these disorders, one or more types of autoantibodies may be synthesized in large quantities. In fact, specific autoantibodies, such as antinuclear antibody (ANA) and rheumatoid factor (RF), have been identified against many body cells and cell components.

ANA forms against cell components such as double- and single-stranded deoxyribonucleic acid (DNA), ribonuclear protein particles, and histones. (See *Immunofluorescent staining for antinuclear antibodies,* page 102.)

ANA is probably not directly cytotoxic since the intracellular nuclear targets are protected by a cell membrane. Instead, it most likely attacks damaged cells, causing their nuclei to swell, extrude, and release chemotaxins. Attracted to the site through chemotaxis, neutrophils and macrophages quickly engulf the severely damaged cell.

RF is antibody synthesized against self immunoglobulin. One or more types of RF appear in classic RA, although they may not be present at the beginning of the illness. RF also appears in other chronic rheumatic diseases, including Sjögren's syndrome and scleroderma.

## Immunopathologic mechanisms

The immune response to these autoantibodies probably involves one or more hypersensitivity reactions as well as the sensitization of lymphocytes to self. Of the four types of immunologic tissue injury (see *Gell and Coombs classification of hypersensitivity reactions,* pages 22 and 23), Type II, III, and IV reactions are implicated in autoimmune rheumatic disorders. Type II and III reactions are mediated by antibodies (humoral response), and Type IV reactions are mediated by T cells and macrophages (cell-mediated response). These reactions may coexist in some individuals. Unfortunately, in many autoimmune disorders, the mechanism of tissue damage is still unclear.

**Type II reactions.** Antibody-mediated Type II reactions involve cytotoxic damage at the tissue level in which antibodies combine with cell-surface antigens.

The target of Type II reactions may be a formed blood element, as in the thrombocytopenia of SLE, in which antibodies form against platelets; or it may be a specific organ tissue, such as kidney or skin, as occurs in scleroderma. Cell damage may then proceed in several ways. Activation of complement may

# SLE: Characteristic immunologic abnormalities

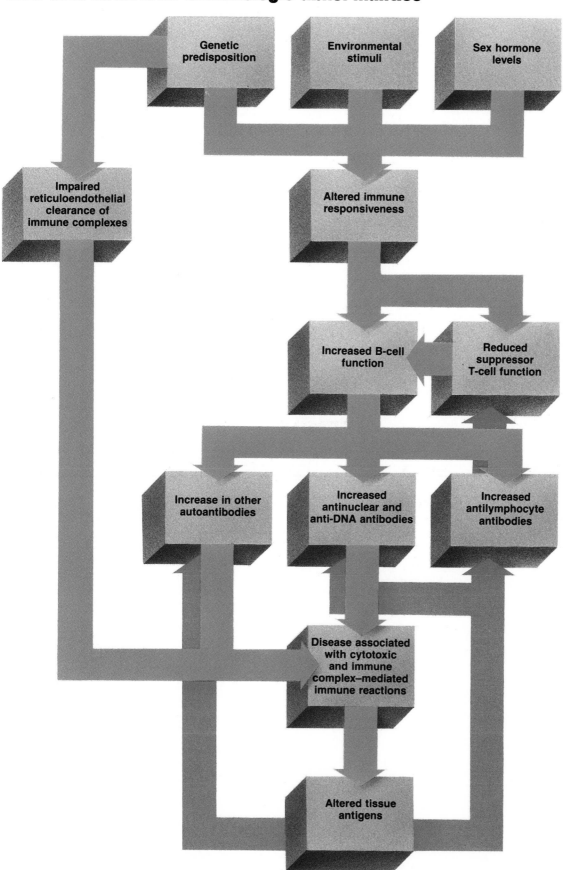

Genetic, hormonal, and environmental influences work together to produce the immunologic abnormalities characteristic of systemic lupus erythematosus.

**Key**

 Forward flow of effect

 Backward flow of effect

## Immunofluorescent staining for antinuclear antibodies

All classes of immunoglobulins can form antinuclear antibodies. These autoantibodies, directed against nuclear constituents, appear in various rheumatic diseases, especially systemic lupus erythematosus (SLE). Immunofluorescent staining reveals one of the following four patterns.

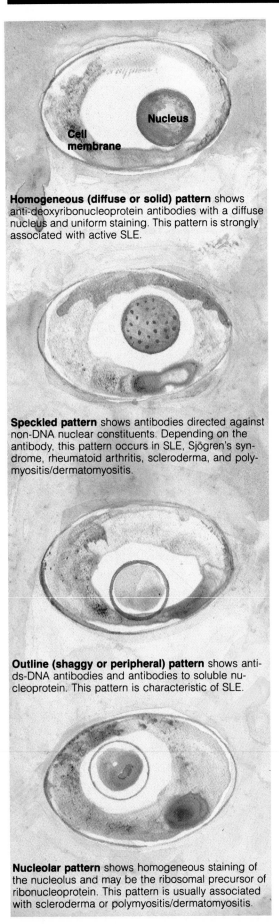

**Homogeneous (diffuse or solid) pattern** shows anti-deoxyribonucleoprotein antibodies with a diffuse nucleus and uniform staining. This pattern is strongly associated with active SLE.

**Speckled pattern** shows antibodies directed against non-DNA nuclear constituents. Depending on the antibody, this pattern occurs in SLE, Sjögren's syndrome, rheumatoid arthritis, scleroderma, and polymyositis/dermatomyositis.

**Outline (shaggy or peripheral) pattern** shows anti-ds-DNA antibodies and antibodies to soluble nucleoprotein. This pattern is characteristic of SLE.

**Nucleolar pattern** shows homogeneous staining of the nucleolus and may be the ribosomal precursor of ribonucleoprotein. This pattern is usually associated with scleroderma or polymyositis/dermatomyositis.

result in the disruption of target-cell membrane, lysis, and cell death. The cell may be destroyed through opsonization and phagocytosis, with or without complement, or through contact with a mononuclear or polymorphonuclear cell, with resulting lysis. Or the cell may not actually be destroyed, but its function may change, thereby changing its usual response to stimuli.

**Type III reactions.** Also antibody-mediated, Type III reactions are inflammatory reactions caused by the formation and localization of immune complexes within the tissue. Immune complexes, a normal product of the humoral immune response, are usually removed from circulation by the reticuloendothelial system. However, when high concentrations of antibody persist for prolonged periods, complexes begin to lodge in tissues, notably the vascular epithelium, the lining of the joints, and the glomerulus of the kidney. Impaired clearance by the reticuloendothelial system may add to deposition of immune complexes in such diseases as SLE.

Once these complexes lodge in the tissues, an inflammatory response results. In this response, complement is activated, chemotactic factors (C5a, C3a) are released, and polymorphonuclear leukocytes infiltrate the area. Lysosomal enzymes released from the polymorphonuclear leukocytes damage vessel walls and lead to hemorrhage, occlusion, and ischemic changes in the tissue and organs served by the damaged vessels. Any organ is susceptible to such damage, which accounts for such varied manifestations in SLE as vasculitis, synovitis, glomerulonephritis, cardiac involvement, and central nervous system (CNS) damage. (See *Results of immune complex formation.*)

**Type IV reactions.** Type IV reactions, also known as delayed hypersensitivity reactions, are cell-mediated reactions. They result from the contact between sensitized T cells and specific antigens. This type of reaction doesn't require complement or antibodies. Instead, it involves the proliferation of T cells and the release of mediators that attract, activate, and maintain macrophages in the area. These macrophages release lysozymal enzymes that damage surrounding tissue. In addition, sensitized T cells can cause direct cell toxicity through cell-to-cell contact, which results in lysis of the target cell. Type IV reactions are thought to be important in temporal arteritis and also may play a role in RA and in Sjögren's syndrome.

# Results of immune complex formation

The formation of immune complexes results in several different processes within the bloodstream. These processes include phagocytosis through complement activation, release of vasoactive substances, and activation of coagulation. Excess circulating immune complexes are deposited in tissues, initiating an inflammatory response. This inflammatory response results in glomerulitis in the renal basement membrane, vasculitis in blood vessels, and arthritis in joint synovia (as shown at bottom right).

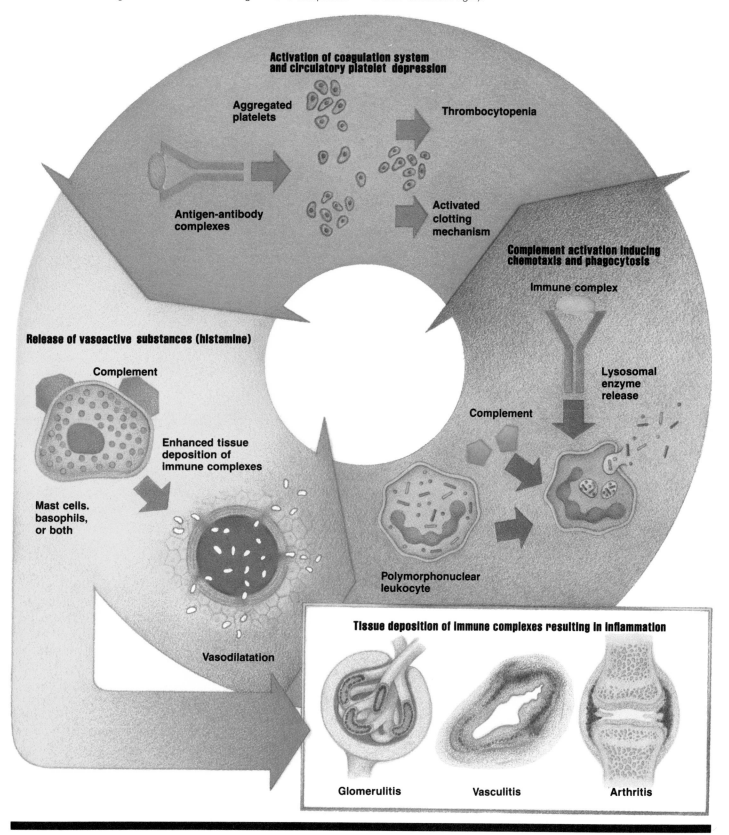

**Activation of coagulation system and circulatory platelet depression**

Aggregated platelets

Thrombocytopenia

Antigen-antibody complexes

Activated clotting mechanism

**Complement activation inducing chemotaxis and phagocytosis**

Immune complex

Lysosomal enzyme release

Complement

**Release of vasoactive substances (histamine)**

Complement

Enhanced tissue deposition of immune complexes

Mast cells. basophils, or both

Polymorphonuclear leukocyte

Vasodilatation

**Tissue deposition of immune complexes resulting in inflammation**

Glomerulitis

Vasculitis

Arthritis

# Ocular effects of autoimmune rheumatic diseases

Autoimmune rheumatic diseases often involve the eyes. In rheumatoid arthritis (RA), Reiter's syndrome, ankylosing spondylitis, and systemic lupus erythematosus (SLE), ocular manifestations may include scleritis (inflammation of the sclera) and uveitis (inflammation of the iris, choroid, and ciliary body). In Sjögren's syndrome, keratoconjunctivitis sicca (lack of tears, resulting in dry eyes and inflammation of the cornea) may occur. In giant cell arteritis and polyarteritis nodosa, ocular manifestations may cause temporal and orbital pain, blurred vision, and scotomas ( blind gaps in the visual field).

## Pathophysiology

How ocular signs occur varies according to the disorder. In RA and SLE, Type III hypersensitivity reactions cause inflammation and tissue damage. In RA, the rheumatoid factor (RF)—antibodies specific for the Fc fragment of altered IgG—and scleral tissue deposits may activate the complement system and release chemoattractants. Then, leukocytes and platelets accumulate, causing occlusive vasculitis, rheumatic nodule formation in the sclera, and scleral collagen destruction.

In SLE, a similar occlusive vasculitis occurs as a result of a Type III reaction involving circulating anti-DNA antibodies. Anti-DNA/DNA complexes deposit in the vasculature of the retinal nerve fiber layer, causing tiny infarcts and subsequent damage to the retina and optic nerve. Characteristic "cotton wool" spots can be seen in the retina.

In Sjögren's syndrome, keratoconjunctivitis sicca may occur. Antinuclear antibodies (ANAs) and RF may be present in Sjögren's syndrome.

In giant cell arteritis and polyarteritis nodosa, Type IV cell-mediated delayed hypersensitivity reactions are thought to cause retinal atrophy. Extensive cellular infiltration of the cornea and retinal vessels causes occlusive retinal vasculitis and tiny choroid infarcts. In giant cell arteritis, the infiltrating cells are giant cells and mononuclear phagocytes. In polyarteritis nodosa, they are polymorphonuclear phagocytes and lymphocytes. Other tissue-damaging mechanisms, such as occur in Type III reactions, may also be involved in polyarteritis nodosa.

## Diagnosis

Serologic tests for RF or ANA help diagnose an immune disorder and rule out infection as the cause of ocular damage. In patients suspected of having ankylosing spondylitis or Reiter's syndrome, human leukocyte antigen (HLA) analysis for identification of the lymphocytic antigen HLA-B27 is significant.

## Treatment

The goal of treatment is to reduce inflammation. The first step is local instillation of corticosteroid drops or ointment. Then, regular oral administration of salicylates appears to modify the intensity and decrease the frequency of attacks. Rarely, immunosuppressive drugs may be helpful.

---

**Common symptoms: Inflammation**

Inflammation is common to all pathophysiologic mechanisms in autoimmune disease. If inflammation can be arrested at an early stage of disease, damaged tissue can often heal and restore normal function. However, chronic inflammation tends to be self-perpetuating and progressively damaging.

Persistent inflammation causes scarring and changes in structure and function that may not be reversible. For example, in SLE, chronic nephritis may eventually cause necrosis, sclerosis, and scarring and may result in renal failure. In RA, continued synovial inflammation involving effusion, cellular infiltrates, and the forming of granulation tissue can ultimately cause destruction of cartilage, erosion of bone, and permanent loss of function.

Although autoimmune disorders may have a sudden acute onset with classic inflammatory manifestations, their onset is more frequently insidious, with recurring periods of remission and exacerbation during which subtle symptoms gradually become more defined. For instance, in early stages of SLE and RA, symptoms generally include joint pain and swelling; generalized fatigue and malaise; and perhaps a few localized signs, such as skin rash, Raynaud's phenomenon, or muscle weakness. These early symptoms may disappear without treatment, leaving the patient symptom-free for months or even years. Autoimmune rheumatic diseases may also affect the eyes. (See *Ocular effects of autoimmune rheumatic diseases.*)

## MEDICAL MANAGEMENT

Because of their overlapping symptoms, insidious onset, and unclear causes, managing autoimmune disorders is a challenge. Accurate diagnosis requires multiple and varied clinical and laboratory evaluations.

## Diagnostic tests

No single criterion confirms or rules out any autoimmune disorder, but certain laboratory tests give supportive diagnostic information. The medical diagnosis may change with changing signs and symptoms.

**General tests.** Initial blood tests can reveal various hematologic abnormalities that accompany rheumatic diseases, including anemia (with any autoimmune disorder), leukocytosis (with RA, polymyositis/dermatomyositis, and vasculitis), leukopenia (with SLE and Sjögren's syndrome), and an elevated erythrocyte sedimentation rate. The latter indicates active inflammation and occurs in all rheumatic diseases.

Urinalysis may reveal elevated red blood cell casts and proteinuria, indicating glomerulonephritis (especially in SLE).

**Serologic tests.** Characteristic serologic abnormalities—notably autoantibodies, circulating immune complexes, and reduced complement—support diagnosis of rheumatic diseases. Other telltale findings include elevated levels of gamma globulins and reduced levels of albumin.

ANAs, anti-DNA antibodies, and many other autoantibodies can be detected in patients with rheumatic diseases. For instance, RF is found in 75% of patients with RA and in 90% of patients with Sjögren's syndrome. A specific antibody to salivary duct autoantigen is found in Sjögren's syndrome, and the LE-cell phenomenon occurs in over 50% of patients with SLE.

In those disorders in which tissue damage results from activation of complement in a Type III reaction, measurement of serum complement shows below-normal levels during active disease. In RA, complement levels in serum may remain normal, but levels in joint fluid are low. Absence of C2 and other complement components may indicate an inherited deficiency that is sometimes associated with SLE.

Abnormal serologic findings become significant when several different tests show abnormalities in the same individual and the titers are significantly above or, in the case of serum complement, below normal.

**Systems tests.** After evaluating clinical signs and symptoms and serologic abnormalities, the next step is assessing affected organ systems. Diagnostic tests for inflammation and immune complex deposition may include joint fluid aspiration; synovial biopsy; skin, muscle, lymph node, or kidney biopsy; and vascular blood flow studies. Immunofluorescent examination of the skin and biopsy tissues can reveal deposits of immunoglobulin and complement components characteristic of SLE, vasculitis, and dermatomyositis. X-rays may detect characteristic erosive changes and deformities. HLA typing may help confirm a diagnosis of ankylosing spondylitis and related disorders.

## Complicated prognosis

Because several of the systemic autoimmune diseases induce potentially fatal multisystemic involvement, researchers have tried to identify predictors of outcome to guide aggressive treatment. So far, their work has produced just one reliable generalization: slowly progressive, undifferentiated disease tends to be controllable; disease that begins acutely, aggressively, and early in life tends to progress rapidly. But even this is far from absolute.

## Treatment

Treatment of autoimmune disorders is difficult because of the unpredictable patterns of remission and exacerbation, the obscurity of pathogenic mechanisms, and the wide variation in individual responses to therapy. Since no single agent or mechanism causes autoimmune disorders, and no known cure exists, treatment generally begins with efforts to reduce inflammation in affected tissues and then proceeds, as necessary, to therapy designed to control the autoimmune response (immunosuppressive therapy). Treatment is also specific to the individual, the disorder, and the organ systems involved.

**Drug therapy.** *Nonsteroidal anti-inflammatory drugs (NSAIDs),* such as aspirin, ibuprofen, and naproxen, relieve pain and stiffness, reduce swelling, and improve function but have no effect on the disease outcome. Aspirin in doses greater than 3.6 g/day is the first drug of choice for RA. Indomethacin and naproxen are more effective in treating ankylosing spondylitis.

*Corticosteroids* have limited usefulness for symptomatic relief because of their potentially severe adverse reactions, but they are used extensively to minimize systemic involvement and to control local inflammation—for instance, by injection into joints or soft tissue. In patients with SLE and polymyositis/dermatomyositis, maintenance doses of corticosteroids sometimes halt progression of the disease and maintain remission. In patients with RA, corticosteroids are not the preferred treatment because the dose required to control symptoms and the chronicity of this disease inevitably lead to serious side effects. When cortico-

## Joint replacement in rheumatoid arthritis

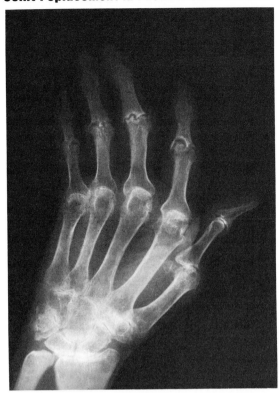

Presurgical X-ray (top) in a patient with rheumatoid arthritis shows deformed joints causing ulnar deviation of the fingers.

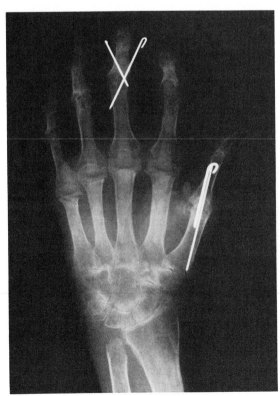

Postsurgical X-ray (bottom) shows Silastic prostheses placed in the metacarpophalangeal joints. Stainless steel Kirschner wires, removed 6 weeks after surgery, hold the new position of the proximal interphalangeal joint in the thumb and middle finger.

steroids are necessary to control acute symptoms, alternate-day dosage schedules may minimize side effects and, in children, may preserve normal growth.

*Antimalarials, gold salts,* or *D-penicillamine* may be given with the NSAID when the NSAID alone or with corticosteroids fails to control the disease. These drugs are not immunosuppressive but seem to be able to halt progression of the disease, especially in RA. Antimalarial drugs, such as hydroxychloroquine, may help in RA and SLE, especially against severe skin disease in SLE. Unfortunately, they have a slow onset of action (1 to 8 weeks) and rarely may cause a progressive retinopathy capable of inducing blindness.

Gold salts and D-penicillamine suppress joint inflammation and are used primarily for treating adult and juvenile RA. D-penicillamine may reduce the rate of new visceral involvement and prolong the survival of patients with scleroderma. However, D-penicillamine and gold salts can cause depressed white blood cell and platelet counts, proteinuria, and skin rashes.

*Immunosuppressive (cytotoxic) drugs* have been used to halt tissue destruction in autoimmune diseases with severe systemic manifestations and to reduce corticosteroid requirements in patients with severe side effects from prolonged use. The most widely used drugs include azathioprine, cyclophosphamide, and methotrexate in dosages much lower than those used to treat cancer. These drugs are commonly administered by either intermittent high-dose I.V. infusion or oral administration, or chronic low oral doses.

Corticosteroids may also be used to control severe autoimmune manifestations since they have immunosuppressive as well as anti-inflammatory effects. However, because of their potentially severe side effects, these drugs require close medical supervision.

**Management of systemic manifestations.** Anti-inflammatory and immunosuppressive drugs can control or halt the inflammatory reaction and autoimmune response of autoimmune disease. Such therapy should also be used with specific treatment of involved organ systems. So, a patient with lupus nephritis may be treated with diuretics, antihypertensives, and other drugs for renal failure. A patient with cardiomyopathy may need digoxin or other cardiac regulatory drugs. A patient with CNS disease may need anticonvulsants.

Joint damage may need surgery. (See *Joint replacement in rheumatoid arthritis.*)

## NURSING MANAGEMENT

The patient with a known or suspected autoimmune disorder requires a nursing approach that acknowledges the broad range of potential signs and symptoms; the variability in clinical presentation; and the impact on the patient and his family of continued uncertainty about diagnosis, prognosis, and the effect of treatment. (See *Rheumatic diseases at a glance*, pages 108 and 109.)

### Nursing history: Look for patterns

Your nursing evaluation should include recent health changes, a systems review for telltale signs and symptoms of autoimmunity, and a family history of related disorders. You should also assess the educational needs of the patient and family and the available resources for coping with chronic illness.

**Present and past illness.** Begin by eliciting biographic information and then the chief complaint. Determine the history of the present illness, including the onset and duration of symptoms and their effect on the patient's normal pattern of activity.

Also ask about recurrent infections, multisystemic diseases, surgery that may have affected the patient's immune response (such as transplantation or thymectomy), and medication (such as hydralazine or procainamide, which may cause drug-induced SLE).

**Family history.** Because of the familial tendency of many rheumatic disorders, ask whether relatives have had any related illnesses. Use the words "arthritis" and "rheumatism," common labels for these disorders.

**Systems review.** Assess the joints, skin, mucous membranes, and muscles, as well as organ systems for a history of multiorgan involvement.

*Joints.* If the patient complains of joint pain, the most common presenting symptom, ask which joints are involved and whether he has any pain (arthralgia) or pain with redness and swelling (true arthritis). Ask if he experiences joint pain or stiffness only in the morning (common in RA) or if exercise, temperature change, or stress provokes it. Find out what relieves it. This information will be valuable, since the number of involved joints and the pattern of onset and resolution are characteristic of different disorders.

When looking for a history of joint involvement, ask if the patient has had any joint or tendon surgery or has any prosthetic joints.

*Skin.* Since so many rheumatic diseases affect the skin, ask for a history of any skin changes, including rashes (especially after sun exposure), ulcers, and changes in texture or character. Also define the type of skin rash, its distribution and duration, and whether it's associated with pain or itching.

*Mucous membranes.* Check for changes in mucous membranes, which often accompany autoimmune disease (especially Sjögren's syndrome). Such changes commonly cause patients to complain of sensations of burning or grittiness in the eyes; "matter" in the eyes on awakening; dryness of the mouth, which may make it difficult to chew or swallow dry food; and the need for frequent drinks of water. Women may complain of vaginal dryness and dyspareunia (discomfort during intercourse).

*Muscles.* Ask the patient if he has difficulty rising from a chair or lifting his arms to comb his hair. These symptoms may stem from muscle inflammation (myositis), a hallmark of polymyositis/dermatomyositis that is usually associated with a history of muscle pain and weakness. These symptoms may also result from muscle wasting associated with chronic arthritis.

*Organ systems.* Find out if your patient has a history of problems with the cardiovascular, respiratory, renal, digestive, and nervous systems, which may involve systemic autoimmune disorders. Common manifestations include chest pain, cardiac dysrhythmias, malignant hypertension, dyspnea, gastroesophageal reflux, menstrual irregularities, and seizures or other neurologic changes.

**Activities of daily living.** Also assess overall functional status, including ability to perform activities of daily living. The patient with a known disability or deformity may require a detailed assessment of his activities of daily living performed by an occupational therapist.

**Resources for coping.** Because autoimmune disorders require lifelong adaptation and coping, a patient's resources often determine his ability to adapt himself to his illness and the many changes it requires. Therefore, you need to assess for personal and financial resources, the availability of supportive family members to help during periods of flare-up, and the patient's home and occupational environments. Your assessment should also address the patient's past behavior during illness, history of compliance with prescribed treatment, level of insight, educational needs, and awareness of community and professional resources.

*(continued on page 110)*

## Rheumatic diseases at a glance

| Disorder | Incidence | Major immunologic features | Pathologic mechanisms |
|---|---|---|---|
| **Rheumatoid arthritis** | Chronic, recurrent systemic inflammatory disease primarily involving the joints; affects three times as many women as men; affects 1 to 3 persons per 100 | • 7S and 19S IgM and 7S IgG rheumatoid factors (RFs) in serum and synovial fluid<br>• Decreased complement and elevated $\beta_2$-microglobulin levels in synovial fluid<br>• ANAs (speckled pattern) | • Type IV (cell-mediated)<br>• Type III (immune complex) |
| **Systemic lupus erythematosus** | Chronic systemic inflammatory disease that follows a course of alternating exacerbations and remissions with multiple organ involvement; affects mainly women—1 per 700 between ages 15 and 64; affects three times as many black women as white | • Positive LE-cell phenomenon<br>• High-titer antinuclear antibodies (ANAs); (homogeneous or outline pattern on immunofluorescence)<br>• Anti–single-stranded and anti–double-stranded DNA antibodies<br>• Depressed serum complement levels<br>• Deposition of immunoglobulin and complement along glomerular basement membrane and at the dermal-epidermal junction<br>• Numerous other autoantibodies | • Primarily Type III (immune complex)<br>• Also Type II (cytotoxic) |
| **Progressive systemic sclerosis (scleroderma)** | Generalized disorder of connective tissue characterized by fibrosis and degenerative changes in the skin (scleroderma), synovium, digital arteries, and parenchyma and small arteries of internal organs; affects twice as many women as men; rarely affects children; affects 4 to 12.5 persons per million, with no racial preference | • ANAs (speckled or nucleolar pattern on immunofluorescence)<br>• Antibodies against the ribonuclease-sensitive component of extractable nuclear antigen (ENA) in patients with mixed connective tissue disease<br>• RF | Unknown; possibly Type III (immune complex) |
| **Polymyositis/ dermatomyositis** | Acute or chronic inflammatory disorder of the skin and muscles, which causes symmetrical weakness; may occur at any age; affects twice as many women as men; affects 1 person in 200,000, with no racial preference; may be associated with malignancy | • Focal deposition of complement, IgG, and IgM in vessel walls of involved tissue<br>• ANAs (speckled or nucleolar pattern on immunofluorescence) | • Unclear; possibly Type IV (cell-mediated) |
| **Sjögren's syndrome** | Chronic inflammatory disorder usually characterized by diminished lacrimal and salivary gland secretions resulting in keratoconjunctivitis sicca and xerostomia; affects mainly women; rarely affects children; occurs in all races; may be associated with rheumatoid arthritis | • Lymphocyte and plasma cell infiltration of involved tissues<br>• Hypergammaglobulinemia, RF, and ANA, including a specific anti-ENA<br>• Autoantibodies against salivary duct antigens | • Type IV (cell-mediated)<br>• Some components of Type III (immune complex) |
| **Vasculitis** | Diverse group of syndromes—polyarteritis nodosa, allergic granulomatosis, angiitis, systemic necrotizing vasculitis—all of which cause a necrotizing inflammation of the blood vessels | • Circulating immune complexes deposited in blood vessels<br>• Possible evidence of hepatitis-B surface antigen (HBsAg) in plasma and in deposits in the arteritic legions | Unclear; possibly all types of mechanisms, but Type III (immune complex) most likely |
| **Spondyloarthropathy** | Diverse group of usually chronic disorders—ankylosing spondylitis, Reiter's syndrome, psoriatic arthritis—all of which involve a particular pattern of joint inflammation and characteristic systemic manifestations; ankylosing spondylitis and Reiter's syndrome more common in males; psoriatic arthritis more common in females | • Associated with HLA-B27 and absence of RF in the serum | • Unclear; possibly strong genetic influence |

| Types of tissue damage | Clinical manifestations |
| --- | --- |
| • Pannus formation (synovial inflammation and proliferation leading to cartilage and bone destruction)<br>• Extraarticular inflammation in virtually any organ | • Symmetric, chronic polyarthritis with erosions and deformity<br>• Extraarticular manifestations, including vasculitis, atrophy of the skin and muscle, subcutaneous nodules, lymphadenopathy, splenomegaly, and leukopenia<br>• Organ involvement of lung and heart rarely symptomatic |
| • Widespread inflammation caused by immune complex deposition in the kidney, skin, joints, pleura, peritoneum, and brain<br>• Vasculitis marked by cellular infiltration of small arteries with possible necrosis and fibrinoid deposits in the arterial wall | • Chronic fatigue and fever<br>• Arthritis, skin rashes, alopecia, serositis, anemia, leukopenia, and nephritis<br>• Raynaud's phenomenon<br>• Disturbances in mentation and aberrant behavior, such as psychosis or depression |
| • Fibrosis and degeneration in the parenchyma and small arteries of the skin, heart, lungs, kidney, and digestive tract<br>• Thickening and sclerosis of the skin, with resultant restrictions in movement and possible deformity | • Raynaud's phenomenon<br>• Polyarthralgia and polyarthritis<br>• Skin abnormalities (pigmentation changes, telangiectasia, subcutaneous calcifications)<br>• CREST syndrome (calcinosis, Raynaud's phenomenon, esophageal dysfunction, sclerodactyly, and telangiectasia) |
| • Muscle inflammation and destruction<br>• Interstitial fibrosis<br>• Lymphocytic and plasma cell infiltration of involved muscle | • Muscle pain and weakness (usually lower extremities first, then atrophy of the muscles of the limb girdles, neck, and pharynx)<br>• Skin rash<br>• Raynaud's phenomenon<br>• Polyarthralgia and polyarthritis<br>• Myocarditis and conduction abnormalities<br>• Dysphagia<br>• Malignant neoplasms (more common than in the general population), most often in the prostate, ovary, breast, uterus, or large intestine |
| • Infiltration and destruction of salivary, lacrimal, and other exocrine glands<br>• Very rarely, vasculitis | • Dry eyes, dry mouth, dry respiratory and reproductive passages<br>• Parotid swelling |
| • Inflammation and damage to large and small blood vessels, with resulting damage to end organs | • Dependent on size of blood vessels and organs involved |
| • Progressive joint fibrosis<br>• Occasional synovitis<br>• Inflammation of skin and mucous membranes<br>• Inflammation at the site of ligamentous insertion into the bone | • Progressive ankylosis of axial skeleton<br>• Possible peripheral arthritis<br>• Possible psoriasis, urethritis, uveitis |

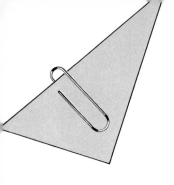

# Rheumatoid arthritis: How to protect your joints

*Dear* _____

Because you have rheumatoid arthritis, you need to conserve your energy and protect your joints from injury. Follow these guidelines.

**Carefully pace your daily activities.** Try to alternate periods of activity with brief rest periods. Be seated for any activity that tires you.

**Simplify your activities.** If you're having a flare-up, simplify your schedule for a while; learn to ask for help.

Use dressing aids, including a long-handled shoehorn, reacher, elastic shoelaces, zipper pull, and buttonhook. And,

when you can, sit down to get dressed. If you have trouble putting your fingers into gloves, wear mittens. Also, be sure to use helpful household items, such as a hand shower nozzle, hand rails, grab bars, and easy-to-open drawers. Keep needed materials, utensils, and tools organized and handy.

**Use good body mechanics.** Use the largest joint available for a given task. Support weak or painful joints as much as possible. Use positions of extension; avoid positions of flexion. Bend your knuckles as briefly as possible to hold objects. Avoid

bending, stooping, or holding the same position for a long time.

Always use your hands near the center of the body. Use your entire body to move heavy objects. Whenever possible, slide objects instead of lifting them. If you must lift something, use both hands with palms turned upward.

**Get adequate sleep.** Use correct sleep posture. Sleep on your back on a firm mattress, using a small pillow. Avoid placing a pillow under your knees, which would encourage flexion deformity.

## Physical examination: Check all systems

Before conducting a systems assessment, observe the patient's overall appearance for general signs of autoimmune disease. In an acute flare-up, the patient is often febrile and prostrated with fatigue. In chronic illness, he may show contracture, deformities, scarring, or signs of Cushing's syndrome from long-term corticosteroid therapy.

**Musculoskeletal system.** A musculoskeletal examination can help determine the extent of old and active joint disease. Gently palpate each joint for pain, swelling, and tenderness—all indicators of current inflammation. Also determine limitations in range of motion, the extent of deformity, and any sensory changes. In many joints, limited extension is an early indication of synovitis in such diseases as RA or SLE.

Muscle atrophy and weakness frequently develop around painful, unused joints. To assess muscle strength, have the patient raise his arms above his head, bend forward and backward, sit and rise from a chair while you observe his ease of movement and gait, and grip two of your fingers.

**Skin and mucous membranes.** Look for skin rashes (SLE and dermatomyositis); symmetrical pitting edema; skin hardening and skin fold loss (scleroderma); rheumatic nodules (RA); digital ulcers, numbness, and color

changes in the fingers in response to cold (Raynaud's phenomenon with SLE, scleroderma, or polymyositis/dermatomyositis); and splinter hemorrhages around the nails (vasculitis).

Also look for bruises, which may result from thrombocytopenia or as a side effect of corticosteroid therapy; and telangiectasias, purpural lesions, and nodules on the extensor surface of the forearm, which may accompany RA. Inspect the inside of the mouth and nose for the mucosal ulcerations of SLE.

**Other organ systems.** After examining the skin and musculoskeletal system, also perform a thorough assessment of cardiovascular, respiratory, renal, and neurologic status. Look for signs of cardiac dysrhythmias and conduction abnormalities; chest pain and pericardial rub characteristic of pericarditis (common with SLE); malignant hypertension (from renal involvement in SLE); mild to severe dyspnea; and seizure disorders, memory loss, and cranial nerve abnormalities (from neuromuscular involvement in SLE).

## Nursing diagnoses: Remain flexible

After you've completed a nursing history and physical assessment, formulate your nursing diagnoses. Your care plan must be flexible because of the unpredictable course of most autoimmune disorders and the systemic problems that may arise. It probably will include these typical nursing diagnoses.

**Activity intolerance related to joint immobility and pain.** To help the patient attain the highest level of mobility within the limitations of his illness, first assess his current ability to perform activities of daily living. This will provide a baseline for activity tolerance. In your assessment, determine factors that increase or decrease tolerance.

Then, medicate for pain before a planned activity. Allow for sufficient rest periods before and between activities. (See *Rheumatoid arthritis: How to protect your joints.*) Remember that the patient with a rheumatic disease often requires 8 to 10 hours of sleep at night and a 1- to 2-hour rest period during the day. Increase activity gradually, and assess the patient's physiologic response to each increase, using baseline information for comparison. Have him perform daily passive and active range-of-motion exercises, which prevent deformity and muscle atrophy and increase circulation, joint mobility, and activity tolerance.

To foster self-esteem and prevent exhaustion, provide assistance and care, as needed, while promoting independence. Refer the patient to a physical therapist, as indicated, to obtain maximum activity tolerance. Provide positive reinforcement and explore possible motivations to encourage activity—for instance, a desire to return to work or social activities.

Consider your interventions successful when the patient has reached his goal for full functioning.

**Alteration in comfort related to bone, joint, and muscle involvement.** To help control pain, first assess its level by asking the patient what activities are impossible because of pain. You may also use one of the common pain scales. Support the patient throughout his pain. Explore different methods of pain relief to help him find the one that provides maximum comfort. Identify factors that aggravate or alleviate pain, and help the patient use this information. Determine the family's perception and understanding of the patient's pain and its treatment.

Consider your interventions successful if the patient reports a decrease in his pain level and satisfaction in his ability to function.

**Knowledge deficit related to home management during an acute flare-up.** To help the patient manage effectively at home during an acute flare-up, emphasize to him that remis-sions and flare-ups are expected in autoimmune disease. Help him design a flexible plan for unexpected bad days, especially regarding work and family obligations. Make sure he allows himself to rest when he is feeling the fatigue and pain of active disease. Enlist the help of the patient's family in these difficult periods.

Tell the patient that care for acute arthritis involves rest of the affected joint in a functional position, often facilitated by immobilization with a splint. Let him know that comfort measures, such as applications of heat and cold, anti-inflammatory therapy, and the judicious use of analgesics, give additional relief. Tell him to begin passive range-of-motion exercises as the inflammation subsides.

Consider your interventions successful if the patient effectively manages his home care.

**Inadequate nutrition related to pain, nausea, or fatigue.** To ensure adequate oral nutrition, assess the patient's nutritional status to determine the severity of the present nutritional deficiency and to give a baseline for future monitoring. Assess his ability to eat, and identify factors such as pain or change in taste that may affect it. To encourage eating, provide a pleasant environment, medicate for pain before meals, schedule uncomfortable and unpleasant activities so that they don't interfere with meals, give oral hygiene before and after meals, and encourage the supportive family to be with the patient at meals.

Encourage a high-protein, high-calorie diet to prevent further weight loss. Schedule the patient for a consultation with the dietitian to incorporate the patient's preferences into the prescribed diet.

Consider your interventions successful if the patient maintains an adequate nutritional oral intake, as measured by caloric count, and maintains a stable body weight.

## Total patient involvement

Your nursing role in autoimmune disorders includes all management phases. Your understanding during the usually long and difficult diagnostic procedure can ease patient and family frustration. Your extensive role in patient and family education assures that the patient and family have the knowledge and skills to manage these chronic illnesses. Your central position during supportive therapy makes you the coordinator among patient, doctor, and other health-care team members. Throughout, your sensitivity can help the patient's adjustment to a permanent disability.

**Points to remember**

- Possible contributing factors to autoimmune disorders include genetic, viral, hormonal, and environmental factors.
- Many autoimmune disorders have overlapping characteristics, many produce similar autoantibodies, and more than one autoimmune disorder may affect one person.
- The basis of tissue damage in autoimmune disorders appears to be an alteration in, or loss of, the immunoregulatory control that normally sustains self-tolerance.
- Loss of self-tolerance stimulates B-cell differentiation and a proliferation of autoantibodies, the immunoglobulins formed against self.
- Tissue damage results from one or more types of hypersensitivity reaction; the immune components and processes involved may differ, but the common result is inflammation.
- Diagnosis of systemic autoimmune disorders is difficult. No single criterion establishes or rules out a given diagnosis or disease, and the medical diagnosis may change as additional manifestations occur.
- These disorders are difficult to treat. Treatment includes anti-inflammatory, corticosteroidal, and immunosuppressive drugs; and surgical replacement of deformed joints.
- You provide the coordinating link between the medical management of the specific disorder and the health-care team members interacting with the patient to provide comprehensive care.

# 8 UNDERSTANDING TUMOR IMMUNOLOGY

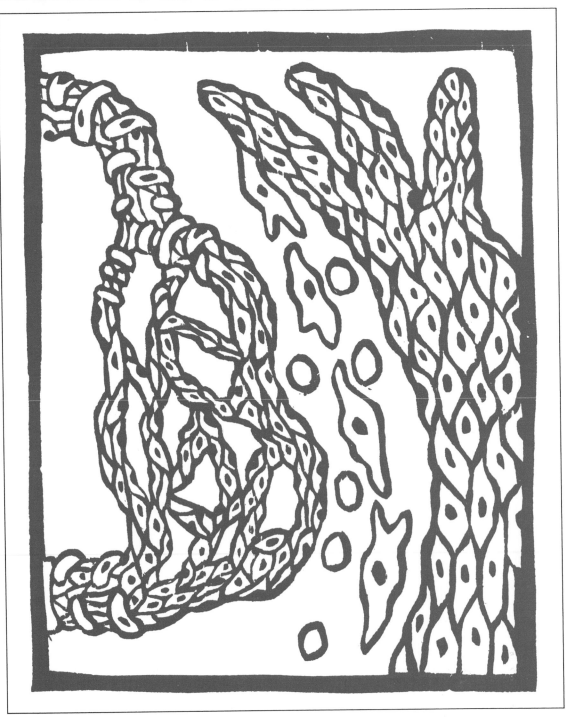

Lymph and circulatory system with malignant cells

The body's immune system has been called the first line of defense against cancer. Unless and until its defenses are breached, immune surveillance apprehends and annihilates malignant or premalignant cells before they can proliferate.

But if something (such as congenital immunodeficiency) interferes with this immune surveillance mechanism, cancer *can* develop— and often does. Researchers believe that when certain external and host influences—such as viruses, industrial chemicals, aging, and abnormal genetic factors—coexist, they can disturb the immune system, creating a cellular environment that allows tumor growth. Once that environment has allowed growth of poorly differentiated, rapidly dividing tumor cells, invasion of adjacent normal tissue and metastasis to distant sites can occur.

This concept of immune surveillance is still unproven, but the role of the immune system in protecting the body from disease isn't. So the more you know about tumor immunology and the treatment and management of immunoproliferative diseases, the better you'll be able to care for patients with cancer.

## Cancer-promoting factors
Various factors believed to affect immune system function may predispose to cancer.

**Genetic influences.** Patients with mild forms of inherited or acquired immunodeficiencies have a high incidence of leukemia, lymphoma, and other malignancies originating in the lymphoid tissue and elsewhere. Genetic susceptibility is related to the human leukocyte antigen (HLA) system.

**Age.** A young child's immature immune system, thin skin, and inadequate inflammatory responses promote susceptibility to cancer (Wilms' tumor, neuroblastoma); an elderly person's diminished immune function, when combined with disturbances in metabolism and the cardiovascular and other systems, has a similar effect.

**Metabolic changes.** Hyperthyroid patients may be cancer-prone.

**Structural and physiologic changes.** These changes interfere with the body's natural defense mechanisms, increasing the risk of cancer. For example, extensive burns can predispose to skin cancer. Chronic irritation and infection also increase the risk of cancer. For example, chronic venous stasis ulcers in the legs may lead to squamous cell carcinoma.

**Viruses.** Herpesvirus Type 2 is linked to cervical cancer; Epstein-Barr virus is linked to lymphoma, Hodgkin's disease, and nasopharyngeal cancer. HTLV I and II, clearly identified as oncogenic viruses in man, cause T-cell lymphomas and leukemias. Investigators suggest that viruses are the ultimate cause of all forms of cancer and that radiation, carcinogens, and other agents simply activate latent viruses.

**Chemicals.** Vinyl chloride, benzene, zinc, copper, arsenic, and other air pollutants increase cancer risk. So, of course, does cigarette smoking, which releases carcinogenic chemicals into the body.

**Environmental factors.** Inadequate, unsanitary living conditions, leading to poor health practices, are associated with high exposure to pathogens. And certain geographic areas are associated with higher cancer rates (Burkitt's lymphoma, Africa; tall lymphoma, southern Japan). Higher rates are also linked to poor nutrition in infancy, which can cause incomplete immune system development.

**Stress.** Physical or psychological stress stimulates production of endocrine hormones, especially adrenal glucocorticoids and adrenocorticotropic hormone. These may suppress the immune system. Stress can also interfere with such cancer-resisting factors as production and maturation of B and T lymphocytes, immunoglobulin synthesis, macrophage transformation, and interferon production.

**Drugs.** Drugs linked to higher cancer rates include hydantoin anticonvulsants such as phenytoin (lymphoma); androgens and oral contraceptives (breast cancer); estrogens (endometrial cancer in premenopausal women); and diethylstilbestrol (clear-cell carcinoma of the genital tract in children whose mothers took the drug while pregnant). Long-term use of immunosuppressive drugs, such as cyclophosphamide (Cytoxan), nitrosoureas such as carmustine (BCNU), and azathioprine (Imuran), are also linked to cancer.

**Radiation.** Therapeutic radiation for a primary tumor sometimes causes a *second* primary tumor. Irradiation of a fetus increases the risk of leukemia; neck irradiation in a child can result in a benign or malignant thyroid tumor 10 to 30 years later.

## PATHOPHYSIOLOGY
Many researchers believe malignant cells develop constantly within the body. These malignant cells produce antigens drawn from the destruction of normal tissue.

*(continued on page 116)*

## Cellular oncogenes
Cancer genes, called oncogenes, which are altered versions of normal genes, have been found in the chromosomes of tumor cells. About 20 different oncogenes have been identified so far. Researchers hope to develop screening tests for oncogenes in people at risk for cancer.

### Proto-oncogenes
In normal cells, oncogenes exist in a repressed state, when they're known as proto-oncogenes. They may be activated by many factors, including genetic accidents, such as abnormal gene transpositions in chromosomes; chemical carcinogens; radiation; or certain viruses. When activated, oncogenes interfere with normal gene expression, causing the host cell to become malignant.

### Myc
One such oncogene has been implicated in Burkitt's lymphoma, a childhood cancer affecting B lymphocytes. A proto-oncogene labeled *myc* exists on a B lymphocyte's chromosome 8. This chromosome sometimes cleaves at the *myc* oncogene and attaches to chromosome 14, next to an immunoglobulin gene (*imm*), which in B lymphocytes is very active. This abnormal gene combination is thought to activate *myc*, stimulating the lymphocyte to abnormal proliferation, eventually resulting in a malignant mass in the patient's jaw or abdomen.

### Other chromosome defects
Chromosome defects such as translocations (as in Burkitt's lymphoma), deletions, or extra genes are common in tumor cells. These defects may or may not occur close enough to a proto-oncogene to activate it and cause disease. Researchers don't know whether such chromosome defects are random or hereditary.

# How oncogenic viruses attack host cells

## Oncogenic DNA virus activity in the host cell

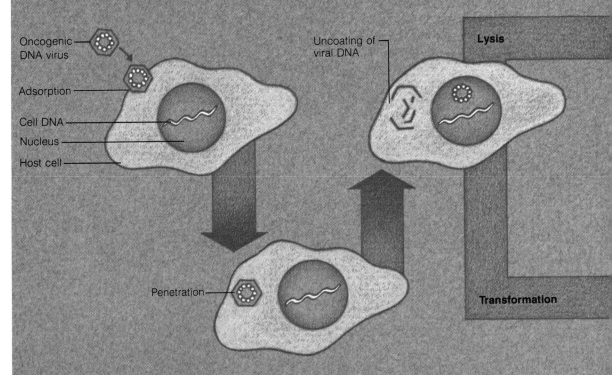

## Oncogenic RNA virus activity in the host cell

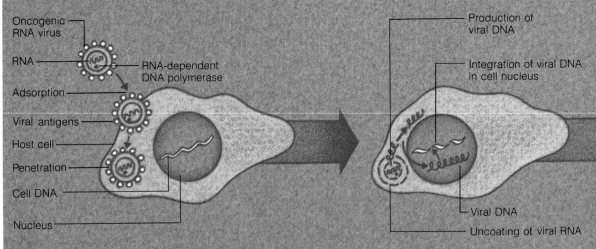

uring infection, DNA- and RNA-based viral proto-oncogenes (repressed cancer genes) are incorporated into the genetic material of an invading virus, where they remain repressed until the virus takes over the biosynthetic function in another host cell. Upon release into the host cell, these activated viral oncogenes induce malignancy.

**Oncogenic DNA.** When an oncogenic DNA virus approaches a host cell, it's adsorbed by, then penetrates, the cell's membrane. Upon reaching the cell's nuclear membrane, the virus loses its protein coating. In host cells permissive for infection, replication and transcription of viral DNA cause formation of viral mRNA. Translation of mRNA then forms viral capsid and other proteins. Finally, the

virus assembles in the host cell's nucleus, causing it to lyse and release new virions.

In nonpermissive host cells, viral DNA is integrated into host DNA. But new viral DNA, capsid proteins, and new virions aren't produced, and the host cell doesn't lyse. However, viral DNA integrated in the host genome transforms the cell and is replicated upon subsequent host-cell division. The new ge-

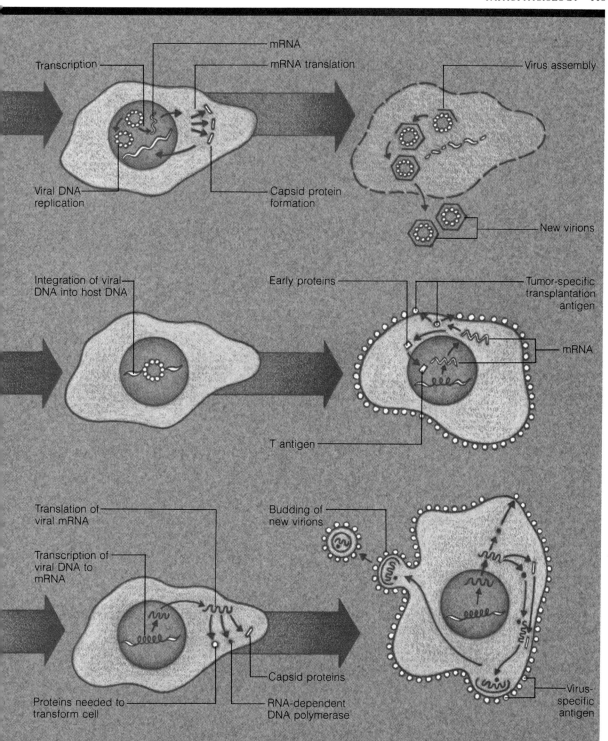

Transcription

mRNA

mRNA translation

Virus assembly

Viral DNA replication

Capsid protein formation

New virions

Integration of viral DNA into host DNA

Early proteins

Tumor-specific transplantation antigen

mRNA

T antigen

Translation of viral mRNA

Budding of new virions

Transcription of viral DNA to mRNA

Capsid proteins

Proteins needed to transform cell

RNA-dependent DNA polymerase

Virus-specific antigen

nome then alters the properties of the host cell, changing it to a cancer cell.

In transformed cells, a virus-specific tumor antigen—T antigen—which is thought to stimulate DNA synthesis, is produced. A tumor-specific transplantation antigen is also produced on the cell surface and may be responsible for immunospecific rejection of a transplanted tumor in a host animal.

**Oncogenic RNA.** Oncogenic RNA viruses cause cancer by simultaneously transforming host cells and by replication. These oncogenic viruses contain an RNA-directed DNA polymerase (reverse transcriptase), which allows formation of a DNA copy of the viral genome. After adsorbing to and penetrating the host cell, the RNA virus produces its own DNA, which becomes integrated into the host

cell's DNA. Transcription of DNA to mRNA occurs next. This is followed by translation of mRNA to capsid protein, RNA-dependent DNA polymerase, virus-specific antigens, and other proteins. Thus, virus-specific antigens produced on the host-cell wall actually transform the cell. New oncogenic RNA virions assembled within the transformed host cell are continually shed through budding.

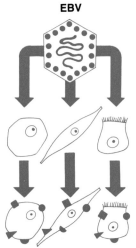
## Tumor-associated antigens

Typically glycoproteins or glycolipids, tumor-associated antigens differ only slightly from the components in normal cells. Those on tumor-cell surfaces are particularly crucial for immunologic recognition and diagnosis and for immunotherapy. Generally, the larger the tumor, the more antigens it produces. A tumor may shed antigens as well as secrete them; shedding may affect antibodies and lymphocytes far from the primary tumor.

**Virally induced antigens.** Such antigens, which manifest themselves identically on all cells they affect, appear on the membranes of infected tumor cells when any viral infection alters deoxyribonucleic acid (DNA).

**Oncofetal antigens.** These antigens are normally produced in large amounts in the fetus and neonate; excessive amounts in maternal blood after delivery may indicate a tumor. Two common oncofetal antigens are carcinoembryonic antigen (CEA) and alpha-fetoprotein (AFP). (See *Oncofetal antigen development.*)

**Antigens present on other tissues.** These are found on tumors and in cells from normal tissues. Cells from acute myeloblastic leukemia (a form of acute nonlymphocytic leukemia), for example, may carry antigens present on normal B cells or monocytes.

**Tissue-specific antigens.** These are present not only in tumor cells but also in all tissues from which the tumor originated. An example is antigens present on sarcomas.

**Tumor-specific antigens.** Specific antigens have been identified in multiple myeloma.

Antigens should normally activate the ongoing immune response. Tumors develop with failure of the immune response.

## Why immune response fails

Researchers have several theories to explain why antigens may fail to evoke a normal immune response.

**Familiar-appearing antigens.** Some tumors look *familiar* to the immune system; that is, they contain no recognizably foreign antigens. This is rare, however—most tumors elicit at least weak immunogenicity when tested.

**Weak antigens.** Some antigens are too weak to elicit a strong immune response. Weakly immunogenic tumors produce cancer cells faster than the body can kill them.

**Antigen-antibody complexes.** Tumors sometimes shed extra antigens, and these antigen-antibody complexes can "blindfold" lymphocytes so they don't recognize the tumor.

These complexes also suppress lymphocyte toxicity to tumor cells by absorbing into lymphocytes' surfaces. This phenomenon—known as enhancement—is associated with large, progressive tumors; disappears when the tumors are removed; and recurs when the tumors recur. (See *Enhancement and blocking antibodies,* page 118.)

**Unstable adhesions.** Because tumor cells don't form stable intercellular adhesions, the necessary interaction between them and lymphoid cells might *also* be abnormal, thereby preventing destruction of the tumor.

**Suppressor T lymphocytes.** By interfering with tumor-specific antibody production, suppressor T lymphocytes can short-circuit the immune response.

**Oncogenic viruses and carcinogenic chemicals.** Such agents can inhibit the immune response, at least temporarily. Thus, exposure to a virus in utero or during infancy from mother's milk can contribute to cancer years later when an external stressor releases the latent virus, which the body never recognized as foreign.

## MEDICAL MANAGEMENT

Diagnosis and treatment of tumors related to the immune system must begin with a complete history and physical examination. Also, several tests help evaluate immune function and definitively diagnose a tumor.

### Tests confirm diagnosis

One key test measures the number of B and T lymphocytes in the blood; another key test is immunoelectrophoresis. (These tests are described in Chapter 3.) Other important tests include tissue biopsies and skin tests.

**Lymph node biopsy.** Before starting definitive cancer treatment, diagnosis must be confirmed through tissue biopsy of an enlarged, accessible lymph node. Needle biopsy doesn't yield enough material for an accurate diagnosis and shouldn't be used. Frozen-section material shouldn't be used either because slightly crushed lymphoid tissue can be mistaken for other types of malignancies.

**Bone marrow aspiration and biopsy.** This test reveals the number and type of abnormal cells. Special staining techniques, chromosomal analysis, and cytochemical studies all contribute to a more exact diagnosis.

**Skin tests.** These include tuberculosis and dinitrochlorobenzene (DNCB) skin tests to determine the host's ability to mount a cell-mediated immune response. In many lymphomas, these tests reveal cutaneous anergy.

Once tumor diagnosis has been established, special blood tests, skeletal surveys, and computerized tomography scans evaluate how far the disease has progressed.

**Tumor markers.** These are tumor-associated antigens whose presence in body fluids, particularly blood, helps to pinpoint the primary tumor site, to evaluate and monitor a patient's response to cancer therapy, and to identify recurrence of a tumor. The level of tumor markers in any body fluid reflects the rates at which cancer cells are growing, dying, and creating and secreting markers; the rate at which the host destroys and excretes markers; and the specific interactions between cancer cells and normal tissue.

*The glycoprotein CEA* occurs normally in minute amounts in serum. However, a tumor in the large intestine secretes large amounts of CEA. Higher-than-normal serum levels of CEA are also associated with tumors of the pancreas, stomach, lung, breast, prostate, endometrium, cervix, and ovary and with cigarette smoking, alcoholic cirrhosis, pancreatitis, and inflammatory disorders.

*The glycoprotein AFP* is a normally synthesized major plasma protein of the early human fetus. Synthesis occurs mainly in the liver and also in the GI tract and yolk sac. Malignant liver cells secrete large quantities of AFP. High serum levels occur in fetuses with neural tube defects and in adults with hepatoma; in germ cell tumors of the testes and ovaries; in endometrial sinus tumors of the ovaries; and occasionally in cancer of the pancreas, stomach, colon, or lung.

## Major cancer treatments

The major cancer treatments—surgery, radiation, chemotherapy, and immunotherapy— may be used alone or in combination.

**Surgery.** Surgery may be the treatment of choice, depending on the stage of the disease, the growth rate and anatomic boundaries of the tumor, the patient's health and treatment preference, and the degree to which surgery may be mutilating. Surgical excision of a solid tumor with a wide margin can remove most of the tumor, reducing the number of malignant cells and thereby facilitating the effectiveness of chemotherapy, radiation therapy, and the immune system.

Surgery is usually the most efficient treatment for oncologic emergencies in immunosuppressed patients. For example, acute bleeding from pulmonary hemorrhage, esoph-

### Oncofetal antigen development

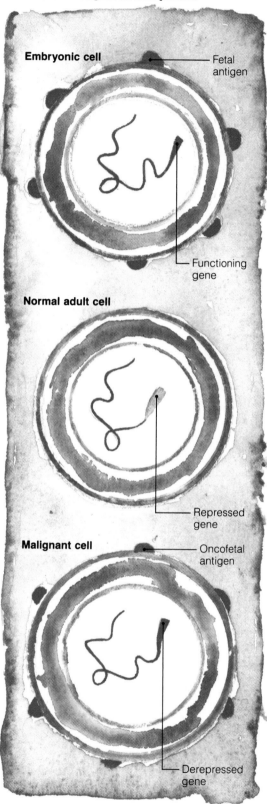

The cell surfaces or serum secretions of many tumors display oncofetal antigens that are thought to result from gene derepression. Normally, functioning genes in the embryonic cell produce fetal antigens, which are repressed in the adult's genes. In malignancy, however, derepression of new genes causes reappearance of fetal antigens—oncofetal antigens.

## Enhancement and blocking antibodies

Enhancement—progressive growth of tumors in tumor-specific serum—may occur when blocking antibodies shield tumors from the activity of T lymphocytes. B lymphocytes transfer blocking antibodies to tumor cells. As a result, T lymphocytes fail to recognize and respond to these foreign cells.

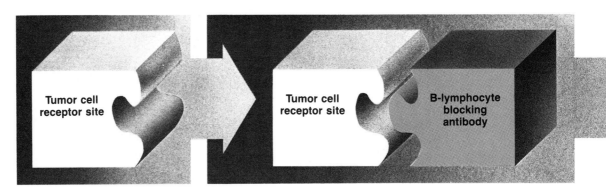

ageal varices, or gastritis may require surgery to ligate a vessel or to remove part of an organ. Another such emergency is perforation of the GI tract resulting from tumor extension or destruction after systemic therapy; surgery typically includes resection, drainage, and direct or delayed anastomosis. Intracranial bleeding or pericardial effusion also necessitates emergency repair; abscesses require drainage to supplement antibiotic therapy.

Surgery may also establish access for other cancer treatments. Surgery is needed for placement of indwelling ports, pumps, permanent catheters, and applicators for internal radiation implants.

Surgery (excision of hormone-producing organs) is also indicated for patients with hormone-dependent tumors. This approach is used most often to combat estrogen-dependent breast cancer: an oophorectomy, adrenalectomy, or hypophysectomy may be done to suppress the breast tumor's growth.

Finally, surgery to interrupt neural transmission of pain impulses is indicated for relief of otherwise intractable pain. The approach selected depends on the patient's prognosis and the location of his pain: unilateral, caudal pain is the easiest to relieve surgically.

**Radiation.** This treatment is used for cure, palliation, and as adjuvant therapy. The effectiveness of radiation therapy in killing tumor cells or inhibiting their reproduction depends on their radioresponsiveness—the tendency to degenerate after radiation. Radioresponsiveness is determined by the cells' mitotic potential, the extracellular environment, the radiation dosage, and the tissue where the tumor originated.

Unfortunately, radiation therapy attacks malignant *and* normal cells—especially rapidly dividing blood cells and platelets, skin cells, and the GI tract mucosa. Consequently, radiation commonly induces bone marrow suppression, causing immunosuppression, skin changes, and mucositis, depending on the

area irradiated.

**Chemotherapy.** Chemotherapy destroys cancer cells or checks their growth while minimizing adverse effects on normal cell function. It interferes with cell reproduction or starves cells by mimicking normal nutrients.

To slow tumor growth, hormones and antihormones are sometimes administered. Corticosteroids such as prednisone have been used for leukemia, lymphoma, and multiple myeloma. Tamoxifen (Nolvadex), an antiestrogen, is used to treat breast cancer because it keeps estrogen from nourishing tumor cells.

Chemotherapy can produce a cure in patients with Hodgkin's disease, choriocarcinoma, testicular cancer, or childhood leukemia; and remission in patients with breast cancer, small-cell carcinoma of the lung, and adult leukemia. It can shrink the tumor and, after surgery or radiation, eradicate microscopic residual disease. Chemotherapy can also be palliative in patients with pain from bone metastasis or from pressure on lymphatic or vascular systems or nerves.

Because chemotherapy can produce some adverse effects, it requires careful consideration of its benefits against risks. Effectiveness relies on the receptiveness of cell type to drugs used, the drug's capacity to reach the tumor (depending on the blood supply to the tumor or whether the drug can cross the blood-brain barrier), the extent of the disease, the patient's nutritional and hydrational status, and his compliance with the regimen. Good bone marrow function is also critical because these drugs can suppress bone marrow production.

**Immunotherapy.** Antigens and other materials are introduced into the patient's body to stimulate an immune reaction to a tumor. Although the effectiveness of immunotherapy has yet to be proven, cancer *does* sometimes go into spontaneous remission, apparently as the result of an immune system response.

In *active specific immunotherapy,* antibody

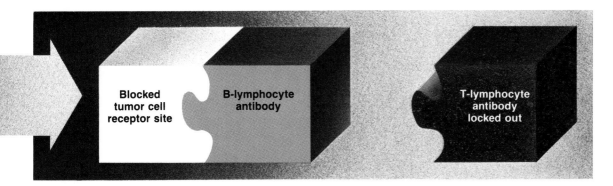

Blocked tumor cell receptor site

B-lymphocyte antibody

T-lymphocyte antibody locked out

production is activated by giving a whole-tumor vaccine of living cells from the patient himself or another source. Antigens are given intradermally, in small doses.

In *active nonspecific immunotherapy,* the immune response—specifically by T lymphocytes—is activated by giving a variety of antigens intradermally, including bovine tubercle bacillus and DNCB.

In *passive immunization,* immunity is transferred from one person to another via serologic agents (substances produced from T lymphocytes). Transfer factor, a water-soluble, dialyzable extract of lymphocytes, shows the best results. However, its effects are only temporary because of serum breakdown and elimination.

In *adoptive immunotherapy,* active immune lymphocytes are transferred via a vaccine into the patient's immune system. These agents may be administered intradermally, orally, through superficial skin lesions, or through body cavities and organs.

### New treatments

Interferon and monoclonal antibody therapy are currently under investigation.

**Interferon.** This agent, derived from human lymphocytes, is thought to work either by preventing cell proliferation or by stimulating the immune system. It's given intramuscularly or intravenously. Interferon strengthens cytotoxic activity of macrophages and sensitized lymphocytes and changes cell surfaces; it also has antiviral characteristics.

It's still being tested for effectiveness against renal cell carcinoma, melanoma, lymphoma, leukemia, mycosis fungoides, and ovarian cancer. The drug's side effects include fever, chills, muscle aches, fatigue, and decreased blood cell production.

**Monoclonal antibodies.** Derived from the cloned cells of mice, these agents—"tagged" to radionuclides—are used experimentally in diagnostic scanning and in the treatment of cancer patients. Monoclonal antibodies selectively locate and destroy cancer cells. Their side effects include fever, chills, hypotension, and allergic reactions.

## NURSING MANAGEMENT

Cancer patients with immunosuppression are commonly seriously ill, so the importance of performing a comprehensive nursing assessment can't be overemphasized.

### A comprehensive history first

Ask the patient to describe his chief complaint. Then ask about his signs and symptoms. When did they start? Are they better or worse now? General weakness, lack of energy, depression, fatigue, fever, and weight loss or gain may indicate cancer.

Next, working from head to toe, ask the patient about skin color or texture changes, such as easy bruising (due to bone marrow suppression or capillary wall defects from malignancy) or itchiness (possible in leukemia or Hodgkin's disease); vision changes; sore throat, white patches in the mouth, difficulty swallowing, painful urination, urinary frequency, or changes in urine appearance (due to infection); or past respiratory or cardiac problems that could compromise future treatment. Also ask the patient if he's experienced lymph node swelling, pain, or tenderness; or nausea, vomiting, loss of appetite, or a change in bowel habits (due to possible lymph node involvement). Weakness, trembling, or palsy may indicate leukemia or central nervous system involvement.

Ask about past hospitalizations and surgeries; allergies; current medications and treatments; on-the-job exposure to chemicals; and family members' illnesses, especially cancer. Ask the patient and his family about their home environment, finances, and emotional support systems. Assess their knowledge of the patient's disease so you'll know what areas to emphasize in your teaching.

## Assessing physical status

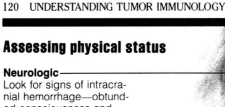

**Neurologic**
Look for signs of intracranial hemorrhage—obtunded consciousness and headache—which may result from a decreased platelet count.

**Lymphatic**
Look for swollen or tender lymph nodes, indicating infection or lymphoma.

**Cutaneous**
Check for poor skin turgor, bruises, petechiae, or bleeding, indicating dehydration and bone marrow depression; and small, red vesicles of early herpes simplex and herpes zoster, commonly occurring in immunocompromised patients.

**Genitourinary**
Check the genitalia for discharges, which may indicate infection. Examine the urine for hematuria or cloudiness, also indicating infection.

**Eye, ear, nose, and throat**
Note conjunctival inflammation or sore throat with white plaques, which may indicate infection. Note visual changes, which may indicate bleeding. Note whitened mucous membranes or bleeding gums, which may indicate bone marrow depression.

**Respiratory/ cardiovascular**
Check for respiratory or cardiovascular abnormalities, which may indicate tumor infiltration or underlying conditions suggesting poor tolerance to surgery or chemotherapy.

**Gastrointestinal**
Note liver or spleen enlargement, indicating leukemia or lymphoma; and rectal bleeding or infection, indicating bone marrow depression.

### A head-to-toe physical examination
First, record the patient's height, weight, and vital signs. These baseline data will also give you clues to his nutritional and hydrational status. Focus on the warning signs of infection and bleeding—the major complications of cancer in an immunosuppressed patient. (See *Assessing physical status.*)

### Typical nursing diagnoses
Use the information gleaned from your patient history and physical examination to develop nursing diagnoses and a care plan. See Chapters 5 and 10 for diagnoses related to controlling infection and Chapter 11 for interventions related to bleeding; other typical diagnoses might include the following.

**Alterations in skin integrity, mucous membranes, and GI tract related to immunosuppression, immobility, and cancer treatment.** Your goal is to prevent skin breakdown, redness, and tenderness at pressure points, as well as trauma to the mucous membranes and GI tract.

To accomplish this, avoid taking rectal temperatures and inserting indwelling (Foley) catheters, and be sure the patient's diet is low in fiber. Remember chemotherapy's side effects, too—nausea, vomiting, diarrhea, constipation, and gastritis, which can irritate the mucous membranes and GI tract and lead to tissue breakdown, infection, and bleeding. To minimize side effects, give antiemetics, antidiarrheals, stool softeners, antacids, and $H_2$ antagonists, as ordered. And to combat rectal skin breakdown from severe diarrhea, keep the patient's skin clean and dry, and apply lotion to prevent cracking. (Wash the skin over irradiated areas with mild, nonabrasive soap, and pat it dry. Don't apply lotion without the radiologist's okay—irradiated skin is very sensitive.) To treat rectal abscesses and promote patient comfort, keep the area clean and dry and give sitz baths several times a day, especially after bowel movements.

Also reposition the patient frequently, massage pressure areas, use pressure-relieving devices (air mattress, fluidized bed) when indicated, record his fluid intake and output, teach him active range-of-motion exercises, and help him walk several times a day.

**Alterations in nutritional or hydrational status related to cancer or cancer treatment.** Loss of appetite and weight often accompanies cancer and its treatments. Your goal is to ensure adequate nutrition and hydration so the patient either gains weight or maintains his present weight and avoids infection.

To accomplish this, give him small, frequent feedings and monitor his diet. (Exclude hard, hot, spicy, or acidic foods or liquids and alcohol.) Because chemotherapy can affect taste buds, the patient may find certain foods too sweet or salty. Ask the family to bring in favorite foods. If necessary, give him commercial dietary supplements. (If possible, avoid feeding tubes—they increase the risk of infection and tissue irritation.)

Consult the hospital dietitian for the patient's daily nutritional requirements and a list of foods he should and shouldn't eat. Help the patient choose palatable, nourishing meals. Keep a calorie count to evaluate his nutritional intake.

Also monitor his fluid intake and output to prevent urinary tract infection and tenacious respiratory secretions and to maintain tissue turgor.

**Patient and family knowledge deficit related to procedures, treatment, or care.** Although cancer is sometimes curable, most patients go home with the disease they had on admission. Your goal is to help the patient and his family understand cancer and its diagnosis and treatment so they'll be more compliant with diagnostic tests, follow-up procedures, and treatment and so they'll know when to seek medical help after the patient's discharged.

To accomplish this, start your teaching on admission and continue throughout the patient's hospitalization. How much you teach at a given time depends on the patient's and family's anxiety level and on their level of understanding. Repeat or rephrase information as necessary, and encourage questions. Prepare the patient for discharge by emphasizing the importance of good nutrition, adequate fluids, skin integrity, rest, and comfort.

Teach the patient and family any procedures they'll need to do at home, and explain the patient's medication regimen. Before discharge, give the patient a written list of signs and symptoms of potential problems, and tell him to seek medical help immediately if any occur. Document everything you teach and the patient's and family's responses.

**Patient's and family's potential inability to cope with cancer and role changes.** A diagnosis of cancer can put tremendous stress on the patient and his family. Your goal is to form a relationship of caring and communication to help them develop effective coping mechanisms.

To promote effective coping, encourage the patient and his family to express their fears and anxieties. Depending on the patient's previous role in the family, suggest new ways for doing household tasks, and discuss which other people or organizations—friends, relatives, church groups, community agencies—are available for support. Recommend self-help and support groups ("Make Today Count" and "I Can Cope"), and contact a public health nurse for information on free equipment and services (home health aides and Meals on Wheels).

Identify the patient's present coping mechanisms and encourage him to use them, if they're not detrimental. Show the patient and his family *you* care by touching, talking, and most important, *listening*.

### Evaluate your care
Your care plan and interventions were successful if you can answer "yes" to the following questions.
• Are the patient's mucous membranes free of infection and his skin intact? Does he have minimal GI tract irritation?
• Did the patient maintain or not lose more than 10% of his body weight? Is he tolerating a preset caloric level without nausea or vomiting?
• Do the patient and his family respond correctly when questioned about information you've taught? Can they correctly demonstrate necessary care procedures? Does the patient recognize signs and symptoms of potential problems and respond to them by seeking medical help?
• Do the patient and his family seem to understand and accept the patient's diagnosis? Have they adapted successfully to life-style changes?

### A final word
Like all seriously ill patients with cancer, the immunosuppressed patient relies on you to recognize new or potential problems and to act decisively before they intensify. He also looks to you for advice, information, and emotional support. A firm knowledge of the treatment and management of tumor immunology ensures that you won't let him down.

**Points to remember**

• The theory of immune surveillance proposes that the immune system identifies malignant and premalignant cells as foreign and destroys them before cancer can fully develop.
• Tumors develop when malignant cell growth exceeds what the immune surveillance system can control or when the immune response fails.
• Investigators have suggested that viruses are the ultimate cause of all cancers and that radiation, carcinogens, and other agents simply activate latent viruses.
• Before definitive cancer treatment can begin, diagnosis must be confirmed through tissue biopsy.
• Infection and bleeding are major complications of cancer in an immunosuppressed patient.

# 9 ANTICIPATING TRANSPLANT REJECTION

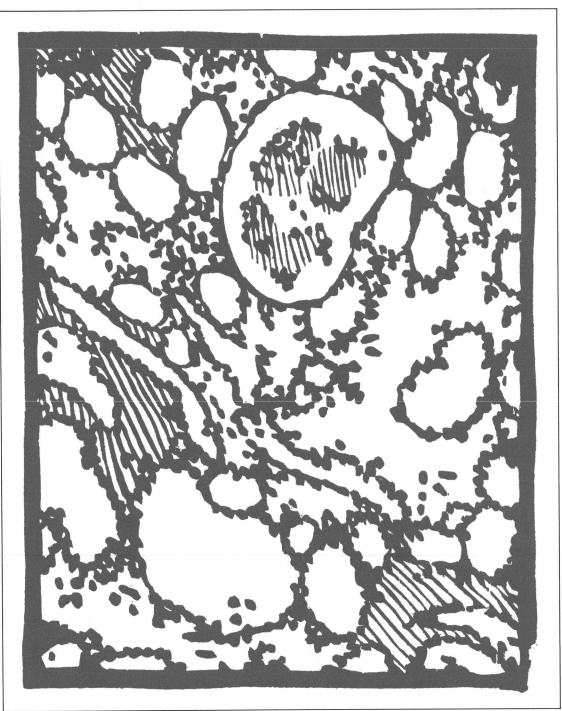

Renal tissue in transplant rejection

n scarcely more than 25 years, organ transplantation has progressed from an idea to a surgical specialty. In the United States, surgeons now perform several thousand kidney, heart, lung, liver, pancreas, bone marrow, and cornea transplants annually.

Patients undergoing transplantation need specialized nursing care before and after surgery and during long-term follow-up. To provide the best possible care, you must understand how the complex immune system operates in transplantation. Also, you must be aware of the legal and ethical problems that organ transplantation poses for the patient and for society as a whole.

## A mixed blessing

Although organ transplantation may be the only means to prolong or improve life, it's not necessarily an easy solution. Despite remarkable advances, organ transplantation is still somewhat unpredictable; its complications are frequent, and success is not guaranteed.

Success rates obviously vary with the specific organ. Renal transplantation usually makes possible a relatively full and normal life. In fact, renal transplantation is the treatment of choice in end-stage renal disease. In the United States, graft survival at 1 year is 60% with a cadaver kidney. Use of cyclosporine improves graft survival to 77%. Graft survival with a kidney from a living donor is even better—roughly 80% to 85% at 1 year and over 90% when donor and recipient are well matched. Graft survival rates decrease with time, however, whether the organ comes from a living donor or a cadaver.

Bone marrow transplantation is the treatment of choice for aplastic anemia. It's also commonly used to treat severe combined immunodeficiency (SCID), various leukemias, and genetic hematopoietic disorders. Although the cure rate varies with the specific disorder, patient survival has been promising.

One-year survival rates for liver transplantation approach 70%. With conventional immunosuppression, 5-year survival rates for heart transplantation approach 50% and are expected to improve with the current use of cyclosporine. Long-term complications of heart transplantation, such as increased incidence of myocardial fibrosis, are yet to be determined.

Combined heart and lung transplantation has been successfully performed in California. Because of the high incidence of pathology simultaneously affecting these organs, this transplantation will probably be performed more frequently than lung transplantation alone.

Segmental or whole pancreas transplantations have been largely unsuccessful, even with the use of immunosuppressives.

Although skin transplantation is widely used in severe burn patients, vigorous rejection is the norm. In contrast, corneal transplantation is infrequently rejected.

## Transplant candidates

Assuming a donor organ is available, who is an appropriate candidate for organ transplantation? The answer depends on the specific organ.

**Kidney.** Typically, candidates for this transplantation have end-stage renal disease. Other qualifying factors include the absence of systemic infection or concurrent major complications, such as pulmonary, cerebrovascular, or neoplastic disease; and a normal lower urinary tract.

**Bone marrow.** Candidates for this transplantation may have SCID, aplastic anemia, leukemia, or genetic hematopoietic disorders. The candidate's potential for cure is the determining factor.

**Liver.** Candidates for this transplantation may have congenital biliary abnormalities, inborn errors of metabolism, or chronic end-stage liver disease. Cirrhosis is a common indication in adults except when it's alcohol-induced.

**Heart.** Candidates for this transplantation may have intractable end-stage cardiac disease. Most candidates have severe coronary artery disease with diffuse left ventricular dysfunction caused by infarction and associated fibrosis. Some have cardiomyopathy from viral infection, myotonic muscular dystrophy, or idiopathic hypertrophic subaortic stenosis. Contraindications for surgery include infection or severe renal, pulmonary, or liver dysfunction.

**Heart and lung.** Candidates for this transplantation may have terminal heart and lung disease or end-stage cardiac disease associated with severe pulmonary vascular disease. Contraindications for surgery include infection, severe pulmonary hypertension, and other serious organ dysfunction.

**Pancreas.** Candidates for islet cell or segmental pancreas transplantation are usually diabetic patients scheduled for kidney transplants. Surgery aims to stop the progression of

## Understanding grafts

A graft is a tissue or organ transplanted to repair a structural or functional defect. Typically, grafts are classified according to the relationship between donor and recipient.

An *allograft* occurs between genetically nonidentical members of the same species. Sometimes called a *homograft,* it's the most common type of graft performed in humans.

An *autograft* occurs within one person when one part of his body is transplanted to another location.

A *heterograft,* or *xenograft,* occurs between different species.

An *isograft,* or *syngraft,* occurs between genetically identical individuals, such as monozygotic twins or members of the same strain of highly inbred animals.

diabetic complications, such as small-vessel disease, neuropathy, and ocular changes.

**Cornea.** Candidates for this transplantation have poor vision due to corneal opacity. Greatly improved vision follows transplantation if other eye structures are intact.

**Skin.** Candidates for this transplantation typically have severe burns. When extensive burns make autografts impossible, allografts or xenografts are temporary treatments.

## PATHOPHYSIOLOGY

Successful transplantation depends on the body's inability to differentiate the transplanted organ from self or to muster its immune defenses against the foreign tissue. Because genetic influences establish the definition of self, they play a leading role in transplantation.

### The role of genetic factors

A brief review explains how genetic factors shape the immune response to transplantation. *Genotype* refers to a person's genetic makeup; *phenotype* refers to the physical expression of the genotype. *Allele* describes one of two or more alternate forms of a gene that control a specific characteristic and occupy corresponding loci on homologous chromosomes. Expression of a specific allele of the genotype depends on whether the allele is dominant or recessive, homozygous or heterozygous. With the exception of identical twins, no two persons have the same genotype.

Genes carry the code for specific cell surface molecules or antigens that markedly influence transplantation. Important antigens include those of the ABO blood group and the major histocompatibility complex (MHC).

**ABO blood group antigens.** These antigens form the basis of human blood classification and are identified serologically. Natural antibodies to blood-group antigens also exist and may be responsible for hyperacute rejection of a transplanted organ from an ABO-incompatible donor. As in blood transfusion, AB is the universal recipient; O, the universal donor.

**MHC antigens.** A cluster of genes known as the MHC codes cell surface antigens. This complex has been identified in various species; in humans, it's called human leukocyte antigen (HLA) and is located on chromosome 6. This MHC contains five gene loci (HLA-A, HLA-B, HLA-C, HLA-D, and HLA-DR). An individual inherits his HLA genotype through two HLA haplotypes, one from each parent.

The alleles encoding the HLA antigens are inherited codominantly. Therefore, an individual expresses eight HLA antigens, unless they are homozygous at some loci. (See *HLA inheritance.*)

HLA antigens determine the success or failure of many transplants by triggering a strong immune response in the presence of nonself HLA antigens. HLA-A, -B, and -C antigens are called Class I antigens. HLA-D and -DR antigens are called Class II antigens. Found on virtually every cell, Class I antigens are the main antigens recognized by the host during graft rejection. Class II antigens are found chiefly on cells of the immune system, including B cells, macrophages, and activated T cells. These antigens elicit a mixed lymphocyte response in which helper T cells proliferate, activating killer T cells and antibody-producing B cells. Class II antigens also play a role in macrophage presentation of antigen to T cells and in efficient collaboration between immunocompetent cells. The T-cell antigen receptor recognizes antigen in the context of Class II antigens.

### Immune mechanisms of rejection

All transplanted organs are immunogenic. However, some organs are naturally less susceptible to rejection. An example is the avascular cornea, protected from rejection by its lack of lymphoid cells, which carry Class II antigens. The cornea does have Class I antigens, but their low concentration makes rejection unlikely.

Much of what is known about rejection comes from the study of kidney transplant rejection. Antigenic differences between the donor and the recipient are known to cause this rejection. However, the exact immune mechanisms responsible for rejection are still unclear.

### Types of rejection

Rejection is classified by the time elapsed between transplant and rejection and may involve cell-mediated or humoral immunity, or both.

**Hyperacute rejection.** Occurring minutes to a few hours after transplantation, hyperacute rejection destroys the donor organ. This type of rejection develops rapidly because the transplant recipient has preformed cytotoxic antibodies against donor antigens. These antibodies result from presensitization during pregnancy, previous blood transfusions, or previous transplantations; or from ABO in-

## HLA inheritance

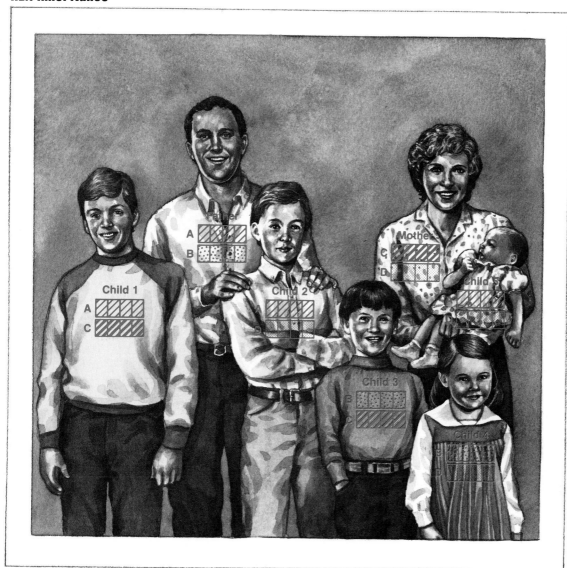

Human leukocyte antigen (HLA), which plays a key role in graft survival, is expressed through two haplotypes: one inherited from the mother and one from the father. The HLA haplotype, or group of alleles inherited as a unit, appears on the short arm of chromosome 6.

In this illustration, paternal haplotypes are A and B, and maternal haplotypes are C and D. A child will inherit one of two possible haplotypes from each parent and display one of four possible genotypic combinations: AC, AD, BC, or BD. Between two siblings, there is a 25% chance that they will be HLA-identical (for example, BD and BD); a 25% chance that they will be HLA-nonidentical (for example, AC and BD); and a 50% chance that they will be HLA–semi-identical (for example, BC and BD). Siblings who are HLA-identical are the optimal match for transplantation.

compatibility. Hyperacute rejection is irreversible and typically begins at the vascular anastomosis in an organ transplant. Removal of the transplanted organ is usually necessary. Fortunately, refined cross-matching techniques have reduced the incidence of this type of rejection.

*Accelerated rejection,* a variant of hyperacute rejection, may occur about 5 days after transplantation. Preformed antibodies and cell-mediated immunity may both contribute to its development. This type of rejection is unresponsive to therapy, but conventional anti-rejection therapy may prevent loss of the graft.

**Acute rejection.** This type of rejection occurs days to months after transplantation as the recipient becomes sensitized to donor antigens. However, it may also appear years later if immunosuppressive therapy is discontinued. Primarily a cell-mediated immune response, acute rejection has a sudden onset known as "first-set rejection," when the recipient becomes sensitized to donor antigens. In a kidney or heart transplant, sensitization may occur in draining lymph nodes or within the graft as circulating immune cells are exposed to the foreign tissue. (See *Renal rejection.*)

Memory cells form during acute rejection and trigger rapid rejection of a subsequent transplant of the same histocompatibility type ("second-set rejection"). The combined cell-mediated and humoral immune responses in acute rejection eventually cause interstitial edema and endothelial damage. But, if the rejection is detected early enough, increased immunosuppression usually reverses it.

**Chronic rejection.** Occurring 6 months to years after transplantation, chronic rejection is characterized by slow, progressive deterioration of transplant function. It's primarily a humoral immune response, involving antibody-mediated damage in the vascular endothelium, which results in graft death.

In chronic rejection, the body's repeated attempts to repair endothelial damage lead to intimal proliferation, necrosis, and collagen deposition, which eventually obliterate the blood vessels. Typically, this deterioration is difficult to treat. However, deterioration varies

## Renal rejection

In *chronic rejection*, antibodies and, possibly, sensitized lymphocytes penetrate the capillaries of the renal allograft, disrupting the endothelium and glomerular basement membrane. The body's repeated attempts to repair these lesions cause accumulation of platelet and fibrin aggregates, endothelial proliferation, and, eventually, vascular obstruction.

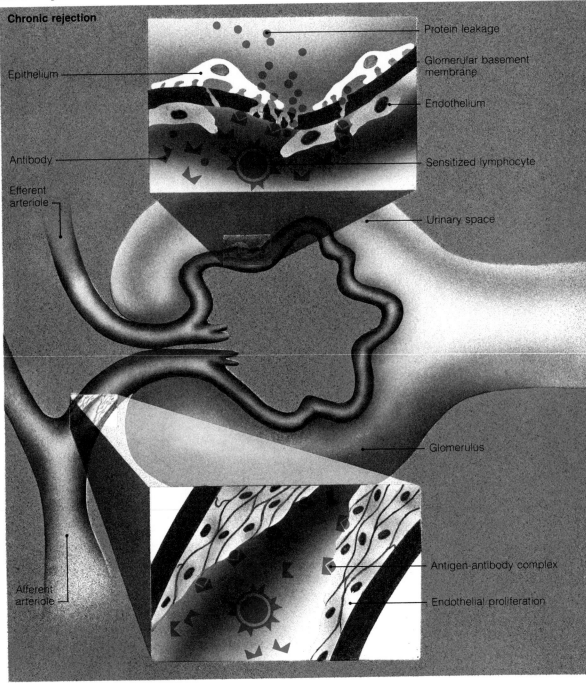

Chronic rejection

Epithelium
Protein leakage
Glomerular basement membrane
Endothelium
Antibody
Sensitized lymphocyte
Efferent arteriole
Urinary space
Glomerulus
Afferent arteriole
Antigen-antibody complex
Endothelial proliferation

in severity; the patient may enjoy adequate transplant function for a few months to years before retransplantation or dialysis becomes necessary.

## MEDICAL MANAGEMENT

Medical management in organ transplantation involves several equally important steps: donor selection, donor evaluation, organ preservation, diagnosis of transplant acceptance or rejection, and prevention or treatment of rejection.

### Donor selection

An indispensable step for successful graft outcome is careful matching of the donor and recipient. Tests of ABO compatibility and histocompatibility, and lymphocyte cross matching may all aid donor selection.

**ABO compatibility.** Evaluating ABO compatibility is the first test for donor selection. Usually, ABO incompatibility eliminates a potential living donor or cadaver for organ transplantation. For example, a donor with A or B antigens would be incompatible with a

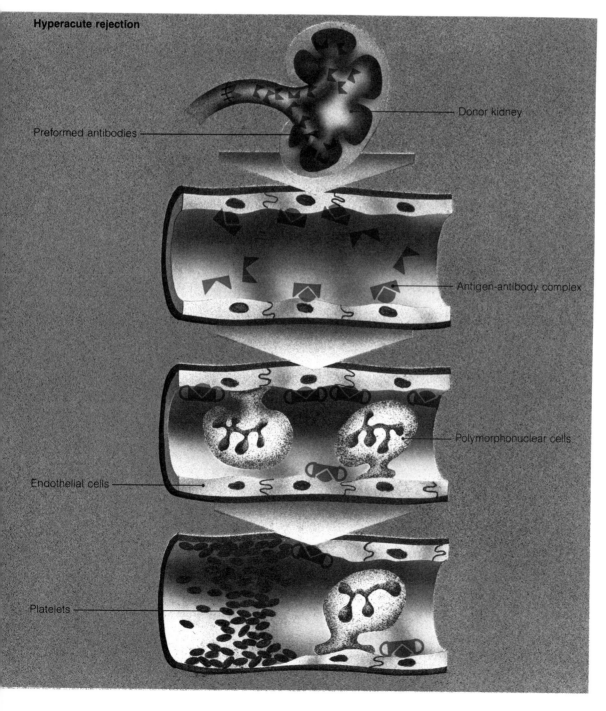

**Hyperacute rejection**

Preformed antibodies

Donor kidney

Antigen-antibody complex

Polymorphonuclear cells

Endothelial cells

Platelets

In *hyperacute rejection,* the recipient's preformed antibodies flood the capillaries of the renal allograft, where they bind to donor antigens. This activates the fibrinogen and complement systems. Platelets immersed in fibrin clots cause vascular occlusion. Complement activation triggers opsonization of the antigen-antibody complex and chemotaxis of polymorphonuclear cells. These cells then infiltrate surrounding tissue, destroying endothelial cells. Vascular occlusion also plays a role in acute rejection. However, in *acute rejection,* antigens from the renal allograft are processed in lymph nodes, where they initiate cell-mediated and humoral immune responses in the nonsensitized recipient. Cytotoxic T lymphocytes are activated, and helper T lymphocytes stimulate antibody production.

recipient with O antigen, who has natural anti-A and anti-B antibodies. However, in bone marrow transplantation, anti-A and anti-B antibodies can now be removed from the recipient to avoid the effects of ABO incompatibility.

**Histocompatibility.** Matching HLA antigens is another test to promote optimal donor selection. Lymphocytes, a rich source of HLA antigens, are used to identify donor and recipient HLA antigens. HLA-A, -B, and -C antigens can also be serologically detected by comparing the reaction of human lymphocyte antigens to a standardized panel of specific antilymphocyte antiserums (tissue typing).

HLA-DR can be serologically detected by the reaction of antigens on B cells with antibodies. HLA-D matching is accomplished through mixed leukocyte culture (MLC) testing. The degree of reaction between the recipient's and donor's lymphocytes estimates histocompatibility. (See *How HLA-D antigen incompatibility promotes graft rejection.*)

Histocompatibility is strongly linked to graft survival. HLA matching with living donor relatives markedly improves graft survival in kidney and bone marrow transplantation. The HLA-A and -B loci are commonly typed for organ matching. Compatibility at HLA-D and -DR loci is also strongly linked to successful transplantation. In contrast, the HLA-C locus is believed to play only a minor role in transplantation. When several donors are available, the one sharing the most HLA antigens with the recipient is preferred. Also, a sibling donor without a haplotype match may have a slightly better advantage than a cadaver.

Whether HLA matching and tissue typing enhance success with cadaver donors is still unclear in liver, heart, and lung transplants. In kidney transplants, reports of success with HLA-A and -B matching have varied. However, matching for the HLA-D and -DR loci improves graft outcome above HLA-A and -B matching alone. An obstacle to HLA-D matching is the length of time required for MLC testing. Currently, cadaver kidneys can be preserved only as long as 72 hours without compromising function.

In cornea transplants, HLA matching and tissue typing are usually not done. Because the cornea is avascular, a graft typically doesn't elicit an immune response. In skin grafts, HLA matching is not routinely done; however, tissue typing may possibly prolong graft survival.

**Lymphocyte cross matching.** Presensitization to donor antigens is readily detected by lymphocyte cross matching. In this test, the recipient's serum is mixed with donor lymphocytes and observed for cell agglutination or lysis; a positive reaction confirms the presence of preformed, circulating antibodies. Lymphocyte cross matching is required whether the donor is a living relative or a cadaver.

## Donor evaluation

Once a well-matched donor has been selected, evaluation of his physical and mental status confirms the decision for organ donation. This evaluation obviously varies between the living donor and cadaver.

**Living donor.** This donor may reasonably offer either a kidney or bone marrow for transplantation. For a potential kidney donor, careful nephrologic study includes the following tests.

*Serum electrolytes* help assess the kidney's regulatory function in acid-base balance.

*Blood urea nitrogen (BUN)* and *creatinine levels* evaluate overall kidney function.

*Glucose tolerance test* helps rule out diabetes mellitus.

*Routine urinalysis* screens for urinary and systemic disorders. Glycosuria and ketonuria may indicate diabetes mellitus or another significant metabolic disorder. Diabetes mellitus may cause nephropathy, which may compromise kidney function. Proteinuria suggests glomerular damage and impaired tubular reabsorption. A positive urine culture indicates infection. However, if appropriate treatment subsequently yields a negative urine culture, the donor may still be considered.

*Creatinine clearance* evaluates the efficiency of glomerular filtration, a chief indicator of renal function.

*Intravenous pyelography* helps evaluate the structure and excretory function of the kidneys, ureters, and bladder and helps detect renovascular hypertension. Functional defects or hypertension may prevent donor acceptance.

*Renography* helps evaluate renal blood flow, nephron and collecting system function, and renal structure. This test involves I.V. injection of a radionuclide followed by scintiphotography, which traces the radionuclide's uptake, transit, and excretion time by each kidney. Slow radionuclide uptake indicates kidney obstruction or renal artery constriction.

*Renal angiography* delineates the arrange-

## How HLA-D antigen incompatibility promotes graft rejection

HLA-D antigen *compatibility*, measured by the mixed leukocyte culture test, helps ensure graft acceptance by the recipient's immune system. A brief look at HLA-D antigen incompatibility explains why this match is vital.

HLA-D antigen *incompatibility* stimulates proliferation of helper T cells (Th). This facilitates activation of cytotoxic T cells (Tc) and antibody-producing B cells (Ba). Both effects promote graft rejection.

ment and patency of the renal vessels. Most transplant centers avoid donors older than age 55 because of increased risk of nephrosclerosis and eventual graft rejection. Nephrosclerosis decreases renal blood flow, which ultimately triggers hypertension.

Besides tests of renal function, a thorough medical history and physical examination—including an EKG and chest X-ray—are essential.

Also, straightforward discussions with the potential kidney donor establish if he's freely willing to donate and if he understands the minimal, but real, operative risk. The same holds true for the potential bone marrow donor: he must be well informed, willing, and in good general health.

**Cadaver donor.** Cadaver organs are taken from brain-dead donors receiving artificial cardiopulmonary support. If the donor failed to sign an organ donation card, permission may be granted by his next of kin. Suitable cadaver donors may be as old as 55 years. The best heart donors are between ages 12 and 50. Vascular or hypertensive disease contraindicates organ donation because poor blood flow contributes to graft rejection. Diabetes is also a contraindication because of premature arteriosclerosis of the donor.

Systemic bacterial or viral infection and cancer also prohibit organ donation. An organ from a cancerous cadaver may seed malignant cells in the recipient, potentially setting the stage for metastatic disease fostered by immunosuppressives. An exception is the cadaver donor with a primary brain tumor, because metastasis does not cross the blood-brain barrier.

Various tests evaluate the status of the cadaver's organs. Measurement of *urine output, urinalysis,* and *serum BUN* and *creatinine levels* helps assess renal function. *Liver function studies,* such as liver enzyme levels, help determine the cadaver's liver status. *Drug screening* and *VDRL testing* help evaluate drug use and rule out infection. Estimation of liver size is also crucial. Adult livers are difficult to use in children. Also, ascites and liver shrinkage from intrinsic disease decrease the space available for a transplanted liver in the recipient. Appropriate *endocrine studies* help evaluate pancreatic function.

The donor's condition just before death determines whether the organ being considered for donation can survive prolonged surgery. For example, heart donors shouldn't have had prolonged cardiac arrest because an extended time between cardiac arrest and organ removal results in increased damage to cardiac tissue. Severe chest trauma or previous heart disease also precludes heart donation, as does a marked difference in organ size between donor and recipient. Pulmonary edema, severe chest trauma, or pneumonia also prohibits heart and lung donation.

**Organ preservation**
Without appropriate organ preservation, successful transplantation is impossible.

The kidney can be preserved for 24 to 72 hours by perfusing physiologic fluids to maintain metabolism and by inducing hypothermia to reduce metabolic demands. Once the kidney is removed, it is immersed in an ice-slush solution, resembling intracellular electrolyte composition, to cool the kidney surface. The renal artery or aorta is also flushed to cool the kidney core.

Next, the kidney may be preserved by either static storage or pulsatile perfusion. Static storage involves placing the kidney in a sterile, solution-filled container, then immersing the container in an ice-slush solution inside a vacuum flask. This method, which keeps the kidney viable for up to 36 hours, is an economical way to preserve kidney function during transport.

Pulsatile perfusion combines hypothermia and membrane oxygenation with a pulsatile flow of perfusate, such as cryoprecipitated plasma. Sophisticated pulsatile perfusion systems like the Belzer machine may preserve the kidney for as long as 72 hours.

Viable for a shorter time than the kidney, the heart and liver are transported in an ice-slush solution. The heart can be preserved for up to 4 hours by combining hypothermia with infusion of an electrolyte solution into the coronary arteries to interrupt myocardial contraction. The liver can be preserved for up to 10 hours, using hypothermia and infusion of an electrolyte solution into the portal vein.

Skin can be preserved for up to 18 hours by placing the tissue in a physiologic salt solution or indefinitely by using controlled freezing in a skin bank.

After removal, the cornea is transported in ice to an eye bank. There, it's flushed with antibiotics, preserved by the tissue culture method, and stored under refrigeration.

Bone marrow is transfused into the recipient on the same day it's aspirated from the donor.

**Transplant acceptance or rejection**
Evaluating transplant outcome focuses on close observation of the organ's function to detect signs and symptoms of transplant rejection. Such clinical findings vary with the type of rejection.

**Kidney.** Accelerated rejection of the kidney typically produces dramatic symptoms. Diminished urine volume, edema, weight gain, and rising blood pressure reflect deteriorating renal function. Elevated temperature, malaise, tenderness, and perhaps kidney swelling accompany intensive infiltration of lymphoid cells and polymorphonuclear leukocytes into renal tissue.

Laboratory findings show decreased creatinine clearance, increased BUN and creatinine levels, proteinuria, and possibly decreased urine sodium excretion.

Technetium scanning may show abnormal distribution of radioactive colloid within the kidney, suggesting tissue damage or dysfunction. Renography usually shows decreased renal blood flow and poor radionuclide uptake in the tubules, indicating decreased glomerular filtration and perfusion.

Renal biopsy can accurately diagnose hyperacute or accelerated rejection; however, it's not routinely done because of the risk of hematoma.

Acute or chronic rejection of the kidney resembles accelerated rejection but tends to be less severe. Again, laboratory findings show decreased creatinine clearance, increased BUN and creatinine levels, and proteinuria.

Biopsy may also diagnose chronic rejection.

**Heart.** Serial endomyocardial biopsy of the right ventricle detects mild cardiac rejection even before clinical signs appear. (See *Endomyocardial biopsy: Detecting heart rejection,* page 132.) The biopsy specimen reveals interstitial edema and mononuclear cell infiltration—signs that typically disappear with increased immunosuppression. Immunologic monitoring may also detect rejection.

At the onset of acute cardiac rejection, 12-lead electrocardiography shows a generalized, progressive decrease in QRS voltage. Atrial dysrhythmias also frequently accompany rejection and confirm the occurrence of some irreversible myocardial damage. Measurement of serum enzymes, such as lactate dehydrogenase, creatine phosphokinase, and serum glutamic-oxaloacetic transaminase (SGOT), is of little diagnostic value since elevated enzyme levels appear long after other signs of myocardial insufficiency. Advanced rejection cripples myocardial function, causing diminished cardiac output.

**Liver.** Although the transplanted liver is not as susceptible to acute rejection as other organs, mild rejection is a risk. Liver function tests help diagnose mild rejection by detecting increased serum transaminase or alkaline phosphatase levels. Increased serum bilirubin levels reflect impaired bilirubin conjugation in the liver, a telling sign of rejection. Increased SGOT and serum glutamic-pyruvic transaminase levels may point to hepatocellular damage associated with rejection.

Liver rejection may be difficult to distinguish from other disorders, such as biliary obstruction and drug toxicity, which may also increase these enzyme levels.

Mild-to-moderate liver rejection may not be clinically apparent. However, in severe rejection, fever, malaise, anorexia, jaundice, pain, and hepatomegaly are characteristic. Technetium scanning shows decreased hepatic uptake.

**Pancreas.** In pancreas rejection, the organ becomes grossly edematous and indurated and shows interstitial hemorrhages. Hyperglycemia is characteristic and may be aggravated by steroids given to reverse rejection.

**Bone marrow.** Progression of the disease that bone marrow transplant was meant to cure signals rejection. (See *Graft-versus-host disease,* pages 134 and 135.)

**Cornea.** In corneal rejection, the organ becomes edematous as lymphoid cells accumulate in the epithelium. A rejection line appears

as these cells move inward from the corneal periphery.

**Skin.** Edema and eventual sloughing off of tissue characterize skin rejection.

## Immunologic monitoring
Along with observation of the transplanted organ's function, monitoring immune activity against donor tissue helps detect rejection early.

Several in vitro tests detect specific antidonor immune activity. Complement-dependent cytotoxins against donor B cells in the recipient's serum are often associated with rejection. A positive antibody-dependent cell-mediated cytotoxicity assay may also indicate rejection by detecting antidonor antibodies. Immunofluorescence may detect antibodies against donor antigens, suggesting rejection and graft loss.

Other tests that evaluate immune activity may also help diagnose rejection. Increased rosette-forming T cells or increased T cells using monoclonal antibodies may be associated with rejection or infection. In addition, markedly increased DNA synthesis in the recipient's peripheral mononuclear cells may indicate rejection or infection. A positive macrophage migration inhibition factor may indicate rejection but is frequently unreliable. A normal quota of helper T cells despite immunotherapy usually indicates rejection. The degree of lymphocyte proliferation in response to mitogens is associated with transplant rejection.

## Transplant rejection: Prevention and treatment
Effective immunosuppression, the key to preventing transplant rejection, may be achieved through drug therapy, radiation, and pretransplant blood transfusions.

**Drug therapy.** Azathioprine and corticosteroids are part of nearly every immunosuppressive regimen. Azathioprine presumably impairs proliferation of immunocompetent cells by interfering with DNA synthesis. Rapidly dividing cells are especially sensitive to its effects. Because its major use is prevention, not treatment, of rejection, azathioprine therapy frequently begins before transplantation.

Corticosteroids may help treat rejection, presumably because of their anti-inflammatory and lymphocytic effects. Corticosteroids limit the production of cytotoxic T lymphocytes apparently by preventing helper T cells from elaborating T-cell growth factor. Long-

## Evaluating the transplant recipient
Thorough preoperative evaluation of the transplant recipient gathers important baseline data and helps ensure a successful graft. In addition to tissue typing and final antibody cross matching, this evaluation includes the following studies.

**Hematology:** complete blood count, platelet count, differential, prothrombin time, partial thromboplastin time, thrombin time

**Chemistry:** serum glucose, blood urea nitrogen, creatinine, calcium, phosphorus, bilirubin, alkaline phosphatase, serum glutamic-oxaloacetic transaminase, serum glutamic-pyruvic transaminase, lactate dehydrogenase, creatine phosphokinase, cholesterol, triglycerides, amylase, lipase, uric acid, total protein, albumin, and globulin levels

**Urinalysis**

**Microbiology:** clean-catch urine culture, blood culture

**X-ray studies:** chest X-ray, voiding cystourethrogram (for kidney recipients), barium enema (for patients over age 40)

**EKG**

**Hepatitis screening**

**Pap smear** (for women who have not had a Pap smear in the last 6 months)

**Gastroscopy** (for patients with positive ulcer history and negative upper GI series)

**Virology:** cytomegalovirus antibody titer, herpes simplex antibody titer, Epstein-Barr antibody titer.

# Endomyocardial biopsy: Detecting heart rejection

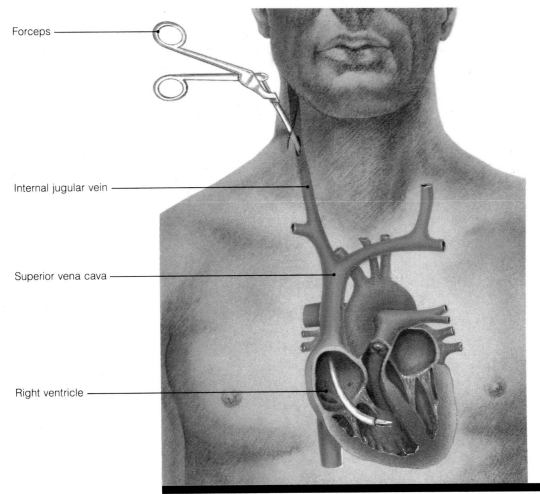

Forceps

Internal jugular vein

Superior vena cava

Right ventricle

To detect rejection of the transplanted heart, endomyocardial biopsy is routinely performed every 3 to 7 days for up to 6 weeks after surgery (when the chance for acute rejection is greatest). It may then be performed annually, as part of the recipient's follow-up care.

In this diagnostic procedure, narrow, flexible biopsy forceps are introduced percutaneously into the internal jugular vein under local anesthetic and advanced through the superior vena cava into the heart. Guided by fluoroscopy, the forceps are directed into the right ventricle, where a small endomyocardial specimen is removed. Microscopic examination of this specimen typically reveals lymphocytic infiltration and damaged endomyocardial cells in heart rejection.

Although this biopsy procedure is relatively safe, the patient must be observed for bleeding at the forceps insertion site and for possible cardiac tamponade.

term use of corticosteroids may also inhibit IgG synthesis, although this is not a major indication for their use.

Prophylactic administration of immunosuppressive drugs aims to delay or even prevent rejection. If rejection does occur, increased dosages of I.V. corticosteroids are usually prescribed. Even after rejection subsides, corticosteroids are continued for life.

Lymphocyte immune globulin, a heterologous serum containing antibodies against lymphocytes, may be given prophylactically or to treat acute rejection. Although it's clearly immunosuppressive, its use is highly controversial. To obtain lymphocyte immune globulin, a suspension of human lymphocytes derived from thymus, spleen, or cultured lymphoblasts is injected into an animal of another species (horse, goat, or rabbit). Serum from the immunized animal is then drawn, and the antibody-containing fraction is isolated, sterilized, and frozen until ready for use. In laboratory animals, an impure form

called antilymphocyte serum is an extremely potent immunosuppressive. Evidently, it acts by selectively depleting lymphocytes responsible for cell-mediated immunity. Cells reacting with the antibody are lysed or phagocytized. Although anaphylaxis is a risk, severe reactions are rare.

Cyclosporine, another potent immunosuppressive, was first used in Europe. It reduces helper-T-cell production of T-cell growth factor, thus impairing initiation of cell-mediated and humoral immunity.

Currently, cyclosporine is widely used in transplantation. It's given before surgery and with other drugs afterward to prevent rejection. In some hospitals, it's being tried to reverse the onset of acute rejection. Reportedly, cyclosporine has improved success rates, particularly in liver, heart, and lung transplants. Although cyclosporine is hepatotoxic and nephrotoxic, its long-term effects have not been well documented. However, it doesn't cause bone marrow suppression, the major drawback of azathioprine. And its side effects can be eliminated by decreasing drug dosage.

**Radiation.** Local radiation to the transplant organ combined with stepped-up immunosuppressive drugs may help reverse rejection. The recommended dose is usually 100 to 600 rads delivered in one or more sessions. Total lymphoid irradiation to induce immunosuppression—a successful method in laboratory animals—is currently being investigated.

**Pretransplant blood transfusions.** By exposing the recipient to donor antigens, pretransplant blood transfusions improve survival. However, the exact mechanism is unclear. Transfusions may improve graft survival by triggering selective production of antibodies against some HLA antigens, but not others, or by inducing cell-mediated immune unresponsiveness. In fact, much controversy still exists about the use of pretransplant blood transfusions. Many argue that the risk of developing antibodies against histocompatibility antigens of potential donors is too great. Although cross matching with potential donor lymphocytes is performed frequently, a positive cross match prevents use of the donor organ. Such wide exposure to multiple antigens could limit the supply of potential donors for a particular recipient.

Still investigational is treatment with monoclonal antilymphocyte antibodies. Produced by hybridomas (hybridized cells), these pure antibodies react with T lymphocytes. Antibodies against specific lymphocyte populations may suppress acute rejection.

## NURSING MANAGEMENT

Whether the patient is awaiting a heart, kidney, or cornea transplant, he's likely to face many difficult questions. "Will this new organ make my life better?" and "What if my body doesn't accept it?" are two examples. As a nurse, you can help by recognizing the patient's special emotional needs and by providing skillful physical care before and after transplantation. Your nursing assessment provides a firm data base for addressing the patient's varied needs.

### Get a thorough history

Begin by obtaining biographic data, such as the patient's name, sex, age, race, religion, occupation, marital status, and number of children and their ages.

Then, determine the patient's chief complaint. When did his present illness begin? How did its progression lead to the decision for transplantation? Find out if the patient understands the surgery and how it will affect his function. Is he anxious about finances, extended absence from work, or the effects of hospitalization on his family? Determine his coping patterns and how he perceives the effect of his illness on his life.

Next, ask the patient what prescription and over-the-counter drugs he's currently taking. Include their dosage and schedule. Has he experienced any adverse effects from these drugs? Note allergies to drugs and other substances.

Review the patient's family history, such as incidence of cancer, hypertension, diabetes, and infectious diseases.

To complete your nursing history, carefully review these body systems.

**Neurologic.** For potential kidney recipients, a neurologic history is especially important because encephalopathy may accompany chronic renal failure. Ask about drowsiness, headache, confusion, tremors, and convulsions.

**Eyes.** Ask about vision changes, discharge, pain, and swelling. Blurred vision may accompany hypertension.

**Ears, nose, and throat.** Ask about earache, nasal discharge, and sore throat. Does the patient frequently experience these signs of infection?

**Cardiovascular.** Because vascular organ transplants involve lengthy surgery and a difficult recovery period, a cardiovascular history is essential. Has the patient ever been treated for hypertension? If so, blood pressure control may be difficult postoperatively when he's receiving corticosteroids, which cause sodium and water retention. Has he ever had a myocardial infarction or been treated for congestive heart failure? If so, he may be a poor candidate for transplant surgery. For the potential heart recipient, low cardiac output is normal as a result of underlying disease. Find out if he has noticed any changes in heart rate or rhythm. How far can he walk? Does he experience chest pain or swelling or pain in his lower legs? What does he use to relieve it?

**Respiratory.** Because respiratory infections are common with postoperative immunosuppression, this history is crucial. Ask about the patient's smoking habits and exposure to environmental pollutants. Does he have a history of respiratory infections or worsening lung disease? Even though both are expected in potential lung recipients, infection must

# Graft-versus-host disease

In graft-versus-host disease (GVHD), immunocompetent donor T lymphocytes attack and destroy vulnerable host cells. Because this disease occurs even with HLA matching, non-HLA antigens may contribute to its development. Occurring most frequently in bone marrow transplants, GVHD affects the skin, liver, intestinal mucosa, and lymph system and may be either acute or chronic.

### Acute GVHD
Acute GVHD shows characteristic skin involvement and is confirmed by skin biopsy. Severe liver involvement also elevates liver enzyme and bilirubin levels.

Symptoms of acute GVHD occasionally appear as early as one week after transplantation, although 30 to 50 days is more typical. An erythematous rash appears first, followed by green, watery diarrhea; abdominal cramps; and, in severe disease, right upper quadrant pain, hepatosplenomegaly, jaundice, and enlarged lymph nodes.

Acute GVHD is graded according to the severity of symptoms and the number of organs involved. (See *Severity of acute graft-versus-host disease.*) Patients with mild disease (grade 1) experience skin involvement alone, whereas those with severe disease (grades 2 to 4) also experience GI or liver involvement, which typically leads to fatal infection. In fact, severe disease has an 85% mortality.

Treatment of acute GVHD includes high-dose corticosteroids, lymphocyte immune globulin, or cyclosporine. These agents may provide symptomatic relief, but their effectiveness in improving survival is still undetermined. In fact, corticosteroid therapy increases susceptibility to infection, the major cause of death in acute GVHD. Use of monoclonal antibodies to destroy donor T lymphocytes is still experimental.

### Chronic GVHD
This form of GVHD may occur whether or not the patient experiences acute GVHD.

Chronic GVHD resembles autoimmune collagen vascular disorders, such as systemic lupus erythematosus. It's characterized by scleroderma-like skin fibrosis and Sjögren's syndrome, in which the mucosa and lacrimal ducts are abnormally dry. Diagnosis of chronic GVHD is confirmed by skin and oral mucosal biopsy. Also, Schirmer's test assesses lacrimal gland function and pulmonary studies measure pulmonary efficiency.

Chronic GVHD appears approximately 100 days after transplantation. It affects the skin, liver, GI system, oral mucosa, eyes, and vagina and causes pulmonary changes and muscle wasting.

Localized skin involvement may resolve without therapy. Treatment of early systemic involvement with combinations of immunosuppressive drugs shows promise but is still investigational.

### Immunosuppression: Key to preventing GVHD
Immunosuppressive therapy against donor T lymphocytes aims to prevent GVHD. Methotrexate, an antimetabolite that inhibits DNA synthesis and has a cytotoxic effect on rapidly dividing cells, is the most commonly used therapy. Irradiation of blood products before they're administered is another therapy to prevent T-lymphocyte replication.

Still experimental is the removal of T lymphocytes from the bone marrow before it's transplanted, either by treating the marrow with monoclonal antibodies or by binding the T lymphocytes to plant substances called lectins.

### Nursing goals
Since patients with GVHD inevitably have some skin involvement, your major nursing goals are to maintain the integrity of the skin and mucous membranes and to prevent infection. Also strive to promote hydration and adequate nutrition to correct marked fluid and electrolyte losses caused by diarrhea and vomiting in severe disease. Monitor the patient with thrombocytopenia for GI blood loss.

Provide comfort measures to ease sore skin lesions, abdominal cramping, and pain. Also provide emotional support to the patient and his family.

---

be resolved before surgery. Progressive lung disease may contraindicate heart, liver, or kidney transplantation. Does the patient ever have difficulty breathing? Is it associated with activity? Has the patient ever noticed blood-tinged sputum? Ask him to describe his sputum.

**Genitourinary.** Does the patient have a history of urinary tract infections? Does he currently have signs of infection? If so, they must be resolved before surgery. If he's undergoing dialysis, ask the date of his last treatment.

**Gastrointestinal.** Because steroid-induced gastric ulcers and postoperative bleeding are significant risks in transplantation, this history is essential. Ask the patient if he has blood in his stools. Has he experienced any abdominal pain, nausea, or vomiting? Are these symptoms associated with food or with stress? Have the patient describe his typical diet.

**Hematologic.** Has the patient noticed any unusual bruising, prolonged bleeding, or fatigue? Expect these signs in potential bone

# Severity of acute graft-versus-host disease

## Stages of GVHD according to organ system

| Skin | | Liver | | Gastrointestinal | |
|---|---|---|---|---|---|
| **Stage** | | **Stage** | | **Stage** | Diarrhea, nausea, and vomiting are also grade +1 through +4 in severity. The severity of GI involvement was assigned to the most severe of the three involvements noted. It is difficult to quantitate most of these manifestations, except diarrhea. |
| +1 | Maculopapular eruption involving less than 25% of the body surface | +1 | Moderate increase of SGOT (150 to 170 IU) and bilirubin (2 to 3 mg/dl) | | |
| +2 | Maculopapular eruption involving 25% to 50% of the body surface | +2 | Bilirubin rise (3 to 5.9 mg/dl) with or without an increase in SGOT | +1 | 500 ml of stool/day |
| +3 | Generalized erythroderma | +3 | Bilirubin rise (6 to 14.9 mg/dl) with or without an increase in SGOT | +2 | 1,000 ml of stool/day |
| +4 | Generalized erythroderma with bulbous formation and often with desquamation | +4 | Bilirubin rise (15 mg/dl) with or without an increase in SGOT (Increases in SGOT were temporarily related to either the onset or the worsening of the skin rash.) | +3 | 1,500 ml of stool/day |
| | | | | +4 | 2,000 ml of stool/day |

## Grades of GVHD

| Grade 1 | Grade 2 | Grade 3 | Grade 4 |
|---|---|---|---|
| +1 to +2 skin rash with or without GI involvement | +1 to +3 skin rash with either +1 to +2 GI involvement or +1 to +2 liver involvement, or both; some patients have fever | +2 to +4 skin rash with +2 to +4 GI involvement with or without +2 to +4 liver involvement; many patients have fever | Similar to grade 3 with extreme constitutional symptoms |

marrow and liver recipients.

**Endocrine.** Ask the patient about changes in appetite, weight, or mental function, such as lethargy or nervousness. Ask about metabolic problems, such as thyroid disorders. Does the patient show signs of diabetes, such as polyuria, polydipsia, or polyphagia? If he's a confirmed diabetic, ask him what control measures he uses. Postoperative corticosteroids may elevate serum glucose levels, so these baseline data are crucial for detecting drug-induced hyperglycemia.

## Perform a systematic physical examination

After noting height and weight, examine the patient from head to toe, giving special attention to those body systems most affected by the diseased organ to be replaced.

**Eyes.** Inspect the patient's eyes for drainage or inflammation. Are inflamed areas tender? Assess the sclera for jaundice. Note corneal opacity in the potential cornea recipient.

**Ears, nose, and throat.** Using an otoscope, inspect for signs of infection—discharge from the ear canal and eardrum inflammation. Using a nasal speculum, inspect the nostrils for discharge and for mucosal swelling or bleeding. Using a tongue depressor, inspect the pharynx for inflammation. Palpate lymph nodes, noting their size and consistency. Are they movable or fixed? Painless or tender? Enlarged lymph nodes may signal infection or neoplasm.

**Cardiovascular.** Check for hypertension, common in patients with renal failure, and for reduced cardiac output, expected in potential heart recipients with severe myopathy. Assess for irregular heart rate and murmurs. Check for peripheral edema and evaluate peripheral pulses. In patients with renal or cardiac failure, specifically note the amount of peripheral and sacral edema. Examine the eyes for retinopathy associated with elevated blood pressure.

**Respiratory.** Auscultate and percuss the lungs to detect progressive lung disease or infection. Measure chest circumference to help match heart size between donor and recipient.

**Genitourinary.** Palpate the kidneys and bladder and examine the genitalia. Inspect the patient's urine, and prepare a specimen for laboratory analysis.

**Gastrointestinal.** Inspect the abdomen for ascites, abnormal skin color, lesions, and scars. Percuss for ascites and tenderness, which may indicate abdominal inflammation. Percuss and palpate the liver to estimate its size. Test the patient's stool for occult blood (guaiac test). Abnormal stool color may result from various GI disorders, such as ulcers, hemorrhoids, or impaired bilirubin excretion.

**Skin.** Observe for unusual bruising and easy bleeding. Signs of infection or poor healing may reflect immunologic incompetence. Assess for jaundice in the sclera and mucous membranes. Also note skin turgor to evaluate hydration.

**Endocrine.** Evaluate the patient's behavior and activity level to help detect metabolic disorders. Assess the thyroid gland. Record height and weight for a baseline to calculate dosage schedules for immunosuppressive therapy.

### Formulate nursing diagnoses

Using the data gathered from baseline assessment, formulate both preoperative and postoperative nursing diagnoses.

**Knowledge deficit related to postoperative recovery and rehabilitation potential.** Your nursing goals are to teach the patient about

transplant surgery so that he understands and accepts the graft outcome and to help him practice measures to reduce postoperative complications. Begin by explaining the transplant procedure. Honestly discuss the probability of success and of postoperative complications. Make sure he understands that transplantation is not an easy cure, that it doesn't guarantee a life free of medical problems and restrictions, and that it requires lifelong follow-up. Give him written information describing follow-up care and the required drug regimen.

Explain what to expect before surgery, including food and fluid restrictions. Have him practice coughing and deep-breathing exercises with an incentive spirometer. Stress the importance of performing these exercises postoperatively.

Inform the family that the patient will be in the intensive care unit for several days, unless he's receiving a cornea or kidney. Describe the complicated equipment necessary for accurate monitoring and, if possible, let them see it beforehand. Inform them about postoperative isolation, if ordered, and describe tests used to detect rejection or such postoperative complications as infection. Also explain the immunosuppressive regimen.

Consider your interventions effective if the patient understands the transplant procedure, accepts its likely outcome, and knows how to perform postoperative measures to prevent complications.

**Knowledge deficit related to self-care after discharge.** Your nursing goal is to help the patient care for himself effectively after discharge. Stress the lifelong need to take corticosteroids and other immunosuppressives, as ordered. Failure to do so will trigger rejection, even of a transplanted organ that has been functioning well for 5 years or more. Because prolonged use of immunosuppressives increases the risk of malignancy, teach the patient about early signs of cancer and about risk factors. Avoid alarming him unnecessarily. Discourage smoking and prolonged exposure to sun. Encourage the female patient to have a gynecologic examination and Pap smear every 6 months.

Describe the signs of infection and rejection specific to the transplanted organ. Make sure the patient realizes that the sooner rejection is detected, the easier it is to reverse. Also emphasize the importance of follow-up care.

Consider your nursing interventions effective if the patient can describe the signs of rejec-

# Clinical findings in graft rejection

Because most patients who receive grafts experience at least one rejection episode, be sure to watch for these signs and symptoms.

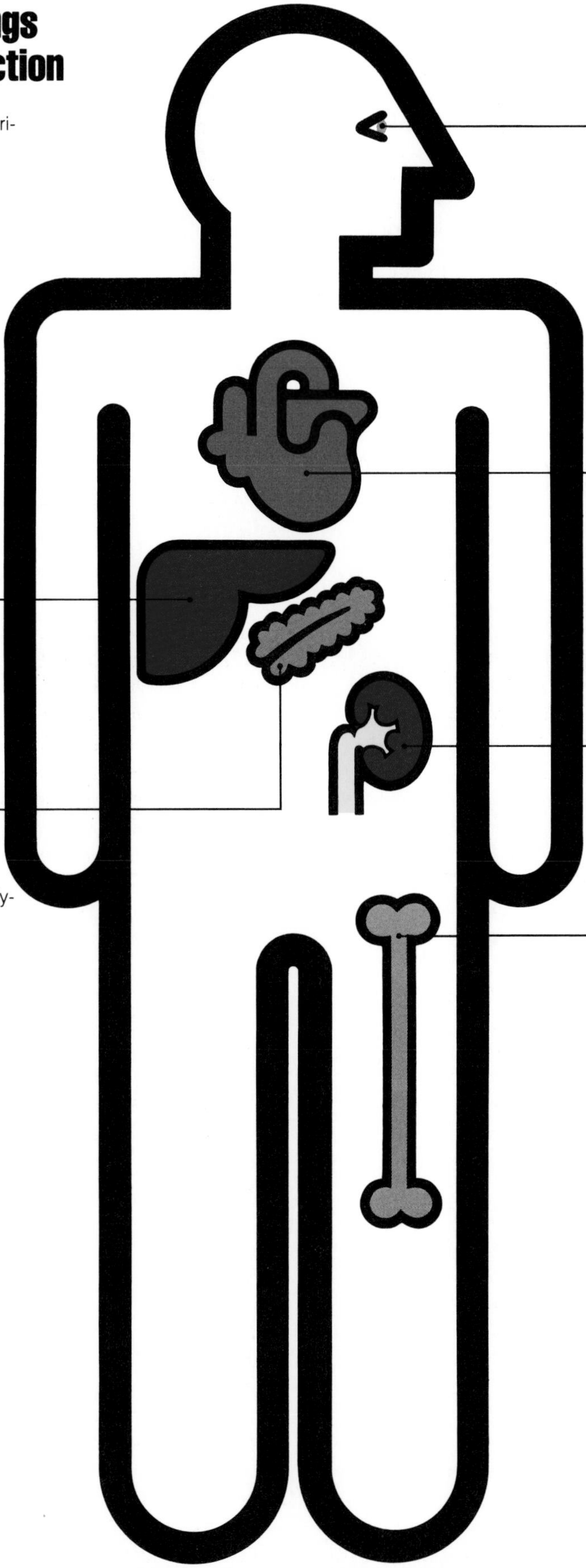

**Corneal rejection**
• Conjunctival hyperemia in perilimbal region
• Cloudy cornea
• Corneal edema
• Accumulation of cells and protein in anterior chamber

**Heart rejection**
• Decreased QRS voltage
• Right axis shift
• Atrial dysrhythmias
• Conduction defects
• $S_3$ gallop
• Jugular vein distention
• Malaise, lethargy
• Fever
• Weight gain
• Right ventricular pump failure

**Liver rejection**
• Altered color of urine or stool
• Jaundice
• Hepatomegaly
• Fever
• Pain (center of back, right flank, or right upper quadrant)

**Pancreas rejection**
• Signs of diabetes mellitus (increased blood glucose levels, polyuria, polydipsia, polyphagia, weight loss)

**Kidney rejection**
• Fever
• Decreased urine output
• Pain or swelling in kidney area
• Elevated blood pressure
• Weight gain
• Malaise

**Bone marrow rejection**
• Severe diarrhea
• Severe jaundice
• Mild-to-severe skin changes
• Graft-versus-host disease

# Environmental control measures: Safeguard against infection

Because immunosuppression increases the transplant patient's risk of infection, environmental control measures are typically part of postoperative care. However, use of such measures varies among hospitals. Many employ temporary *reverse (protective) isolation* when leukopenia follows high-dose immunosuppression, although the Centers for Disease Control maintains it's no more effective than *strict handwashing and aseptic technique.* Review the steps below so that you'll be prepared to follow either procedure.

### Strict handwashing and aseptic technique
• Wear a clean gown and, if required, a mask and gloves when caring for the transplant patient.
• Limit contact with outside staff and visitors. Don't allow visits by anyone known to be infected or ill.
• Carefully wash your hands before, during, and after patient care.
• Observe strict asepsis during daily care of I.V. sites, catheters, and incisions.
• Provide frequent mouth and skin care to prevent skin breakdown.
• Monitor the patient's white blood cell (WBC) count; report a low WBC count and tighten precautions, as ordered.

### Reverse isolation
• After locating the patient in a private room, explain isolation procedures to him to ease anxiety and promote cooperation.

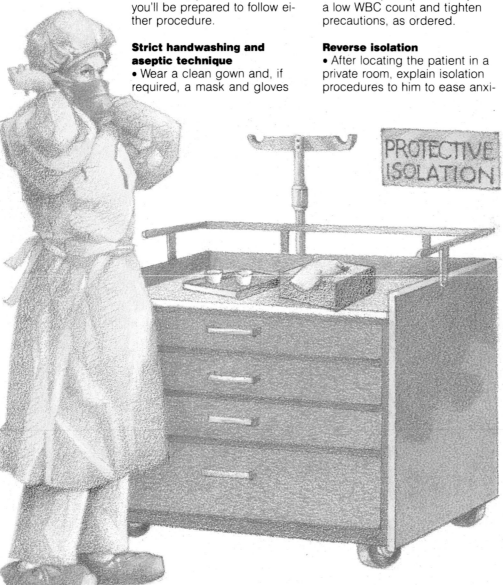

• Make sure the room is cleaned and has new or scrupulously clean equipment. Because the patient doesn't have a contagious disease, articles leaving the room require no special precautions and the room needs no special cleaning precautions after the patient's discharged.
• Keep supplies—gowns, gloves, masks, caps, plastic bags—in a clean enclosed cart or in an anteroom outside the room. Also stock sterile linens and head and shoe coverings for the patient especially susceptible to infection, such as the bone marrow recipient. Keep additional supplies, such as a thermometer, stethoscope, and blood pressure cuff, in the room to minimize trips in and out, and to prevent contaminating the patient with equipment used on other patients.
• Keep the door to the room closed. Post reverse isolation cards on the door.
• Put on a clean gown, mask, cap, and gloves each time you enter the patient's room.
• Wash your hands with an antiseptic agent before putting on gloves to prevent bacterial growth on gloved skin; wash gloves with antiseptic if they become contaminated during patient care; and wash your hands after leaving the room.
• Instruct the housekeeping staff to put on gowns, gloves, caps, and masks before entering the patient's room; advise them not to enter if they're ill or infected.
• Also don't allow visits by anyone known to be infected or ill. Show visitors how to don gowns, gloves, caps, and masks and instruct them to remove them only after they leave the room.
• Don't perform invasive procedures such as urethral catheterization unless absolutely necessary, because their use risks serious infection.
• Avoid transporting the patient out of the room; if he must be moved, put a gown and mask on him first.

tion, infection, and cancer and understands the importance of adherence to treatment and follow-up care.

**Potential for infection related to immunosuppression.** Early after transplantation, when immunosuppression is most intense, infection is the most life-threatening complication. To prevent infection or to intervene promptly to resolve it is the key nursing goal. Recognize that immunosuppressive agents typically mask obvious signs of infection. Watch for more subtle signs, such as temperature elevation above 100° F. (37.8° C.). Obtain sputum, urine, blood, and drainage specimens for culture, as ordered.

Maintain strict asepsis when caring for drainage or incision sites. Also, institute a prophylactic antibiotic regimen, as ordered. Avoid potential sources of cross-contamination, such as the hospital room, staff, or equipment, by instituting environmental control measures, as your hospital protocol directs. After bone marrow transplant, the patient may be placed in a laminar airflow environment to reduce the risk of infection. The kidney recipient who is leukopenic or septic may be placed in strict reverse isolation. Typically, the heart or heart and lung recipient is placed in reverse isolation for up to 4 weeks. The liver recipient is placed in modified reverse isolation because postoperative infection in such patients usually results from endogenous organisms. Since all transplant patients risk hepatitis from large-volume blood transfusions during surgery, institute hepatitis precautions to protect staff and other patients.

Consider your nursing interventions effective if the patient shows no signs of infection.

**Potential alteration in tissue perfusion related to transplant rejections.** Your nursing goal is to promote optimal function of the transplanted organ. Most patients receiving transplants experience at least one rejection episode during postoperative hospitalization. For example, rejection of the transplanted heart or heart and lung is expected once or twice during the first 6 weeks when immunosuppressive therapy is being adjusted. Since early treatment improves the chance of reversing rejection, watch carefully for signs of rejection. (See *Clinical findings in graft rejection,* page 137.) Monitor the transplanted organ's function, assessing physical signs and laboratory results. Adjust immunosuppressive dosage, as ordered, and observe its effects.

Support the patient physically and emotionally if rejection occurs. Make sure he realizes that rejection is the body's normal response against tissue it recognizes as foreign and that acute rejection can be treated successfully without sacrificing organ function.

Consider your nursing interventions effective if the patient's transplanted organ functions adequately.

## A Pandora's box?

Although it has proved to be a lifesaving technique, organ transplantation has opened a veritable Pandora's box for the government, the general public, hospitals, patients and their families, and perhaps for you, too. Consider, for example, the problem of selecting patients for transplantation. Few established guidelines exist to help doctors decide which patients should receive the few available donor organs. However, the U.S. Senate passed the Organ Transplant and Procurement Act of 1984, which supports development of a sound national policy on transplantation, including a coordinated method for distribution of donor organs.

The perennial search for donor organs has caused the definition of death to come under close scrutiny. Currently, the definition of brain death is accepted in the United States. Potential cadaver donors are declared dead when doctors are certain that no brain activity remains and that the patient's life cannot continue without artificial support. However, cadaver organs can be transplanted only if the donor has willed his organs or if his next of kin gives consent when brain death occurs. Some advocate a law to permit removal of viable organs without permission of the donor's family, unless the donor expressed opposition to organ donation during his lifetime. Some religious and cultural beliefs specifically prohibit organ donation.

The limited financial resources of potential organ recipients poses another serious problem because current medical insurance plans typically don't cover the costs of transplantation. However, the federal government does reimburse the living donor or family of the cadaver donor for medical expenses associated with organ donation.

Despite these problems, organ transplantation undoubtedly has a place alongside many other medical miracles. By understanding how the immune system works in organ transplantation and by delivering skillful nursing care before and after surgery, you can help ensure that the patient benefits from this extraordinary technique.

**Points to remember**

- Successful transplantation depends on the body's inability to differentiate the transplanted organ from self or to muster its immune defenses against the foreign tissue.
- ABO or HLA antigen incompatibility commonly initiates transplant rejection.
- Rejection is classified as hyperacute, acute, or chronic, depending on the time elapsed between transplant and rejection. It may involve cell-mediated or humoral immunity, or both.
- Immunologic monitoring after transplantation may detect rejection before clinical signs of transplant organ dysfunction appear.
- Effective immunosuppression, the key to preventing transplant rejection, may be achieved through drug therapy, radiation, and pretransplant blood transfusions.
- Cyclosporine has significantly improved transplantation outcome, but it may cause hepatic and renal toxicity.
- Chief among nursing goals after transplantation is prevention of infection because immunosuppression renders the patient helpless to fight infection.
- Typically, grafts from living donors are more successful than those from cadavers.

# 10 CONTROLLING INFECTIONS

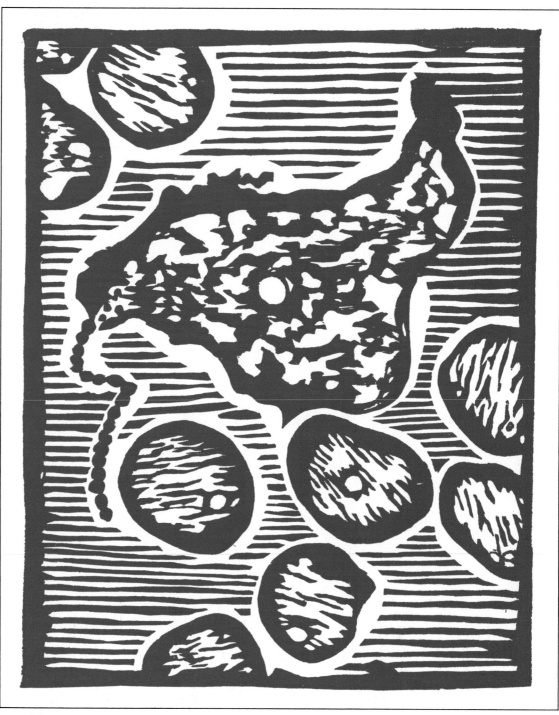

Phagocytosis

Despite improved methods of treating and preventing infectious disorders—complex immunizations, potent antibiotics, and modern sanitation methods—infection still accounts for much serious illness in the hospital as well as outside. Nosocomial (hospital-acquired) infections are a constant problem. Nosocomial infections develop in about 5% of hospitalized patients in the United States. Predisposition to these infections results from immunosuppressant therapy and from invasive procedures.

No matter what your nursing specialty, you can expect to encounter patients with infectious disorders. The infection may be the primary problem or a complication resulting from another condition. To deal effectively with an infectious disorder, you must try to bolster your patient's immune defenses. How? By taking steps to protect him from unwarranted infection; by helping him to an uneventful recovery from an infection; and by keeping an established infection from spreading.

An understanding of the pathophysiology of infection and of how your patient's immunologic and nonimmunologic defense mechanisms operate to combat it will help you manage infection more effectively.

### What is infection?

Simply defined, infection is an invasion of the body by pathogenic microorganisms (viruses, bacteria, fungi, protozoa) that reproduce and spread, causing disease by local cellular injury, secretion of a toxin, or immune (antigen-antibody) reactions in the host. Many factors can increase a patient's susceptibility to infection: extreme youth or old age; inadequate nutrition; substandard living conditions; immunosuppression resulting from chemotherapy, radiation, or steroid therapy; acquired immunodeficiency syndrome (AIDS); diabetes mellitus; debilitation resulting from chronic disease; and use of invasive procedures (such as I.V. lines, endotracheal tubes, or urinary catheters) that provide portals of entry to the body.

To induce clinical effects, pathogens must penetrate many overlapping physical and chemical barriers. Breaching these defenses is no easy task; this is probably why most people are relatively healthy despite continuous exposure to many potential pathogens. Nevertheless, the body's defenses are not impregnable, as we'll see from some examples below.

## DEFENSES: INTERRELATED

What protects the patient (or "host") from the omnipresent threat of infectious disease? Four basic lines of defense—*nonimmunologic host defenses, the inflammatory response, the mononuclear phagocyte system* (also known as *the reticuloendothelial system),* and *the immune system* itself.

If a pathogen breaches the body's nonimmunologic defenses, it is dealt with by the inflammatory response, which involves cellular elements of the mononuclear phagocyte system and cells and substances of the immune system. (For a thorough treatment of these last two systems, see Chapter 1.)

**Nonimmunologic defenses.** The skin normally presents an impenetrable barrier to invasion by microorganisms. Specific body functions, including the respiratory tract's mucociliary elevator, epithelial cell turnover, defecation, urination, salivation, sneezing, and lacrimation, also help eliminate microorganisms.

Some microorganisms defeat these barriers by their superior ability to attach themselves to tissue surfaces. Organisms with such ability include salmonella, which readily attaches to the intestinal epithelium, and *Neisseria gonorrhoeae*, which similarly attaches to the genitourinary tract.

Lysozyme, an enzyme found in tears, saliva, and nasal secretions, eliminates bacteria by attacking the mucopeptides in their cell walls.

Normal body flora stimulate natural antibody formation and help prevent other microorganisms from establishing themselves in the body. For example, *Propionibacterium acnes*, a common skin bacterium, produces lipids that inhibit colonization of *Staphylococcus aureus*.

**The inflammatory response.** When virulent microorganisms penetrate nonimmunologic barriers, chemical mediators released by inflamed tissue attract polymorphonuclear leukocytes (neutrophils) and macrophages to the site of injury via the blood. These cells, known as phagocytes, engulf the invading organisms (*phagocytosis*). In an immunocompetent host, phagocytosis and inflammation localize and destroy potential pathogens. (See *The inflammatory response,* page 143.)

Not all microorganisms fall victim to phagocytes, however. Pathogens such as *Staphylococcus aureus, Streptococcus pneumoniae, Hemophilus influenzae, Neisseria meningitidis, N. gonorrhoeae,* and *Klebsiella pneumoniae* have surface factors on their cell walls that help them resist phagocytosis. Other microorganisms are engulfed, but not harmed, and are carried to sites where they may later proliferate. Organisms with this capacity for intracellular survival include *Mycobacterium tuberculosis, Histoplasma capsulatum, Toxoplasma gondii, Mycobacterium leprae,* and *Chlamydia.*

Still other organisms, such as some staphylococci and streptococci, secrete diffusable substances known as virulence factors or aggressins, mostly enzymes, that impair phagocyte function (membrane disruption, degranulation).

Phagocytosis may also fail to destroy all the invading microorganisms if the host has an inadequate number of neutrophils (neutropenia) or if their function is impaired by genetic defect, chronic disease, or drugs such as steroids.

**The immune response.** If nonimmunologic and inflammatory defenses fail or are inadequate, a specific immune response develops. The presence of microorganisms in the body calls forth *humoral (antibody-mediated)* and *cell-mediated* immune defenses that support the inflammatory response.

*Humoral immune defenses.* Antibodies, secreted by plasma cells, play an important part in the body's defenses against invading pathogens. They provide specific protection in several ways: by neutralizing bacterial toxins; by inducing or enhancing phagocytosis, bacteriolysis, and agglutination through activation of the complement cascade; and by preventing microorganisms from attaching to mucous membranes.

Neutralization is effective against bacteria that produce toxins, such as those causing diphtheria, cholera, tetanus, gas gangrene, and botulism.

Phagocytosis is carried out most importantly by macrophages and polymorphonuclear leukocytes. Complement, functioning as an opsonin, recruits additional phagocytes and lyses bacteria. This action is especially important against capsular organisms, such as *Streptococcus pneumoniae,* that resist phagocytosis.

Bacteriolysis and agglutination involve interactions between antibody and bacterial surface antigens. In bacteriolysis—particularly significant in meningococcal and gonococcal infections—complement and an antibody work together to destroy bacteria extracellularly and intracellularly. In agglutination, specific antibodies (agglutinins) interact with insolu-

ble particles—such as gram-negative bacteria—causing them to localize or clump together, thus becoming more vulnerable to phagocytosis.

*Cell-mediated immune defenses.* Cell-mediated immunity (CMI), involving T cells, is another important means of defense, especially against viruses, mycobacteria, fungi, and intracellular parasites. When stimulated by an antigen to which it's already sensitized, the T cell secretes lymphokines that enhance the effectiveness of macrophages and other phagocytic cells.

**Immune defenses against viruses**
Extracellular viruses may be affected by many of the same immune responses elicited by bacteria. However, since antibodies only work outside cells, they cannot act against intracellular viruses.

Antibodies can help resist viruses by neutralizing antigen receptors on viral surfaces, which prevents the viruses from attaching to and penetrating host cells. Complement enhances the antibody-mediated neutralization process and, by depositing components C5 to C9 on their surfaces, may also lyse some viruses directly. Viruses coated with antibodies (opsonized) are also more susceptible to phagocytosis.

In addition to these antibody-mediated mechanisms, virus-infected cells may be destroyed by three types of cell-mediated immune mechanisms: *natural cytotoxicity, cytotoxic T cells,* and *antibody-dependent cell-mediated cytotoxicity.*

Natural cytotoxicity is mediated by *natural killer (NK) cells,* which consist of specialized T cells and macrophages. These NK cells can lyse target cells coated with antigens to which the immune system has not yet been exposed.

The presence of one type of human interferon seems to increase antiviral activity of NK cells. This interferon protects uninfected cells from infection by stimulating them to secrete protective antiviral substances. Because of its intracellular mode of action, interferon is species-specific but not virus-specific.

Cytotoxic T cells recognize viral antigens and lyse the infected cells.

Antibody-dependent cell-mediated cytotoxicity acts against virus-infected cells coated with antibodies. This type of cell lysis is mediated by cells similar to NK cells; they bind with Fc receptors present on the antibody

# The inflammatory response

Inflammation is a complex sequence of events occurring as a host defense mechanism to such threats as invasion by microorganisms or trauma. The external signs of inflammation are redness, swelling, pain, warmth, and possible loss of function at the site. Inflammation begins as a localized reaction in injured tissue, but, through the release of various chemical substances, it involves systemic changes as well.

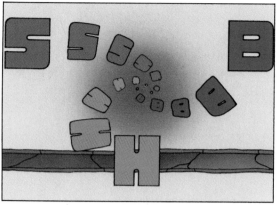

Infection or injury stimulates the release of histamine, bradykinin, serotonin, and other chemical mediators such as prostaglandins from affected tissue.

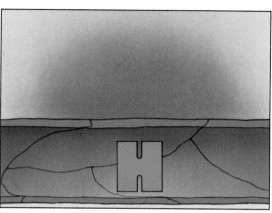

These mediators cause vasodilation and increased blood flow to the area, as evidenced by redness and warmth.

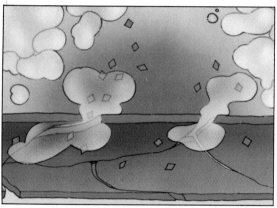

These mediators also cause increased capillary permeability, which allows protein- and fibrinogen-rich fluid to shift from the blood vessels to the interstitial space. Fibrin clots tend to wall off the area of infection, and congestion in the area causes edema, pain, and decreased function.

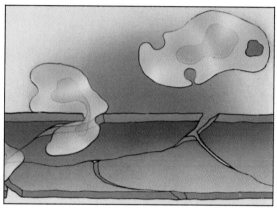

Activation of complement and other components of the immune response triggers migration of polymorphonuclear leukocytes, macrophages, and other inflammatory cells into the inflamed area, as evidenced by pus formation.

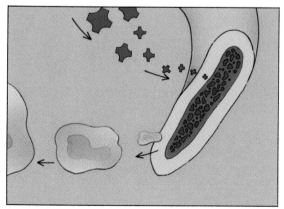

As phagocytosis occurs, other chemical mediators are released. Phagocytic cells release pyrogens, which act on the hypothalamus to increase body temperature, producing fever.

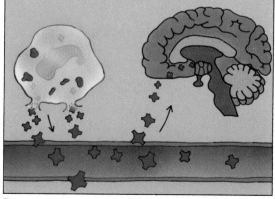

These pyrogens and other substances circulate to the bone marrow, where they increase the production and release of white blood cells. Eventually, when infection is under control, regeneration of the inflamed area occurs with fibrin deposition and scar-tissue formation.

## Modes of viral transmission

At the cellular level, viruses are transmitted in three ways: extracellularly, intercellularly by cell fusion, and intracellularly by incorporation into the cell genome. (The genome is the complete set of chromosomes contributed by one of the male-female pair.)

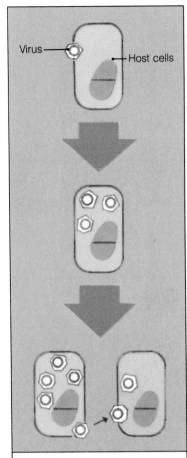

**Extracellular transmission**
In this transmission mode, viruses are released by lysis of an infected cell and spread to other cells. Influenza and adenoviruses are examples of viruses that spread by this route.

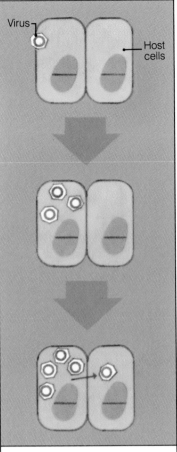

**Intercellular transmission**
In this transmission mode, viruses such as herpesvirus (especially cytomegalovirus, Epstein-Barr virus, and varicella zoster virus) spread intercellularly from host cell to host cell by inducing cell fusion. The viruses then pass through specialized structures in the cell walls (desmosomes), thus avoiding the extracellular environment.

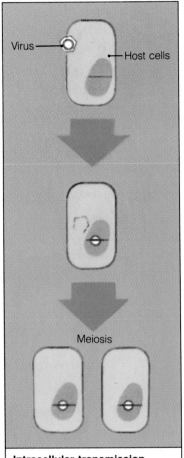

**Intracellular transmission**
In this transmission mode, viruses such as retroviruses spread by incorporating themselves into the cell genome and traveling from the parent cell to the daughter cells during meiosis.

molecules that coat the infected cell, and lyse the cell.

Some viruses, notably the influenzas, can reinfect the same host more than once because they can rapidly change the structure of their surface antigens. This trait, known as serologic plasticity or antigenic variation, enables such viruses to repeatedly sidestep immune defenses.

Other viruses spread intracellularly from host cell to host cell by inducing cell fusion—as a host cell divides, some viruses are incorporated into the new cell. And still others incorporate themselves into the cell genome in the nucleus and then pass onto the new cell during mitosis. (See *Modes of viral transmission.*)

### Immune defenses against parasites
Parasitic infections resulting from protozoa or helminths stimulate a variety of complex antibody-mediated and cell-mediated immune defenses. The specific response depends on the parasite's form and its location within the host's body. Patients with parasitic infections may recover completely with or without protection from reinfection, or they may experience a relapse or exacerbation of ongoing

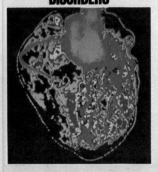
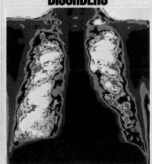
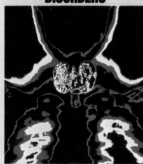
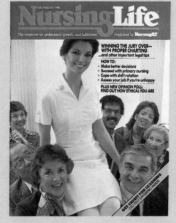

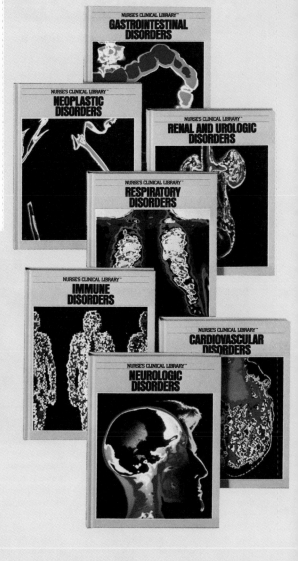

# Introduce yourself to the new NURSE'S CLINICAL LIBRARY™ series.

A comprehensive book for each specific body system disorder. That's what makes this set of books so valuable to nurses. No longer will you have to go to one book for drug information, then another for pathophysiology, and still another for diagnostics. Each book in the NURSE'S CLINICAL LIBRARY is a complete source for each body system disorder. And as a subscriber to the series, you save $3.00 off the single-copy price of each book. Act now. Send the postage-paid card above today!

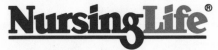
# Mail the card at left to get your trial copy of *NursingLife*.

Send no money now. Just mail the card at left and we'll send you a trial copy of *NursingLife*, the fastest growing nursing journal in the world. You'll discover how to avoid malpractice suits, answer touchy ethical questions, get along better with doctors and other nurses, work better under pressure, and much more. Send for yours today!

signs and symptoms.

Most parasitic diseases stimulate production of antibodies, even though these play a relatively minor role in the defense against parasites. Malaria is one exception; in response to multiple malarial infections, an effective IgG antibody response develops against the malarial parasite's merozoite stage.

Recent studies suggest that CMI may help prevent and control some parasitic infections, such as toxoplasmosis and schistosomiasis. Unfortunately, though, CMI may induce severe complications. For example, in a patient with schistosomiasis, a cell-mediated immune response to helminthic ova lodged within the liver may lead to granuloma formation, cirrhosis, and even death.

### Immune defenses against fungi
Fungal infections, called mycoses, are primary and usually self-limiting in immunocompetent human hosts. However, mycoses may have serious systemic effects in patients with compromised immune systems. Patients with deficient CMI may experience frequent and often life-threatening fungal infections.

### MEDICAL MANAGEMENT
Effective treatment of infectious disorders can begin only after detection of their causative organisms. This requires integration of diagnostic tests with patient history and physical examination findings. Unfortunately, specific diagnosis is often difficult because so many infections share common clinical features. (See *Recognizing common bacterial, viral, parasitic, and fungal infections,* pages 146 and 147.)

### Diagnostic tests
Various cultures as well as an array of hematologic, histologic, serologic, dermatologic, and radioimmunoassay tests are used to help diagnose infectious disorders.

**Cultures.** These tests reliably identify bacteria, fungi and some viruses. Gram's stain quickly distinguishes gram-positive from gram-negative bacteria and helps the investigator select an appropriate antibiotic treatment while awaiting results of other tests.

**Hematologic tests.** The complete blood count, combined with a white blood cell (WBC) differential, is frequently done to help determine the presence of infection. The WBC differential can provide more information about the patient's immune system and about the severity of an infection. A low WBC differ-

ential (leukopenia) may indicate viral infection, such as influenza, measles, rubella, or mononucleosis.

**Histologic tests.** Microscopic evaluation of tissue samples, using special stains and other techniques, can help identify specific pathogens. For example, viruses may cause characteristic changes in host-cell size and shape, which are diagnostic. A Tzanck smear, which involves microscopic evaluation of frozen scrapings from skin lesions, is used to identify herpesvirus.

**Serologic tests.** Based on antigen-antibody reactions, these tests are used to detect the presence of either an antigen or an antibody in the patient's blood and can sometimes identify an infectious disorder directly.

Serologic tests are not without some problems, however. For example, positive results may be delayed until the patient has had sufficient time to produce detectable levels of the antibody. Also, a positive result may only mean that the patient has been exposed to the pathogen at some time in the past. Often, tests need to be done during the acute and convalescent stages of the disorder to demonstrate a rise in the antibody titer and confirm that particular disorder. Bear in mind also that false-positive and false-negative results may occur.

*Erythrocyte sedimentation rate* and *C-reactive protein* tests, both nonspecific, are used to detect inflammation from any source.

*Cold agglutinins* are antibodies that cause red blood cells to agglutinate at low temperatures. They may be found in an infection such as atypical pneumonia (*Mycoplasma pneumoniae*).

*Hemagglutination inhibition tests* demonstrate the presence of rubella, influenza, measles, and several other viruses.

*Immunodiffusion tests can* confirm some fungal infections.

*Complement fixation tests* reveal fungal and rickettsial infections and viral infections such as mumps and influenza.

*Agglutination tests* can help diagnose tularemia, rickettsial and fungal infections, and mononucleosis.

*Precipitation tests* can help diagnose fungal infections as well as the presence of *Hemophilus influenzae* and *N. meningitidis.*

*Radioimmunoassay tests* are commonly used to detect hepatitis B antigens.

**Skin tests.** These tests elicit either a delayed or immediate hypersensitivity reaction. Antigens commonly used in skin tests are *Can-*

# Recognizing common bacterial, viral, parasitic, and fungal infections

| Infection/organism | Immunologic mechanism | Characteristics of disease |
|---|---|---|
| **Bacterial** | | |
| **Brucellosis** <br> *Brucella abortus* <br> *B. suis* <br> *B. melitensis* <br> *B. canis* | • Antibodies ineffective, used diagnostically <br> • Phagocytosis by fixed macrophages <br> • Small number of bacteria may survive macrophages | • Acute or chronic illness manifested by chills, fever, and weakness <br> • Histologic response is granuloma formation; abscesses may appear in some tissues (especially spleen and bones) |
| **Hemophilus influenzae** <br> *Hemophilus influenzae* <br> gram-negative rod | • Capsular polysaccharides are antiphagocytic <br> • Opsonic antibody effective | • Is most common cause of bacterial meningitis in infants and young children; can cause death and mental retardation <br> • Is important cause of otitis media and epiglottiditis <br> • Can cause pneumonia, bacteremia, and meningitis in adults |
| **Neisseria meningitidis** <br> *Neisseria meningitidis* <br> (meningococcus) <br> gram-negative <br> diplococcus | • Capsular polysaccharides are antiphagocytic <br> • Possesses type-specific antigens <br> • Possesses a lipopolysaccharide-endotoxin complex <br> • Pili mediate nasopharyngeal epithelium adherence <br> • Lysed by antibody and complement | • Originates in nasopharynx; ranges from transient asymptomatic bacteremia to fulminating, rapidly fatal septicemia with disseminated intravascular coagulation or Waterhouse-Friderichsen syndrome <br> • In metastatic infection, may involve joints, heart valves, and other loci, but skin and meninges are most common targets |
| **Staphylococcus aureus** <br> *Staphylococcus aureus* <br> gram-positive coccus | • Produces many aggressins, including coagulase, leukocidin, enterotoxins, and hemolysins <br> • Most organisms appear killed once ingested by polymorphonuclear leukocytes <br> • Antigen can be detected | • Can be highly destructive; produces prominent abscess formation in the heart, kidneys, lungs, muscles, joints, bones, and central nervous system (CNS) <br> • Skin infections very common <br> • Occurs in patients with foreign bodies present (for example, sutures, catheters, and heart valves) |
| **Tuberculosis** <br> *Mycobacterium tuberculosis* <br> intercellular aerobic <br> acid-fast bacillus | • Survives and proliferates in mononuclear phagocytes <br> • Lymphocyte-macrophage interaction regulates immunity but may destroy host tissue <br> • Infection well tolerated for several weeks (in non-immune patient) while active immunity develops <br> • Humoral immunity ineffective <br> • Delayed hypersensitivity | • Predominantly pulmonary disease transmitted by aerosol <br> • Secondary infection can develop in any organ system after hematogenous spread <br> • Inflammatory response is granuloma formation with giant cells and caseation necrosis |
| **Viral** | | |
| **Chicken pox** <br> Varicella zoster herpes-virus | • Antibody develops 1 to 4 days after rash <br> • Interferon concentration in vesicular fluid inversely related to severity of disease <br> • Humoral immunity occurs | • Common in childhood <br> • Successive pruritic lesions progress rapidly from macules and papules to vesicles, pustules, and crusts |
| **Cytomegalovirus (CMV)** <br> Cytomegalic virus of <br> herpes group | • Antibodies ineffective <br> • Cell-mediated immunity occurs | • Infects salivary glands <br> • Chronic; may produce hepatitis and mental retardation if acquired in utero; may cause death <br> • In older persons: CMV mononucleosis, hepatitis, rash, Guillain-Barré syndrome <br> • Commonly asymptomatic, unless immunosuppressed |
| **Herpes zoster** <br> Varicella zoster herpes-virus | • Humoral immunity ineffective <br> • Cell-mediated immunity effective but doesn't prevent relapses <br> • Immunosuppression may permit dissemination | • Common in adults <br> • May be a reactivation of a latent varicella infection <br> • Inflamed dorsal root ganglia, neurologic pain, and vesicles clustered on the dermatomes innervated by the affected ganglia <br> • Latent viruses persist in ganglia between attacks |
| **Viral hepatitis** <br> Hepatic B virus | • Immune response ineffective <br> • Persistent antigenemia due to hepatitis B surface antigen ($HB_sAg$) stimulates anti-$HB_sAg$ production, causing circulating immune complexes. If $HB_sAg$ is eliminated, illness is similar to one-shot serum sickness with transient clinical manifestations. If production of $HB_sAg$ continues, $HB_sAg$-antibody complexes are present, causing generalized necrotizing vasculitis. | • Usually subclinical <br> • If clinical, may be mild to fulminant, with fever, headache, anorexia, nausea, vomiting, and right upper quadrant pain; about 10% to 20% of patients have serum sickness with skin rashes, arthralgia, arthritis <br> • Development of necrotizing vasculitis can be life-threatening |

## Recognizing common bacterial, viral, parasitic, and fungal infections (continued)

| Infection/organism | Immunologic mechanism | Characteristics of disease |
|---|---|---|
| **Parasitic** | | |
| **African trypanosomiasis**<br>*Trypanosoma brucei*<br>*T. gambiense*<br>*T. rhodesiense* | • Nonspecific IgM increases<br>• Antigenic variation occurs<br>• Specific antibodies can lyse or clump parasites | • Transmitted by tsetse fly<br>• Sleeping sickness occurs when parasite enters CNS<br>• Intermittent fever, headaches, transient edematous swelling; enlarged lymph nodes become fibrotic; may take months to years to affect CNS; progressive CNS symptoms lead to continuous sleep, coma, and death |
| **Malaria**<br>*Plasmodium vivax*<br>*P. ovale*<br>*P. falciparum*<br>*P. malariae* | • Species-specific IgG antibody produced after multiple infections<br>• Antigenic variation occurs<br>• Reticuloendothelial activity increases<br>• Partial immunity occurs after multiple exposure | • Transmitted by female anopheline mosquitoes<br>• *P. malariae* destroys red blood cells in a 72-hour cycle; other species have 48-hour cycles<br>• Chills-fever-sweat malarial syndrome exhibited<br>• Infective merozoites released from liver cause relapse |
| **Toxoplasmosis**<br>*Toxoplasma gondii* | • IgA, IgG, and IgM antibodies produced (nonspecific)<br>• Specific antibody present<br>• Natural acquired immunity widespread; cell-mediated immunity aided by humoral factors | • Cats may be definitive hosts<br>• Generally asymptomatic; protozoan cysts appear in tissues<br>• Ranges from benign lymphadenopathy to an acute, often fatal CNS infection<br>• Fetus susceptible, especially during first trimester (usually fatal); in later pregnancy, may cause hydrocephalus, blindness, or other ocular or neurologic damage |
| **Fungal** | | |
| **Candidiasis**<br>*Candida albicans*<br>*C. tropicalis* | • Serum anti-*Candida* "clumping factors" cause *Candida* agglutination and may facilitate uptake by phagocytic cells<br>• Polymorphonuclear leukocytes are critical in hematogenous dissemination defense<br>• Renal tubule is immunologically protected focus for *C. albicans* replication | • Overnight growth occurs on mucosal surface when host defenses deficient<br>• Preferred target organs: eyes, kidneys, meninges, skin, and myocardium |
| **Coccidioidomycosis**<br>*Coccidioides immitis* | • Polymorphonuclear leukocytes are destroyed by endospores<br>• Cell-mediated immunity develops in 2 to 3 weeks, enhancing macrophages' effectiveness<br>• Delayed hypersensitivity | • Mostly asymptomatic<br>• May present as a pulmonary disease—pneumonia, abscesses, and thin-walled cysts—or as a disseminated disease process<br>• Most devastating is meningeal involvement, which is usually complicated by hydrocephalus |
| **Histoplasmosis**<br>*Histoplasma capsulatum* | • Cell-mediated immunity effective<br>• Antibodies produced are useful for diagnosis<br>• Delayed hypersensitivity | • Self-limiting pulmonary disease<br>• Systemic dissemination may occur, usually in immunocompromised patients<br>• Granulomatous lesions form; liver, spleen, and lymph nodes enlarge; and high fever occurs |

*dida*, mumps, tuberculosis, coccidioidomycosis, and histoplasmosis. As in serologic tests, skin tests often give false-negative or false-positive results. For example, if a patient is allergic to the diluent in which an antigen is suspended, a false-positive reading is possible unless the diluent is used as a control. Conversely, if a patient is anergic or if the skin test is administered incorrectly, a false-negative reading may result.

### Treatment: Drugs, surgery
Effective treatment depends on the causative microorganism and the associated disease and may involve drug therapy, surgery, or both.

**Drug therapy.** Infection may require antibiotics to combat the pathogen and other drugs to relieve the symptoms of the infection. Sometimes antibiotics alone may provide relief from associated symptoms as they work against the causative agent.

Antibiotics usually control infections if selected correctly. This depends on pathogens' susceptibility to the drug; the ability of the drug to reach or penetrate the infected tissue; and the drug's compatibility with the patient's condition. For an immunocompromised patient, it's often better to use a bactericidal antibiotic rather than one that's bacteriostatic. In kidney or liver failure, the antibiotic chosen should not be toxic to these organs.

Various drugs may be required to relieve distressing symptoms. Some topical and systemic agents help relieve pruritus and pain accompanying rashes in such diseases as measles, chicken pox, and herpes. Cough suppressants may be indicated when coughing interferes with rest and nutrition; but because coughing helps clear the respiratory tract, these suppressants shouldn't be used indiscriminately. Similarly, antidiarrheals are recommended only for diarrhea that isn't self-limiting. Although diarrhea helps remove pathogens or their toxins, persistent diarrhea can lead to severe fluid and electrolyte imbalance.

A mild analgesic may be administered for pain, although most pain resolves quickly after the start of antimicrobial therapy.

**Surgery.** Surgical procedures may be required to drain abscesses, debride necrotic tissue at infection sites, excise anaerobic cellulitis, remove products of conception after a septic abortion, or remove foreign bodies.

## NURSING MANAGEMENT
Effective nursing care of the infected patient requires a careful patient history, followed by a thorough physical examination to help identify the pathogen and plan appropriate intervention.

### Obtain a patient history
Begin by asking the patient about himself; find out about his home, neighborhood, and workplace. This data can provide clues about diseases endemic to particular areas.

Ask the patient if he can recall any exposure he might have had to an infectious disease; remember that some diseases have a long incubation or latent period, so that even exposures that occurred several years ago may provide useful information. Has he contracted any infectious diseases in the past? Does the same infection tend to recur? How often? This may provide clues about the patient's level of immunocompetence.

Ask the patient about recent travel. Since it provides opportunities for exposure to endemic pathogens, find out when and where he went and how long he stayed. Did he briefly visit another area or country, or did he work or live there? While traveling, did he visit cities or rural or wilderness areas? While traveling in endemic areas, did he take prophylactic antibiotics or exercise any other special precautions?

Try to find out about any potential exposure to contaminated food or water. Does the patient consume raw (unpasteurized) milk or milk products, or raw or undercooked meat or fish? In many cultures, people routinely consume raw meat and fish, so define the patient's dietary habits in detail.

Does his water supply come from a municipal system, a well, or a surface source? Does he swim in lakes or streams or use them as water sources during camping or hiking trips? Such activities may risk exposure to the parasite *Giardia lamblia.*

Ask the patient about any contact with animals, including insects and birds. Explain that animals can transmit pathogens to humans. Find out if he has any pets or has had any close contact with someone else's pets. Has he ever spent time on a farm or worked with animals? Has he ever been exposed to animal excrement, handled dead animals, or been bitten by any animals?

Ask about any other circumstances that suggest a pathogen; for example:
• Immunosuppressive agents, such as corticosteroids, radiation, or chemotherapy, increase the patient's susceptibility to infection. Therefore, a patient undergoing treatment for cancer, or one who has had a tissue transplant, must be watched very closely. Even the transplanted tissue itself may transmit infectious agents.
• Use of other drugs, especially aspirin, indomethacin, and other anti-inflammatory drugs, as well as alcohol or heroin abuse may impair the inflammatory response.
• Transfusions of contaminated blood or blood products can transmit syphilis, hepatitis, malaria, or AIDS.
• Past accidents, trauma, or surgery may provide entry sites for microorganisms. Hormones associated with pregnancy may also suppress the immune system.
• Chronic diseases, such as hyper- and hypothyroidism, diabetes mellitus, renal failure, and hepatic malfunction, can compromise the body's immune response and its ability to heal traumatized tissue.
• Certain human leukocyte antigen types are associated with increased susceptibility to some diseases.
• A psychosocial history may reveal substandard living conditions or exposure to health hazards. Determining sexual practices (including number and sex of partners) may identify patients exposed to sexually transmitted diseases, such as gonorrhea, syphilis, or AIDS.

**Look for signs and symptoms.** Ask the patient about characteristic signs and symptoms linked to infectious diseases. First ask about general symptoms, such as malaise, listlessness, inability to concentrate, apathy, uneasiness, light-headedness, weakness, and aching joints. Then ask about specific symptoms as you examine the patient thoroughly. Infectious diseases can affect the GI, neurologic, and hematopoietic systems. Anorexia, nausea, vomiting, and diarrhea are common; anxiety, confusion, delirium, or convulsions may result from infection of brain tissue or from metabolic abnormalities caused by the infection. Leukocytosis usually occurs during an infection; anemia, in prolonged infections. Alterations in coagulation factors can result in disseminated intravascular coagulation.

## Perform the physical examination

Because most infectious diseases produce varied and widespread signs and symptoms, your examination must include all of the patient's body systems. Remember that some signs and symptoms develop later in the course of his infection. For this reason, routine patient reassessment is critical.

**Assess vital signs.** Note the presence of fever, a hallmark of infection. Only a few infections—notably gonorrhea, syphilis, and lepromatous leprosy—fail to induce fever.

Check the pulse for tachycardia, which commonly accompanies fever; septic shock can cause cardiovascular collapse. Check for hypotension, which may occur without shock in severe infections.

Check the patient's respirations for rate, depth, and rhythm, and auscultate his heart and lungs for signs of dyspnea and respiratory distress. Dyspnea, sneezing, coughing, sputum production, hemoptysis, or night sweats suggest pulmonary infections.

**Inspect the skin.** Check for rashes, lesions, sores, ulcers, and changes in color, temperature and moisture. Don't forget to look between fingers and toes and under the breasts or scrotum. Also, assess the mouth and throat. Sore throat may occur in many infections. Sores on the tongue or on mucous membranes, as well as dental caries, may provide entry sites for microorganisms.

Any lesions or open areas, regardless of size, can be significant. Ask the patient when the lesion first appeared and if it has changed in any way, and ask if it itches. Note the appearance, location, size, and number of all lesions.

If drainage is present, record its color and consistency. Take care to avoid direct contact with lesions or with drainage, which may be infectious.

**Examine the eyes.** Look for redness, swelling, itching, tearing, and drainage. Abnormal findings may suggest cellulitis, corneal infection, or endophthalmitis.

**Perform palpation.** Palpate the abdomen for organomegaly or masses, and listen for bowel sounds to evaluate peristalsis. Palpate all lymph nodes for signs of enlargement and other changes.

**Inspect the musculoskeletal system.** Key findings on inspection include tenderness or pain affecting the ears, nose, fingernails, or toenails. Also, check for muscle weakness and limitations in range-of-joint movement. Note the presence and location of joint tenderness, erythema, or swelling.

## Formulate nursing diagnoses

When you've completed the patient history and physical examination, you're ready to formulate nursing diagnoses and to establish an appropriate care plan. In patients with infectious disease, your nursing diagnoses may include the following:

**Alteration in body temperature secondary to an infectious disorder.** Your goal is to help the patient achieve a stable or declining body temperature. Keep in mind that, although fever usually results from infection, the degree of fever may not accurately reflect the infection's severity. Neonates, very young infants, and very elderly patients may have subnormal temperatures during an infection. Also, immunocompromised patients may manifest only a slight fever response to even a severe infection.

Common neurologic signs and symptoms of fever include lethargy, irritability, headache, and photophobia. Monitor the patient's mental status for signs of decompensation, such as confusion or disorientation.

Take the patient's temperature every 4 to 6 hours at the same times each day and by the same route (axillary, oral, or rectal.) If the infection responds to the appropriate antibiotics, the patient's temperature should decline within 48 hours of starting the drugs. Note the administration of antipyretics on the fever chart, and be aware of antipyretics in other drugs, such as analgesics.

If necessary, reduce the patient's temperature; make sure the room isn't overheated, remove unnecessary clothing and covers, ad-

### EMERGENCY MANAGEMENT

# Treating septic shock

Septic shock is caused by septicemia, a potential complication of urinary, intestinal, biliary, and female genital tract infections.

Researchers believe septic shock is triggered by the effects of microbial toxins on host cells. In many cases, it is caused by the endotoxin in the gram-negative cell wall, although gram-positive bacteria as well as other microorganisms may also be responsible.

Immunosuppression is a risk factor and is usually present when viruses, parasites, or fungi cause shock. Other risk factors include diabetes mellitus, cirrhosis of the liver, and burns.

Signs and symptoms of septic shock are nonspecific and subtle. If undetected, they rapidly progress to cardiovascular failure. Mortality is about 50%.

Signs and symptoms of early (warm) shock include warm, dry skin; normal or slightly elevated blood pressure; widening pulse pressure; bounding pulse; chills and fever; moderate tachycardia; increased respirations; and mental confusion.

Signs and symptoms of late (cold) shock include pale, moist skin; chills and fever; marked disorientation; tachycardia; and increased respirations.

If you suspect septic shock, immediately notify the doctor and follow these guidelines.
• Give oxygen as ordered. Monitor arterial blood gases.
• Establish an I.V. line. If your patient already has one in place, check and maintain its patency. Prepare the patient for insertion of a central venous or pulmonary artery catheter.
• Insert an indwelling (Foley) catheter to monitor urine output.
• Draw blood culture specimens and collect body fluid specimens, as ordered. Be sure to obtain all blood and culture specimens before administering the first dose of an antibiotic.
• Give fluids and drugs I.V., as ordered. Usually, the doctor orders rapid infusion of Ringer's lactate solution or normal saline solution with sodium bicarbonate to prevent circulatory col-

lapse from third-space fluid shift.
• Monitor vital signs every 30 minutes or more frequently, as indicated.

• Document your findings.
*Important:* If these interventions fail to reverse warm shock, prepare your patient for transfer to the intensive care unit.

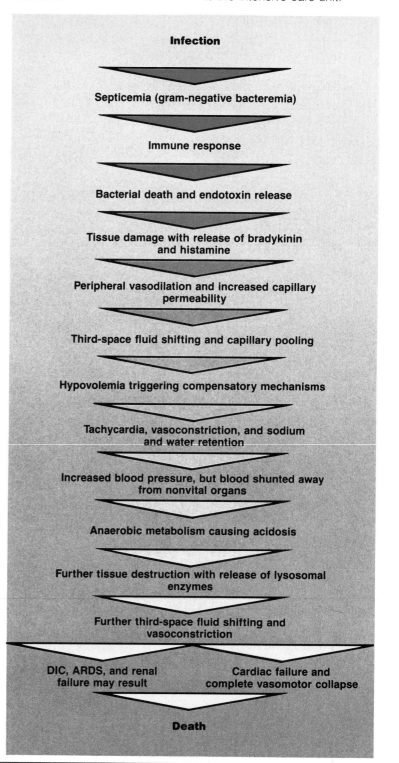

**Infection**

**Septicemia (gram-negative bacteremia)**

**Immune response**

**Bacterial death and endotoxin release**

**Tissue damage with release of bradykinin and histamine**

**Peripheral vasodilation and increased capillary permeability**

**Third-space fluid shifting and capillary pooling**

**Hypovolemia triggering compensatory mechanisms**

**Tachycardia, vasoconstriction, and sodium and water retention**

**Increased blood pressure, but blood shunted away from nonvital organs**

**Anaerobic metabolism causing acidosis**

**Further tissue destruction with release of lysosomal enzymes**

**Further third-space fluid shifting and vasoconstriction**

**DIC, ARDS, and renal failure may result**          **Cardiac failure and complete vasomotor collapse**

**Death**

minister antipyretics, and give the patient a tepid sponge bath.

Monitor the patient's heart and respiratory rates, blood pressure, urine output, electrolyte levels, and blood gases to determine if he can tolerate the increased metabolic rate that accompanies fever. Remember that fever increases metabolic rate about 15% for every 1-degree (Centigrade) rise in temperature.

**Alteration in nutrition due to increased metabolic rate from fever.** Your goal is to meet the patient's increased nutritional needs. This is often difficult due to symptoms such as nausea, vomiting, diarrhea, and lethargy.

To help reduce the metabolic rate, schedule adequate rest and fewer activities.

Monitor the patient's weight and his fluid intake and output. Also, if necessary, consult the dietitian to help plan meals with adequate calories and protein.

**Potential for fluid volume deficit due to an infectious disease.** Your goal is to maintain adequate fluid volume. Some symptoms (sore mouth and throat, nausea, and lethargy) may prevent adequate fluid intake, whereas others (diarrhea, vomiting, and sweating) increase fluid loss. In sepsis, fluid may shift to intravascular spaces. Monitor the patient's intake and output from all sources. Also check pulse and respiration rates, blood pressure, and urine specific gravity to help evaluate his fluid status.

**Potential for nosocomial infection related to hospitalization.** Your goal is to protect your patient from acquiring a nosocomial infection during his hospitalization. Practice good infection-control procedures, such as washing your hands before and after patient contact. Reduce accumulated secretions in the patient's lungs by encouraging coughing and deep breathing, promoting early ambulation, and elevating the head of the bed.

Prevent bowel flora from gaining access to the blood by helping the patient avoid constipation and hard stools. Keep a stool chart; encourage adequate fluid intake; provide a diet high in roughage; promote early ambulation; and administer stool softeners and laxatives, as needed.

To help prevent skin breakdown in the bedridden patient, change his position frequently. Also, provide meticulous care of the mouth, perineum, invasive lines, tubes, and catheters. In a patient with a compromised immune system, provide protective precautions.

Remember that antibiotics used to treat one infection may not protect the patient against other infections.

**Potential for transmitting contagious disease.** Your goal is to help prevent the spread of a contagious disease to visitors, hospital personnel, or other patients. Question the patient about any contacts he has had with family, friends, and others. If necessary, isolate the patient as directed by your hospital's policy or according to precautions established by the Centers for Disease Control.

Familiarize yourself with the procedure for reporting certain infectious diseases to the state health department. Examples of reportable diseases are tuberculosis, hepatitis, gonorrhea, poliomyelitis, syphilis, measles, and rubella. Reporting the patient's disease will help ensure that the patient's family, friends, and other contacts receive appropriate prophylactic treatment.

**Knowledge deficit regarding infection management and prevention.** Your goal is to help the patient understand his disease and its management. Develop an individualized teaching plan to help the patient achieve this goal. Explain the infection, its mode of transmission, and its signs and symptoms. Review the basics of good nutrition and hygiene.

Instruct the patient about medications and their possible adverse effects, and emphasize the importance of promptly reporting adverse effects. Be sure he knows how to perform any special procedures, such as dressing changes, before leaving the hospital.

### Evaluate your interventions

Consider your nursing interventions successful if the patient's vital signs, mental status, and urine output remain stable; if his fever remains stable or subsides; if his weight remains stable; if electrolyte, protein, and albumin levels remain normal; if no new infections develop and contagious infections don't spread to visitors, hospital personnel, or other patients; and if the patient recognizes the signs and symptoms of his disease and understands all aspects of its management.

### Keys to care: Monitoring and support

Detection and management of infectious disorders have improved in recent years. Your careful assessment techniques can often help to correctly diagnose an infectious disorder early on. And your care plan to combat fever and the spread of infection, your monitoring of the treatment's progress, and your ongoing psychological support should ensure an uneventful recovery for your patient.

**Points to remember**

- The immune system prevents or controls infectious disease in the host by mobilizing four levels of defense to turn aside or destroy pathogens.
- Humoral and cell-mediated immune defense mechanisms protect the intact host against most bacterial, viral, parasitic, and fungal infections.
- Many kinds of microorganisms escape host-initiated immune reactions by producing antiphagocytic surface factors and by using intracellular modes of transmission.
- Correct pathogen identification is critical to effective management of infectious disease.

# 11 RECOGNIZING HEMATOLOGIC DISORDERS

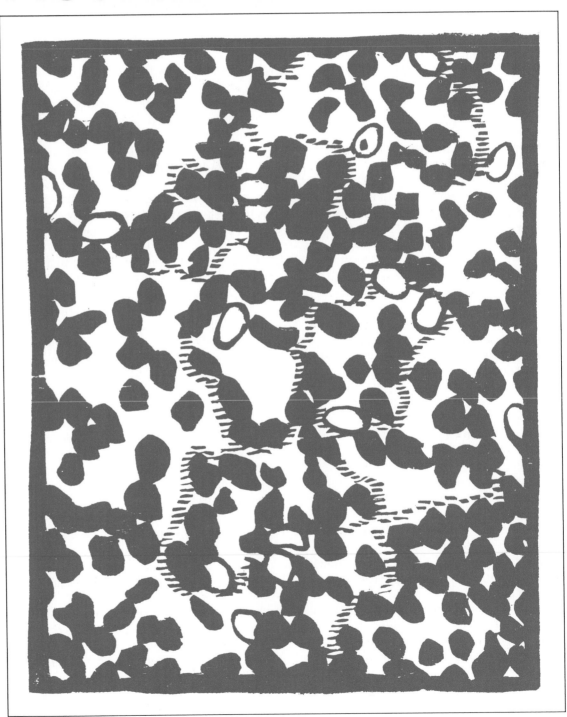

Lymphoma cells

The hematologic and immune systems are closely related because they share a functional unit—the leukocyte (white blood cell, or WBC), one of the three formed elements of blood and an integral part of the immune response. Immune dysfunction can affect leukocytes, as well as erythrocytes (red blood cells, or RBCs) and thrombocytes. When this happens, disruption of both immunologic and hematologic systems can result in a limited, self-stabilizing condition or a progressive, overtly destructive disorder.

Because of the complex interaction of these systems, immune-related hematologic disorders are commonly difficult to identify and to manage. Patients with these disorders may present diverse signs and symptoms, as in complicated multiple myeloma. Others may show no signs or symptoms at all, as in chronic lymphocytic leukemia. Still others may develop complications from bleeding and infection, producing medical emergencies. With a thorough understanding of the pathology and current treatment of these disorders, you can confidently manage such patients.

## PATHOPHYSIOLOGY
Immune-related hematologic disorders vary considerably in symptomatology, clinical course, and prognosis and can be broadly classified into two groups: diseases involving destruction of blood cells and diseases involving the abnormal proliferation of WBCs. (See *Classification of immune-related hematologic disorders,* page 154.)

### Destructive blood disorders
These disorders, including immune hemolytic anemias, immune thrombocytopenias, and immune neutropenias, follow sensitization of blood cells with antibody. Their specific immunologic mechanisms vary.

**Immune hemolytic anemias.** Excessive destruction of RBCs (hemolysis) following RBC sensitization with autoantibodies characterizes these disorders. Signs and symptoms vary and may include fatigue, dyspnea, palpitations, jaundice, and, in severe disorders, shock. In *autoimmune hemolytic anemia,* sensitization can occur two ways: through a warm reacting antibody (generally an IgG that reacts with RBCs at 37° C. [98.6° F.]) or through a cold reacting antibody (generally an IgM that reacts with RBCs below 37° C.). Each may be secondary to other autoimmune diseases or to infections but may also be idiopathic.

Several mechanisms can cause *drug-induced immune hemolytic anemia.*
• Preformed immune complexes that occur between drug and drug antibody sensitize RBCs. (This is known as the "innocent bystander" mechanism.)
• The drug binds to RBC membranes, acting as a hapten and causing a high titer of drug antibodies.
• The drug may modify the RBC membrane, making the cells more susceptible to lysis.
• Other drug actions, which are not yet understood, may also occur.

*Alloantibody-induced immune hemolytic anemia* occurs when self-immunization triggers hemolysis. For example, in hemolytic anemia of the newborn, maternal IgG antibodies cross the placenta and react with antigens on fetal RBCs. Another type of alloantibody-induced hemolytic reaction sometimes occurs after a blood transfusion, when the transfused blood contains an antigen for which the patient has an antibody.

**Immune thrombocytopenias.** Thrombocytopenias involving platelet destruction result from platelet sensitization by autoantibodies. Classic signs are bleeding and purpura.

*Idiopathic thrombocytopenic purpura (ITP)* results from autoantibody destruction of circulating platelets and subsequent removal of these cells by macrophages of the spleen (and sometimes of the liver) and by other parts of the monocyte-macrophage system. It typically affects children (often after a viral infection) and young adults.

*Drug-induced immune thrombocytopenia* occurs through one of the mechanisms described under drug-induced immune hemolytic anemia. (See *Drugs that cause destructive hematologic disorders.*)

*Neonatal thrombocytopenic purpura* can occur when maternal antiplatelet antibodies cross the placenta.

*Posttransfusion purpura* occurs about 1 week after transfusion of a blood product. Its cause is usually an alloantibody in the transfused blood that's generally directed against the platelet $PLA_1$ antigen. It occurs almost exclusively in women.

**Immune neutropenias.** Immune-related neutropenias result from a deficiency of circulating neutrophils caused by increased neutrophil destruction or decreased neutrophil production. Signs and symptoms vary and may include painful buccal or pharyngeal mucosal ulcers, fever, chills, weakness, and extreme prostration.

## Drugs that cause destructive hematologic disorders

**Immune thrombocytopenias:**
Aspirin
Carbamazepine
Cephalothin
Digitoxin
Methyldopa
Phenytoin
Quinidine
Quinine
Rifampin
Thiazide diuretics
D-penicillamine

**Immune hemolytic anemias:**
Aminosalicylic acid (PAS)
Chlorpromazine
Insulin
Isoniazid
Levodopa
Mefenamic acid
Melphalan
Methyldopa
Penicillin
Quinidine
Quinine
Rifampin
Sulfonamides
Sulfonylureas
Cephalosporins
Thiazide diuretics
Acetaminophen

**Immune neutropenias:**
Sulfonamides
Tolbutamide
Chlorpropamide
Phenylbutazone
Propylthiouracil

# Classification of immune-related hematologic disorders

### Destructive disorders

**Thrombocytic**
- Idiopathic (autoimmune) thrombocytopenic purpura
- Autoimmune thrombocytopenias secondary to autoimmune disorders such as systemic lupus erythematosus (SLE) and to proliferative white blood cell (WBC) disorders and infections
- Drug-induced immune thrombocytopenias
- Posttransfusion purpura
- Alloantibody-induced immune thrombocytopenias from maternal sensitization during pregnancy or from sensitization due to previous transfusions

**Erythrocytic**
- Autoimmune hemolytic anemias, such as warm-antibody types and cold-antibody types
- Drug-induced immune hemolytic anemia
- Alloantibody-induced immune hemolytic anemias, such as hemolytic transfusion reactions and hemolytic disease of the neonate

**Neutrocytic**
- Autoimmune neutropenia secondary to autoimmune disorders such as SLE or rheumatoid arthritis
- Drug-induced neutropenia
- Isoimmune neonatal neutropenia

### Proliferative disorders

**Leukemias**
- Acute lymphocytic leukemia
- Acute nonlymphocytic leukemia
- Chronic myelogenous leukemia
- Chronic lymphocytic leukemia
- Hairy-cell leukemia

**Lymphomas**
- Hodgkin's disease
- Non-Hodgkin's lymphomas

**Plasma cell dyscrasias**
- Multiple myeloma
- Waldenström's macroglobulinemia
- Others

*In autoimmune neutropenia,* production of autoantibodies with specificity for antigens NA$_2$ and ND results in neutrophil destruction. This disorder sometimes accompanies an underlying autoimmune disease, such as systemic lupus erythematosus (SLE) or rheumatoid arthritis. When this happens, the causative mechanism may be the neutrophils' adsorption of immune complexes.

*Drug-induced neutropenia* may result from bone marrow suppression or the innocent bystander mechanism (attachment of drug-antibody immune complexes to neutrophils).

*Isoimmune neonatal neutropenia* probably results when fetal neutrophils enter maternal blood, stimulating antibody production there; these antibodies presumably reenter fetal blood and agglutinate circulating neutrophils during the neonatal period.

## Proliferative WBC disorders

Abnormal proliferation of WBCs, the primary cells of the immune system, results in a wide range of disorders generally classified as leukemias, lymphomas, and plasma cell dyscrasias. (See *Classification of malignant lymphoproliferative diseases by lymphocyte type.*)

**Leukemias.** As you probably know, these diseases—classified as acute or chronic—involve proliferation of WBCs through abnormal maturation. These abnormal cells accumulate in the peripheral blood, bone marrow, and body tissues. General signs and symptoms include anemia, bleeding, and infection.

In *acute leukemia,* cell maturation is blocked at the primitive blast stage. Immature leukemia cells collect in the bone marrow and in other tissue, destroying normal hematopoietic function. Clinical features vary, depending on the type of acute leukemia, but generally include weakness, fever, weight loss, anemia, bleeding, and infection.

*Chronic leukemias* are characterized by abnormal accumulation of cells that are better differentiated than those of acute leukemia. In chronic myelogenous leukemia, abnormal myeloid cells accumulate in the blood, bone marrow, spleen, and other organs. This disease may progress to acute leukemia. In chronic lymphocytic leukemia (CLL), small lymphocytes with abnormally long life spans accumulate in blood, lymph nodes, and bone marrow and in the liver, spleen, and other organs. In some patients, this condition remains asymptomatic and benign for years; in others, it progresses rapidly.

**Lymphomas.** These solid malignant tumors of the immune system involve abnormal proliferation of lymphoid stem cells or their lymphocytic or histiocytic derivatives. Signs and symptoms generally include painless lymph node enlargement, pruritus, fever, weight loss, infection, and bone and central nervous system (CNS) involvement.

In *Hodgkin's disease,* proliferative cells include lymphocytes, histiocytes, eosinophils, and Reed-Sternberg cells. Relative predominance of lymphocytes varies according to the type of Hodgkin's disease. Types in which lymphocytes predominate (often affecting younger patients) have the best prognosis.

*Non-Hodgkin's lymphoma* involves lymphocytic, histiocytic, or mixed types. The affected cells may demonstrate incohesive aggregation or no aggregation, but they characteristically cause effacement and subsequent enlargement of lymph nodes.

**Plasma cell dyscrasias.** These disorders can occur when a single clone of plasma cells normally involved in immunoglobulin synthesis proliferates disproportionately, causing an overabundance of various immunoglobulins. The monoclonal immunoglobulin (or paraprotein), which can be found in the patient's serum or urine, characterizes plasma cell dyscrasias.

*Multiple myeloma's* characteristics include marrow plasma cell tumors and the presence of serum or urine paraprotein (IgG, IgA, IgD, or IgE paraproteins or Bence Jones protein). Signs and symptoms include anemia, recurrent infections, skeletal pain, and sometimes CNS involvement or renal failure. Infiltration of bone produces osteolytic lesions, predisposing patients to spontaneous fractures. Prognosis is better for patients with IgG-type myeloma proteins and for patients who respond slowly and steadily to drug therapy. Patients with multiple myeloma sometimes develop acute leukemia.

*Waldenström's macroglobulinemia* is marked by excess production of IgM, the direct cause of the resulting—and characteristic—hyperviscosity syndrome. Raynaud's phenomenon and recurrent bacterial infections may occur.

## MEDICAL MANAGEMENT
Correct management requires diagnosis based on a battery of appropriate tests. Treatment, of course, is aimed at minimizing or eradicating the disorder's cause.

### Diagnosis
Laboratory investigation of immune-related hematologic diseases begins with routine blood tests and proceeds to immunologic tests; specific tests are selected according to the suspected diagnosis.

**Blood tests.** Abnormal findings on standard blood tests can be the first clue to diagnosis. General studies ordered include complete blood count with WBC differential, RBC indices, reticulocyte count and differential, platelet count, peripheral cell smears, and erythrocyte sedimentation rate.

Results of these tests may suggest hemolytic disease in a patient who hasn't suffered blood loss when a normochromic, normocytic anemia is apparent with a substantial reticulocytosis. In a patient with severe hemolysis, reticulocyte production may be four to eight times above basal level or even higher.

In ITP, the *platelet count* is usually below 100,000 µl; a peripheral cell smear may show no platelets; and anemia, if present, is secondary to blood loss or due to combined hemolytic anemia and ITP.

A *granulocyte count* below 1,500/mm³ may indicate neutropenia (except in infants less than 1 month old).

Leukocytosis classically indicates not only leukemia but also a variety of other disorders, such as infections. Diagnosis of leukemia requires histologic examination of bone marrow.

**Bone marrow and lymph node histology.** Bone marrow aspiration and biopsy provide valuable information about blood disorders, aiding the diagnosis of thrombocytopenia, leukemia, Hodgkin's and non-Hodgkin's lymphomas, and plasma cell dyscrasias.

In thrombocytopenia, bone marrow megakaryocytes are abnormal and more numerous but are not surrounded by platelets.

In acute leukemia, bone marrow biopsy shows an increased number of blast cells; in chronic myelogenous leukemia, results show myeloid hyperplasia with immature myeloid cells. In plasma cell dyscrasias such as multiple myeloma, biopsy shows more plasma cells in bone marrow.

Analysis of lymph node tissue is instrumental in the diagnosis and classification of lymphomas. (See *Histologic classification of lymphomas,* page 156.)

**Bleeding and clotting times.** Coagulation tests evaluating these factors are sometimes used to evaluate bleeding disorders, especially immune thrombocytopenias, in which bleeding time is prolonged. Partial thromboplastin time (PTT) and prothrombin time (PT) are normal, but clot retraction is poor and, in severe illness, prothrombin consumption is low. A positive capillary fragility test also characterizes thrombocytopenia.

**Compatibility testing.** This is done for all patients before blood transfusions to prevent the development of alloantibody-induced immune hemolytic anemia. Compatibility testing includes determining ABO type and Rh factor (see *Routine ABO typing,* page 157); testing blood serum for alloantibodies; and testing the patient's serum with the donor's RBCs (cross matching) to ensure compatibility and to check for alloantibodies not present in reagent blood cells.

**Immunologic tests.** The specific immunologic tests ordered for a patient generally depend on blood test results and on the type of disorder the doctor suspects.

Immunologic tests are vital when hemolytic anemia is suspected because diagnosis of

## Classification of malignant lymphoproliferative diseases by lymphocyte type

**B lymphocyte**
Chronic lymphocytic leukemia (CLL)
Multiple myeloma
Waldenström's macroglobulinemia
Heavy chain diseases
Most lymphomas with favorable histology
Burkitt's lymphoma
Immunoblastic sarcoma of B cells
B-cell variant of acute lymphoblastic leukemia (ALL)

**T lymphocyte**
T-cell variant of CLL
Mycosis fungoides-Sézary syndrome
Some lymphomas with unfavorable histology
T-cell ALL
Immunoblastic sarcoma of T cells

**Monocyte, macrophage**
Histiocytic medullary reticulosis
Hodgkin's disease (possible)

**Undefined, uncertain**
Common ALL of childhood
Leukemic reticuloendotheliosis (hairy-cell leukemia)
Hodgkin's disease

## Histologic classification of lymphomas

### Hodgkin's disease (Rye conference)

Lymphocyte predominance
Nodular sclerosis
Mixed cellularity
Lymphocyte depletion

### Non-Hodgkin's lymphomas (Rappaport)

Nodular
  Lymphocytic, well differentiated
  Lymphocytic, poorly differentiated
  Mixed lymphocytic-histiocytic
  Histiocytic
Diffuse
  Lymphocytic, well differentiated
  Lymphocytic, poorly differentiated
  Mixed lymphocytic-histiocytic
  Undifferentiated
  Histiocytic

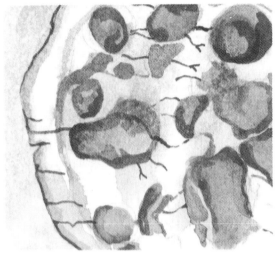

*Hodgkin's nodular sclerosis*

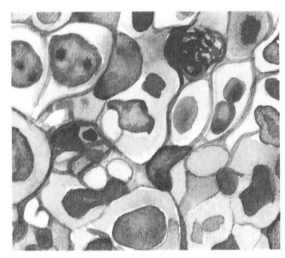

*Non-Hodgkin's diffuse histiocytic*

this disease depends on detecting immunoglobulins (antibodies) on the surfaces of RBCs. One way to do this is with the Coombs' test, which assesses antibody activity at various temperatures to evaluate the patient for cold- or warm-antibody types.

To evaluate a patient for ITP, a variety of immunologic tests may be done to determine the presence of antiplatelet antibodies. These tests include radiolabeled Coombs' reagent assay, antiglobulin consumption assay, and radioactive staphylococcal protein A–binding assay.

Immunologic tests often used to detect immune neutropenias include the microleukocyte agglutination test, antiglobulin consumption assay, and alveolar macrophage test, as well as granulocyte cytotoxicity assays.

Other specific immunologic tests may be needed to diagnose diseases such as SLE, which may underlie autoimmune hemolytic anemia or ITP in some patients. Autoimmune diseases associated with immune neutropenias can be detected with serum antinuclear antibody or neutrophil cell-surface immune complex tests.

Serum protein electrophoresis and immunoelectrophoresis aid in the diagnosis of proliferative WBC disorders (paraproteinemia). They identify paraproteins seen in malignant plasma cell dyscrasias.

**Other tests.** Diagnosis may also require urinalysis, routine chemistries, serum viscosity tests, and such procedures as chest X-rays, skeletal bone surveys, and bone scans.

### Treatment

Treatment of immune-related hematologic disorders depends, as you'd expect, on the cause. For example, treatment of a hemolytic reaction during drug therapy or a blood transfusion requires discontinuation of the drug or the transfusion and appropriate symptomatic therapy. (See *Immediate reactions to blood transfusions,* page 158.)

The main goal in treating proliferative WBC disorders is mass destruction of abnormal cells.

**Drug therapy.** Corticosteroids (most commonly prednisone) are generally effective for patients with the warm-antibody type of autoimmune hemolytic anemia. When corticosteroids aren't effective, splenectomy may be performed.

Immunosuppressive drug therapy with cytotoxic drugs may be used for postsplenectomy patients with ITP; if a patient with ITP doesn't respond to splenectomy or isn't a candidate for it (see below), vincristine may be effective. Most patients with multiple myeloma respond well to cytotoxic drug therapy.

In a large percentage of patients with acute lymphoblastic leukemia (ALL), especially children, initial therapy with drugs produces primary remission.

Antimicrobial drug therapy is necessary for patients with neutropenia who develop fevers above 100.4° F. (38° C.). The recommended therapy is I.V. administration of ticarcillin disodium and gentamicin.

Drug therapy may also be necessary for some patients with Waldenström's macroglobulinemia who need frequent plasmapheresis.

**Splenectomy.** This surgical procedure may be used for patients with the warm-antibody type of autoimmune hemolytic anemia when corticosteroids are ineffective or when hemolysis persists after 2 to 3 months of corticosteroid therapy. However, splenectomy is ineffective for patients with cold-antibody types of autoimmune hemolytic anemia and for those with the warm-antibody type of immune hemolytic anemia in which erythrocytes are coated only with complement or with IgM and complement.

For adult patients with persistent and symptomatic ITP that hasn't responded to steroids, splenectomy is the treatment of choice. It produces complete, prolonged remission in most such patients.

**Plasmapheresis.** This procedure, used for patients with Waldenström's macroglobulinemia, removes excess IgM antibodies.

**Transfusions.** Paradoxically, blood transfusions can be the cause of, or cure for, hemolytic reactions. Of course, when a transfusion is the cause, it should be stopped immediately and replaced with appropriate therapy. But in immune hemolytic disease occurring in neonates, transfusions may correct the disorder. If amniocentesis and antibody determination indicate that the neonate has a severe hemolytic disorder, intrauterine transfusions of compatible blood can be given during the last trimester by injecting the abdominal

cavity of the fetus with compatible blood. Immediately after delivery, if blood-type tests and a direct Coombs' test confirm severe hemolysis, treatment includes exchange transfusions.

In neonatal thrombocytopenic purpura, treatment may involve exchange transfusions, platelet transfusions from the mother, or corticosteroids.

For patients with multiple myeloma as well as other leukemias and lymphomas, blood transfusions may be given to treat symptomatic anemia.

**Other treatments.** Patients with multiple myeloma also generally require supportive treatment, including administration of analgesics for pain, maintenance of adequate hydration for kidney function, and local radiation treatments (avoiding active bone marrow sites) to help reduce pain and tumor size.

Besides chemotherapy, immunotherapy and bone marrow transplantation may be used to treat patients with acute leukemia.

In some immune hemolytic disorders, *minimal treatment,* or no treatment at all, is actually preferred. For example, when patients

## Routine ABO typing

Cellular agglutination, the clumping of cells in the blood, is a major risk of blood transfusions. To prevent this complication, routine ABO typing is performed. This test has two parts: forward typing and reverse typing.

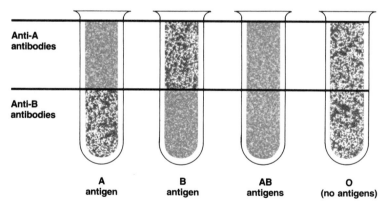

**Forward typing** tests cells with anti-A and anti-B serum antibodies. A saline solution of red blood cells with specific antigens is mixed first with anti-A antiserum and then with anti-B antiserum. Agglutination will occur if A antigens and anti-A antibodies or B antigens and anti-B antibodies are tested together.

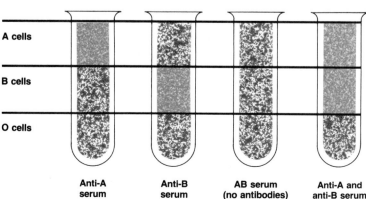

**Reverse typing** is performed to confirm the results of forward typing. The serum is tested against A, B, and O cells. (O cells serve as a control and help detect agglutinating materials unrelated to antigen-antibody reactions.) Agglutination will occur if the serum and the cells are mismatched.

**Key**

 Agglutination

 No agglutination

## Immediate reactions to blood transfusions

As you probably know, immediate reactions can occur during, immediately after, or up to 96 hours after any blood transfusion. Primary causes are incompatibility, contaminated blood, or too-rapid infusion. Study this chart: you'll learn what to look for, how to treat the reactions, and how to prevent them from happening again.

| Reaction and causes | Signs and symptoms | Nursing interventions | Prevention |
|---|---|---|---|
| **Hemolytic reaction** Uncommon, possibly fatal; due to ABO or Rh incompatibility or to improper storage | Chills, fever, low back pain, chest pain, hypotension, nausea, vomiting, and bleeding abnormalities | • Keep the vein open by connecting a secondary line of normal saline solution to the blood line. • Correct shock by administering oxygen, fluids, and epinephrine, as ordered. • Maintain renal circulation by administering mannitol or furosemide, as ordered. • Collect blood and urine samples for analysis. • Record intake and output after transfusion. Watch for diuresis and oliguria. | Minimize the risk of hemolytic reaction by: • double-checking the patient's identification and blood type to make sure the blood is compatible • beginning the transfusion slowly • remaining with the patient for the first 20 minutes of the transfusion. |
| **Febrile reaction** Common, not serious; caused by the presence of bacterial lipopolysaccharides | From mild chills and fever to extreme signs and symptoms resembling hemolytic reaction | • For mild cases, administer antipyretics and antihistamines, as ordered. • For severe cases, treat like hemolytic reaction. | • Keep the patient covered and warm. • Use normal saline–washed red blood cells (RBCs) or frozen, normal saline–washed packed cells. • Administer antipyretics with the blood. IMPORTANT: Never add antihistamines to the blood bag. |
| **Allergic reaction** Common, not serious; due to an atopic substance in the blood | Pruritus and urticaria, occasional facial swelling, chills, fever, nausea, vomiting | • Notify the doctor. • Administer parenteral antihistamines or, for seriously ill patients, epinephrine or corticosteroids, as ordered. | • Determine if the patient reacted allergically to previous transfusions. If so, he has a two-in-three chance of recurrence. |
| **Plasma protein incompatibility** Uncommon, not serious; caused by IgA incompatibility | Flushing, abdominal pain, diarrhea, chills, fever, dyspnea, hypotension | • Treat for shock by administering oxygen, fluids, and epinephrine, as ordered. • Sometimes corticosteroids are administered. | • Transfuse only IgA-deficient blood or well-washed RBCs. |
| **Blood contamination** Uncommon but serious; due to presence of gram-negative *Pseudomonas*, coliform, or achromobacteria | Chills, fever, vomiting, diarrhea, shock | • Treat with antibiotics and corticosteroids, as ordered. | • Use air-free methods to draw and deliver blood. • Maintain strict storage control and use aseptic technique. • Change the filter and tubing every 4 hours and the blood at least every 4 hours. |
| **Circulatory overload** Common and treatable; due to a too-large infusion | Engorged neck veins; constricted chest, with breathing difficulties; flushed feeling; moist rales; eventually, acute edema | • Keep the primary line open with dextrose 5% in water (not saline solution). • Notify the doctor immediately; he may order administration of diuretics, rotating tourniquets, or phlebotomy therapy. | • Use packed RBCs instead of whole blood. • Infuse at a reduced rate if the patient's at high risk for a reaction. • Keep the patient warm and in a sitting position. • Use a diuretic when you begin the transfusion. |
| **Air embolism** Rare; possibly fatal; due to air entering blood via tubing | Blood foaming in the heart; subsequent pumping impairment leads to shock | • Treat for shock. • Turn the patient on his left side, with his head down. | • Expel air from the tubing before starting the transfusion. • Don't allow the blood bag to run dry. |

have cold-antibody types of autoimmune hemolytic anemia, keeping them warm is the only effective treatment. Children with mild or moderately severe ITP may be observed without therapy. (If thrombocytopenia becomes severe, though, or if bleeding occurs, corticosteroids may be given; however, platelet count doesn't respond to corticostereoids as effectively in children as it does in adults.) Splenectomy should be considered only when severe thrombocytopenia lasts for 3 to 6 months; after that time, spontaneous remission is unlikely in children. Treatment may also be unnecessary for asymptomatic patients with CLL.

## NURSING MANAGEMENT
Immune-related hematologic disorders can affect different body systems. Consequently, you should take a thorough history and perform a careful physical examination.

### The nursing history
Begin by collecting biographic data. Remember these points:
• Autoimmune hemolytic anemia, ITP, and autoimmune neutropenia affect women more commonly than men.
• ALL chiefly affects children under age 10, whereas Hodgkin's disease rarely does.
• CLL most commonly strikes men between ages 50 and 70.
• Multiple myeloma chiefly affects patients over age 40.
• Macroglobulinemia primarily affects the elderly.

Next, assess the patient's chief complaint. Because of the widespread effects of immune-related hematologic disorders, patients' complaints vary—but the most common are abnormal bleeding, lymphadenopathy, pain, fatigue and weakness, dyspnea, and fever.

Fatigue and weakness may be associated with any of the immune-related hematologic diseases. Pain may occur in some of the proliferative WBC disorders: unexplained skeletal pain, especially in the back or thorax, sometimes accompanies multiple myeloma, whereas sternal pain sometimes accompanies acute myelocytic leukemia. Abnormal bleeding is a classic sign of ITP and may also be a factor in leukemia, along with fatigue and dyspnea. Dyspnea also frequently develops in late hemolytic anemia. Fever may signal infection in leukemia or in neutropenia. Lymphadenopathy is a very likely, but not invariable, sign of most proliferative WBC disorders.

Now explore the patient's past medical history and the course of his present illness. Ask about bleeding problems; complications of wound healing or previous surgeries; adverse experiences with blood transfusions, drug therapy, chemotherapy, or radiation; and known allergies, including incidents of anaphylaxis. Obtain a history of past surgeries, noting especially splenectomy or tumor removal.

Finally, do a complete systems review, looking for clues to hematologic dysfunction, which—as you know—can affect any body system.

### The physical examination
Your examination of the patient, like your history taking, should cover all body systems. Keep in mind that certain seemingly nonhematologic physical findings can actually stem from hematologic disease. For example, a decreased level of consciousness may be from intracranial hemorrhage caused by ITP; and absent bowel sounds, from abdominal hemorrhage, also caused by ITP.

If the patient hasn't experienced complications, your physical findings may be minimal. Some key areas to assess include the skin, mouth, eyes, and lymph nodes.

Check the patient's skin color. Pallor results from decreased hemoglobin content; jaundice, from accumulated bile pigment due to rapid or excessive hemolysis; and petechiae or ecchymoses, from hemorrhage into the skin.

Inspect the mouth for swelling, redness, or bleeding of the gums and for creamy white patches of exudate (candidiasis)—all commonly found in leukemic patients.

Inspect the eyes for jaundiced sclera or pallor in the conjunctiva. Funduscopic examination of the eyes in a patient with thrombocytopenia and anemia may reveal retinal hemorrhages.

Palpate lymph nodes for enlargement and tenderness. Palpate the liver and spleen as well. Hepatomegaly and splenomegaly occur in leukemia and neutropenia; splenomegaly also accompanies lymphoma.

When you conduct the cardiovascular examination, be alert for signs attributable to anemia—for example, tachycardia from a compensatory effort to increase cardiac output. Also assess for systolic murmurs or bruits (especially carotid bruits)—both related to disorders affecting blood volume and viscosity. Check for widened pulse pressure from increased stroke volume.

### EMERGENCY MANAGEMENT

# Bleeding in patients with low platelet counts

Decreased platelet counts result from malignant disease or treatment procedures. Concern for bleeding begins when the count falls below 50,000 µl and intensifies when it falls below 20,000 µl.

The most serious bleeding usually occurs in the brain or the lungs. Intracranial bleeding can begin spontaneously; the patient is most likely to complain of a headache and may report vision changes (suspect occipital lobe bleeding). If this occurs, do a neurologic assessment and report the information to the doctor immediately. If he suspects intracranial bleeding, he may order a platelet transfusion and possibly computerized tomography. He may also recommend withholding pain medication so signs of intracranial bleeding won't be masked. During this time, continue to do frequent neurologic assessments.

Bleeding in the lungs in a patient with a low platelet count usually occurs in conjunction with an infectious process.

Frank blood in the pleural space, or hemothorax, indicates hemorrhagic pleural effusion, which restricts chest or lung expansion. Suspect hemothorax when a patient with a low platelet count and a history of fever, malaise, or purulent sputum complains of dyspnea, shortness of breath, pain, or anxiety. If this happens, alert the doctor, monitor vital signs, and assess lung sounds and mental status. The doctor will probably order a chest X-ray and arterial blood gases. A patient with large amounts of pleural blood may need thoracentesis; if pleural bleeding persists, he may require surgery and platelet transfusion.

Another possible bleeding site is the abdomen; however, the frequency of severe abdominal bleeding has dropped as a result of increased use of antacids, prophylactic platelet administration, and the development of $H_2$-antagonist medications. Be alert for the signs and symptoms of abdominal bleeding: hematemesis, melena, occult fecal blood, hypovolemia, and anemia.

As a precaution against bleeding in patients with low platelet counts, avoid invasive procedures and I.M. and S.C. injections when possible. If you must perform an invasive procedure, apply pressure to the area for a full 5 minutes postprocedure (or longer if signs of bleeding continue).

Monitor the patient's vital signs every 4 hours, and routinely check his urine, stool, sputum, and vomitus for blood. Check his needle insertion sites for signs of bleeding and his skin for petechiae and ecchymoses.

Teach patients to observe bleeding precautions, too. Advise them to avoid anything, such as sharp-edged furniture, that could puncture or bruise their skin. Tell them not to strain during bowel movements and to avoid abrasives, such as hard-bristled toothbrushes.

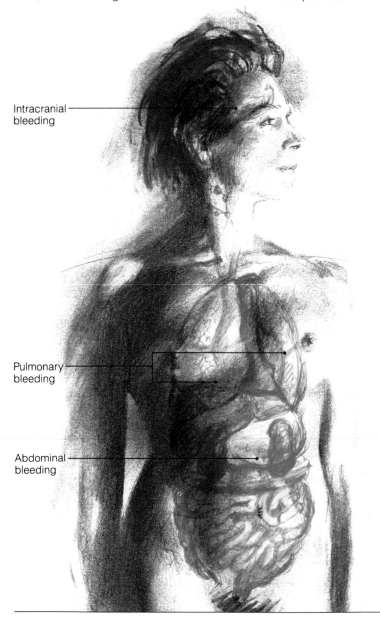

Intracranial bleeding

Pulmonary bleeding

Abdominal bleeding

During the neurologic examination, watch for abnormal reactions to pain or touch stimuli, to changes in position and vibratory sense, and to tendon reflex testing. These may indicate nerve compression by a mass, as in lymphoma; or intracranial bleeding, as in ITP.

## Formulate nursing diagnoses

When you've completed the physical examination, correlate your assessment results to form nursing diagnoses.

**Potential for injury related to altered hematologic status.** A patient with a WBC disorder is vulnerable to infection. So assess him at least daily, observing for such signs and symptoms of infection as redness, swelling, localized pain, and fatigue or weakness.

Monitor his body temperature closely, too, especially if he has neutropenia or a proliferative WBC disorder. Notify the doctor at once if his temperature rises—remember, an infection can quickly become lethal in such a patient. Administer cool sponge baths and antibiotics and antipyretics, as ordered. (If the patient is severely neutropenic, he may require reverse isolation.) Perform all nursing procedures using strict aseptic technique.

Bleeding can pose a serious threat if your patient has a decreased platelet count. Observe him for hemorrhagic tendencies, and report any evidence of spontaneous bleeding or increased bruising. (See *Emergency management: Bleeding in patients with low platelet counts.*) Assess the patient frequently for internal bleeding, too. Use a small-gauge needle when you inject medication.

If bleeding occurs, keep the patient quiet and on bed rest until the doctor orders otherwise. Apply gentle pressure or cold compresses to the bleeding sites, as indicated. Be careful not to disturb any clots. If the patient is bleeding from his mouth or throat, have a tracheotomy set handy for emergency use, and keep his head turned to the side.

If the patient's treatment includes blood transfusions, use extreme care in administering blood units for transfusion to prevent hemolytic anemia. Be sure you're prepared to manage transfusion reactions. (See *Immediate reactions to blood transfusions,* page 158.)

Consider your interventions effective when the patient is free of injury.

**Alterations in comfort related to the disease or treatment.** In your daily patient care, remember that most patients suffering from immune-related hematologic disorders, especially those receiving drug therapy and radiation treatments, are weak and easily fatigued. Plan your care to conserve the patient's strength. For example, minimize his activities so he gets plenty of rest. (A patient with multiple myeloma, however, *should* be encouraged to ambulate to prevent hypercalcemia and further bone loss.)

If an anemic patient experiences dyspnea, elevate the head of his bed, and administer oxygen as indicated. Use pillows to support him in the orthopneic position. Encourage him to rest, and watch his diet to exclude gas-forming foods; these can cause abdominal distention, which prevents full lung expansion.

If the patient is on drug therapy, instruct him to avoid foods and beverages that can irritate mucous membranes, which commonly become ulcerated during chemotherapy. Encourage him to rinse his mouth with mild, cool solutions before and after meals and to use applicators or a soft-bristle toothbrush to prevent irritation and bleeding. Keep his lips well lubricated to prevent cracking.

Encourage fluid intake (unless contraindicated) to replace fluid loss from diaphoresis. Maintain a cool environmental temperature.

If the patient has bone or joint pain, administer hot or cold compresses, as ordered. If necessary, provide for joint immobilization, or relieve pressure by using a bed cradle.

Consider your interventions effective when the patient tells you he's feeling comfortable.

**Fear related to an uncertain future.** To help the patient and his family understand and cope with the patient's disease, try to ease the fear and anxiety they may feel. Explain the nature of the disease—including any discomfort and activity limitations associated with it and with its diagnosis and treatment—so they'll be prepared to respond appropriately.

Don't underestimate the importance of listening to the patient. Promote his relaxation, comfort, and dignity, and encourage his family to participate in his care. Consider your interventions effective when the patient's able to express his fears.

## Support is the key

Many immune-related hematologic diseases take patients through alternating courses of despair and hope, depending on whether their disease is acute or in remission. And the lack of cures for most such diseases only adds to their fear and confusion. Your attentive, informed support can do much to help patients cope with these disorders and to give them hope despite an uncertain future.

**Points to remember**

- Immune-related hematologic disorders are broadly classified as destructive or proliferative.
- Destructive blood disorders follow sensitization of blood cells with antibody.
- Abnormal proliferation of white blood cells, the primary cells of the immune system, results in a wide range of disorders classified as leukemias, lymphomas, and plasma cell dyscrasias.
- Compatibility testing is done for all patients before transfusions to prevent alloantibody-induced immune hemolytic anemia.
- Laboratory investigation of immune-related hematologic disorders begins with routine blood tests and proceeds to immunologic tests.
- Infection and bleeding are medical emergencies in the leukemic patient.
- Drug therapy is the treatment of choice for many of these disorders.

# 12 COMBATING GLOMERULONEPHRITIS

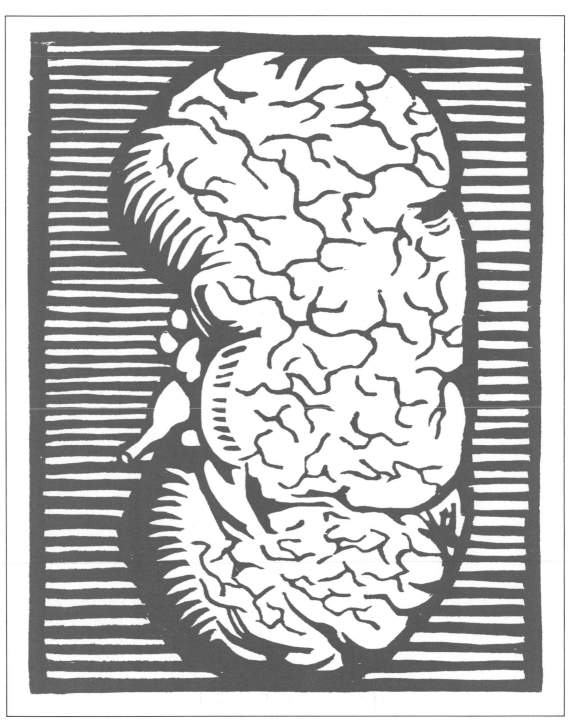

Enlarged kidney with granular surface

You may understand glomerulonephritis as a synonym for renal failure, with all the complications and distress that entails. But you may not realize that it often evolves via immunologic dysfunction as the major cause of chronic renal failure. One of several immune mechanisms may result in glomerular damage that's difficult, if not impossible, to stop.

Glomerulonephritis requires that you help a patient deal with an unexpected, uncertain, and often grim prognosis. You'll do this best if you understand what causes glomerulonephritis and how to combat it.

## PATHOPHYSIOLOGY

Renal dysfunction generally occurs as a result of an immune reaction. This reaction can affect the tubules and surrounding interstitial tissue, causing tubulointerstitial nephritis; but it usually affects the glomerulus, causing glomerulonephritis. In glomerulonephritis, immune-inflammatory reactions generally result from disease or from the presence of immune complexes in the glomeruli.

### How immune complexes form in the glomeruli

Commonly, antibodies react with nonglomerular antigens to form immune complexes. The antigens may be exogenous (from bacteria, viruses, chemicals, or drugs) or endogenous (derived from body tissues). The resulting immune complexes are scattered along the glomerular basement membrane. Occasionally, immune complexes result from antibodies to endogenous antigens in the glomerular basement membrane (as in Goodpasture's syndrome). These antibodies, called anti-GBM antibodies, may also cross-react with antigens in the tubular basement membrane.

These immune mechanisms activate complement in the glomeruli, causing an increase in polymorphonuclear leukocytes, the release of histamine, and in turn glomerular damage from inflammation and coagulation. In glomerulonephritis, these immune-inflammatory reactions change the capillary endothelium, the glomerular basement membrane, the visceral epithelium of the tuft, and the parietal epithelium of Bowman's capsule. The severity of these changes varies with the type and duration of the immune-inflammatory reaction. Initial changes may be focal, affecting a few glomeruli, or widespread. Usually, focal changes later become widespread.

### Characteristic signs and symptoms

Signs of glomerulonephritis can occur in many combinations. They usually include the following abnormalities: *proteinuria* from loss of epithelial foot processes with increased glomerular permeability to protein; *oliguria* from loss of functional nephrons; *edema* from increased reabsorption of sodium and water and diminished glomerular filtration rate; *hypertension* from increased blood volume or increased secretion of renin and aldosterone; *elevated blood urea nitrogen (BUN) and serum creatinine levels* from decreased excretion of waste products; and *excretion of red blood cells (RBCs), white blood cells (WBCs), and granular casts*. Glomerulonephritis (especially membranous, membranoproliferative, and chronic glomerulonephritis) may progress to nephrotic syndrome (marked by proteinuria exceeding 3.5 g/day, hypoalbuminemia, edema, and hyperlipidemia).

## MEDICAL MANAGEMENT

The course and treatment of glomerulonephritis can vary with the prognosis, the rate of renal deterioration, and the mechanism of immunologic dysfunction.

### Thorough diagnostic workup essential

Diagnosis of glomerulonephritis rests heavily on the results of blood tests, urine studies, and complement assays but requires renal biopsy with immunofluorescent microscopy and possibly electron microscopy to identify the cause of immunologic dysfunction.

**Laboratory tests.** Significant blood work includes creatinine clearance tests, a serum creatinine test, and a BUN test. An elevated creatinine with increased BUN level suggests renal failure. Further tests, such as renal biopsy, must be done to determine the type of renal disease. Urinalysis screens for hematuria; proteinuria; and the presence of RBCs, WBCs, or granular casts.

A throat culture positive for group A beta-hemolytic streptococcus and an elevated anti-streptolysin O titer indicate streptococcal infection as a possible source of acute glomerulonephritis.

**Immune tests and renal biopsy.** In glomerulonephritis resulting from immunologic dysfunction, serum complement assays are diagnostically valuable. Levels of C3 and C4, detected in radial immunodiffusion tests, are decreased during acute glomerulonephritis.

Renal biopsy with immunofluorescent and possibly electron microscopy is the most use-

## Classification of glomerulonephritis

**Primary glomerulonephritis**

Antiglomerular basement membrane disease

Acute postinfectious glomerulonephritis

Idiopathic rapidly progressive or crescentic glomerulonephritis

Membranoproliferative glomerulonephritis

Focal glomerulonephritis
IgA nephropathy

Idiopathic membranous glomerulonephritis

Chronic glomerulonephritis

Lipoid nephrosis

Focal glomerular sclerosis

**Secondary glomerulonephritis**

Systemic lupus erythematosus

Polyarteritis nodosa

Wegener's granulomatosis

Henoch-Schönlein syndrome

Goodpasture's syndrome

Bacterial endocarditis

Malignancy

**Poststreptococcal glomerulonephritis** is an example of renal disease mediated by immune complexes. *Renal biopsy* (at right) shows diffuse proliferative glomerulonephritis with a variable number of neutrophils and other leukocytes in glomeruli. *Immunofluorescence* (see inset) shows IgG and C3 as granular deposits along the glomerular capillary loops.

**Goodpasture's syndrome** is an example of renal disease mediated by antibody to the basement membrane. *Renal biopsy* (at right) shows cellular or fibrocellular crescents in most glomeruli and fibrin deposits in Bowman's space. Often the glomerular tuft is collapsed, and capillary walls are disrupted. *Immunofluorescence* (see inset) shows immune reactants, mostly IgG and C3, as continuous linear deposits along the glomerular basement membrane.

## Identifying renal biopsy and immunofluorescence results

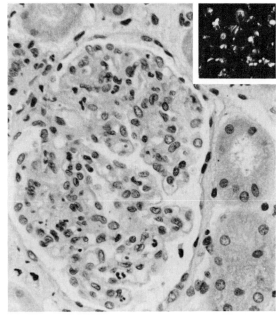

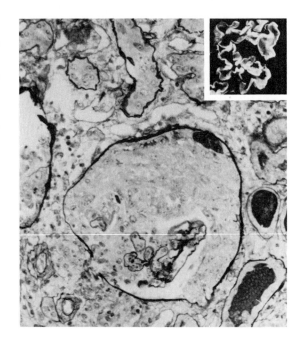

ful test for immune-induced glomerulonephritis. Renal biopsy identifies the type of renal disease and secures tissue specimens for microscopy; immunofluorescence detects immune complexes directly, using cellular substrates. Positive results of renal biopsy and microscopy for glomerulonephritis reveal deposits of immune complexes along the glomerular basement membrane. Characteristic patterns of immune complex deposits differentiate exogenous from endogenous antigens: antibody response to nonglomerular (exogenous) antigens causes deposits that appear

as granular areas that look bumpy; antibodies to basement membranes (endogenous) cause deposits in continuous linear patterns (see *Identifying renal biopsy and immunofluorescence results*).

### Treatment addresses the source of dysfunction

For example, antibodies to nonglomerular antigens require treatment that centers on removing the antigen; an autoimmune response requires treatment that inhibits antibody production. Thus, glomerulonephritis that results from infection, such as streptococcal pharyngitis, may respond to antibiotics.

Glomerulonephritis may be associated with neoplasm. Nephrectomy is sometimes appropriate for severe pulmonary hemorrhage associated with Goodpasture's syndrome. This last-resort treatment, although sometimes lifesaving, is controversial because it rules out recovery from Goodpasture's syndrome, which occasionally occurs. However, treatment for glomerulonephritis is generally supportive. It may include anti-inflammatory and immunosuppressive drugs, such as corticosteroids, cyclophosphamide, and azathioprine. But use of such drugs is controversial primarily because they don't work in all patients, though they do work well in some.

### NURSING MANAGEMENT

Because glomerulonephritis commonly produces a confusing array of physical and psychological symptoms, your careful attention to the patient's problems can make all the difference in his care. As always, useful nursing diagnoses begin with a thorough history and complete physical examination.

### Background information first

Take a detailed patient history, including biographic and medical data. For example, the patient's age may be important; poststreptococcal glomerulonephritis usually occurs in children (but all age-groups are susceptible). Ask about exposure to anything that could cause glomerulonephritis, such as microbial or viral infections, immunizations, and some drugs. Get a complete medical history, including questions about underlying immune-related disorders, such as systemic lupus erythematosus, vasculitis, and cryoglobulinemia.

Determine the patient's chief complaint. Although chronic glomerulonephritis may be initially asymptomatic, acute glomerulonephritis may show abrupt symptomatology, such as oliguria and possibly hematuria at onset. Also, if you suspect Goodpasture's syndrome, find out if hemoptysis is present.

**Physical examination next**
Examination should focus on signs of renal dysfunction and on complications of acute or chronic renal failure.

**Examine the skin.** Look for signs of dehydration or fluid overload. Signs of dehydration include poor skin turgor and dry mucous membranes; signs of fluid overload include peripheral edema, tachycardia, and rales. If you find peripheral edema, determine if it's pitting or nonpitting, and note its exact location. Look for skin discoloration, such as pallor from anemia, that commonly occurs in renal failure. Also look for skin excoriation that may occur as a result of severe itching, a common symptom of uremia.

**Assess cardiovascular status.** Hypertension often accompanies glomerulonephritis. Also, congestive heart failure may be present if the patient is experiencing fluid overload. To assess for congestive heart failure, check for tachycardia, the presence of an $S_3$ heart sound, rales, and hypoxia.

**Assess neurologic status.** Watch for confusion, the result of accumulating waste products in the blood in azotemia or uremia. Uremia also produces neurologic changes, such as changes in sensory and motor function. Consider that a diminished level of consciousness may also result from hypoxia secondary to congestive heart failure.

Because patients respond to chronic illness differently, you should also assess the patient's psychological state. Note any defense mechanism the patient may use to cope with illness, such as denial, regression, or displacement.

**Plan the patient's care**
Nursing care addresses specific symptoms as stated in appropriate nursing diagnoses.

**Fluid overload related to sodium and water retention.** Your goal is to prevent fluid overload and its signs and symptoms. Give fluids according to the patient's fluid loss and daily weight. Remember to include insensible fluid loss through the respiratory system and gastrointestinal tract in the daily measurement. Generally, the insensible loss is estimated at 500 to 1,000 ml. Teach the patient to maintain a record of his fluid intake and output to ensure accurate measurement. Because hypertension may result from fluid overload, monitor the patient's blood pressure closely. Also, re-

alize that fluid overload may cause changes in patterns of urination, impaired ventilation, and metabolic imbalances.

Consider your interventions successful if the patient avoids fluid overload and its symptoms.

**Potential for impaired skin integrity related to weakened tissue at edematous sites or skin trauma from relentless itching and scratching (caused by uremic buildup).** Your goal is to avoid skin breakdown and to minimize itching. Be sure to turn the bedridden edematous patient frequently. Also, use a bed cradle and a special mattress to relieve pressure. Control uremic itching by keeping the patient's skin clean and by using nonirritating soap, sodium bicarbonate in bathwater, oatmeal baths, bath oil, or lotion. If itching is intense, encourage the patient to rub lotion into his skin instead of scratching.

Consider your intervention effective if the patient avoids skin breakdown and if itching is minimized.

**Activity intolerance related to bed rest during the acute phase of glomerulonephritis.** Bed rest may be encouraged until hematuria and hypertension are resolved and BUN and creatinine levels normalize. Your goal is to prevent hazards of immobility (such as decubiti and pneumonia). Take preventive measures: pad all bony prominences, turn the patient frequently, and encourage frequent coughing and deep-breathing exercises. Remember, too, that restriction of dietary protein increases the risk of decubiti. So, encourage liberal ingestion of carbohydrates to provide energy and to reduce protein catabolism.

Consider your interventions successful if the patient has avoided hazards of immobility.

**Disturbance in self-concept and anxiety related to knowledge deficit and body changes.** Your goal is to teach the patient about the physiology and effects of his disease. Schedule time with the patient to talk about his feelings and concerns. Answer his questions openly and honestly. Explain all procedures and any changes in his treatment regimen. Encourage family participation in his care.

Consider your interventions effective when the patient expresses decreased anxiety.

**Updating care**
By frequently monitoring the patient's condition and being alert to physical and emotional changes, you can offer care that closely addresses his symptoms and offers necessary reassurance and support.

**Points to remember**

- Glomerulonephritis, which usually results from an immunologic reaction, is the leading cause of chronic renal failure.
- Two mechanisms of antibody-induced injury can initiate glomerular damage—immune complex deposits or formation of antibody to the glomerular basement membrane.
- Usual symptoms of glomerulonephritis include proteinuria, hematuria, oliguria, edema, and hypertension.
- Renal biopsy is most useful for confirming immune-induced glomerulonephritis.
- Nursing care should address specific physical symptoms, such as problems of fluid overload, and provide emotional support.

# 13 MANAGING FUNCTION IN NEUROLOGIC DISORDERS

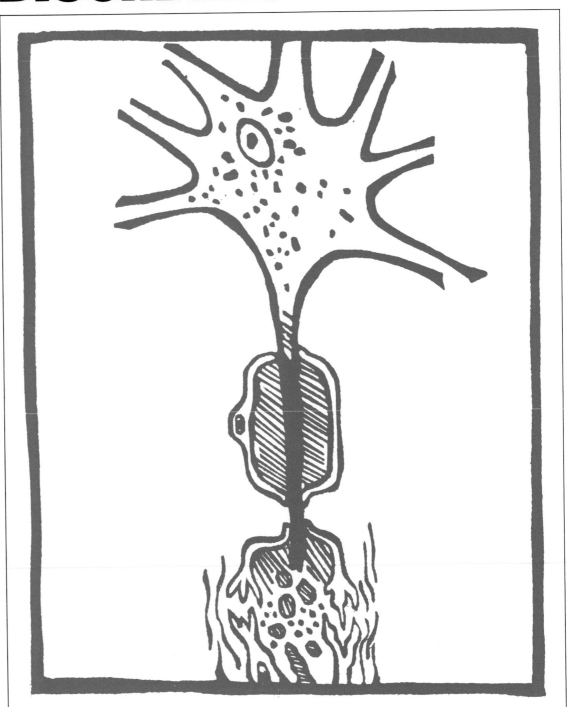

Wallerian degeneration of peripheral nerve

Certain diseases of the central and peripheral nervous systems display features suggesting immunologic dysfunction. The primary four are acute disseminated encephalomyelitis (ADEM), multiple sclerosis (MS), Guillain-Barré syndrome (GB), and myasthenia gravis (MG). Immunologic dysfunctions may also occur in other neurologic diseases (subacute sclerosing panencephalitis, myotonic dystrophy, and amyotrophic lateral sclerosis), but the pathogenetic link is less clear.

In any case, dysfunction in the immune and nervous systems induces wide-ranging and often variable clinical effects that require skilled nursing care. You can offer such care if you learn to recognize the clinical features of these diseases and know what treatments and supportive measures are most helpful in managing them.

## PATHOPHYSIOLOGY
Of the four primary immune-related neurologic diseases, all but MG are classified as demyelinating diseases, involving inflammatory destruction of the myelin sheath surrounding nerve fibers. (See *The physiology of neuromuscular disturbances,* page 168.) The immunologic mechanisms at work in these diseases are not clearly understood, but research suggests they may play a significant role as causative factors.

### Acute disseminated encephalomyelitis
A demyelinating disease of the central nervous system (CNS), ADEM usually follows infectious disease or immunization although it may occur concomitantly with a natural infection such as measles or influenza. Evidence suggests that various infectious agents trigger an autoaggressive attack on myelin, producing a single type of CNS lesion. Such evidence includes signs of cell-mediated, but not humoral, immune response to the basic myelin protein that measures highest during the acute phase of the disease and declines thereafter.

ADEM lesions occur mainly in the perivascular regions of cerebral, and occasionally spinal, white matter. As the disease progresses, the lesions become decreasingly inflamed and increasingly sclerotic. Symptoms of ADEM begin suddenly, with neurologic symptoms following systemic symptoms within 24 to 48 hours. Incidence appears to bear no relation to race, sex, or age. Mortality ranges from 1% to 27%, a higher rate being associated with measles.

### Multiple sclerosis
In MS, another demyelinating disease of the CNS, the immunologic mechanisms may involve an autoimmune response to axonal myelin or to oligodendrocytes, the synthesizers of CNS myelin. Suppressor T-cell levels are known to decline just before an MS attack and to rise at the end of an attack. This change may allow a latent autoimmune reaction to occur. Or an MS antigen may be present on suppressor T cells and oligodendrocytes. Other unexplained changes that accompany MS attacks include hyperfunctioning of circulating B cells and excessive IgG levels within the CNS, suggesting B-cell stimulation or an immunoregulatory defect.

MS lesions (plaques) occur in CNS white matter in patchy, sporadic patterns in areas of myelin and oligodendrocyte loss (especially in the brain stem, spinal cord, cortex, and optic nerve). These plaques contain increased levels of immunoglobulin, suggesting local production. The resulting symptoms, course of the disease, and prognosis vary greatly. In most patients, prolonged remissions occur; in some, rapid progression leads to death within months of onset.

Environmental and age factors seem to determine the risk of MS. Incidence varies in temperate climates; peak onset occurs at age 30. Because geographic residence up to mid-teenage years is significant, some factor occurring during adolescence possibly influences risk.

### Guillain-Barré syndrome
This demyelinating disease, also called acute idiopathic polyneuritis, affects the peripheral nervous system (PNS). Like ADEM, GB often follows viral infection or immunization, with the viral antigen possibly triggering an autoimmune reaction to myelin. This disease may also follow physical stress such as surgery or, rarely, malignant lymphoid disease.

GB involves segmental demyelination of inflamed peripheral nerves; in areas of severe damage, this may include axonal destruction and wallerian degeneration. Evidence of cell-mediated immune response during GB may include serum specimens containing antimyelin antibodies, low levels of immune complexes, and complement components.

GB usually begins with weakness in the feet and legs, followed closely by paralysis and progressing within anywhere from 24 hours to 3 weeks to the hands and arms and then to respiratory musculature. Sensory function is

## The physiology of neuromuscular disturbances

**Disruption of myoneural transmission**

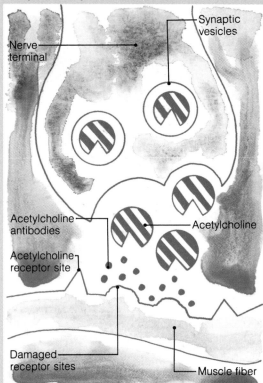

In MG, destruction of 70% to 90% of acetylcholine receptor sites at the myoneural junction disrupts transmission of nerve impulses. This destruction reduces acetylcholine-receptor interaction.

**Demyelination**

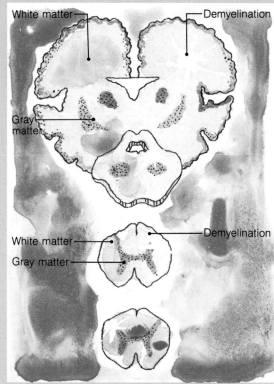

In MS and ADEM, destruction of the myelin sheath surrounding the nerve axon occurs in CNS white matter. This demyelination impairs conduction of nerve impulses, causing partial loss or dispersion of the muscle action potential.

spared. Usually, progression takes 3 to 7 days. GB may affect the cranial nerves (especially the seventh). Incidence of GB disregards race, sex, and age. Mortality is low.

### Myasthenia gravis

Like ADEM, MS, and GB, MG impairs transmission of nerve impulses, but not because of demyelination. Rather, MG is thought to result from an autoimmune deactivation of acetylcholine receptor sites, which are necessary for normal impulse transmission to muscles. Antibodies to acetylcholine receptors block and remove these receptor sites from the postsynaptic membrane. These antibodies may also activate the complement system, leading to further myoneural junction damage.

MG may be associated with thymomas; other autoantibodies; and other autoimmune diseases such as systemic lupus erythematosus and rheumatoid arthritis.

MG causes muscle weakness aggravated by exertion, eventually, in some patients, causing respiratory failure from progressive involvement of respiratory muscles. MG most often strikes women in their thirties and men in their sixties or seventies. Mortality is 5% to 10%, most often affecting elderly patients.

### MEDICAL MANAGEMENT

Because tests for these immune-related neurologic disorders rarely prove conclusive, diagnosis centers mostly on the patient's history and on clinical findings. However, certain diagnostic tests offer helpful supportive information. (See *Diagnostic tests.*)

### Treatment: Symptomatic and supportive

Most forms of therapy for these disorders aim at controlling symptoms, and most long-term treatment remains supportive.

**Drug therapy.** Corticosteroids may be pre-

### Wallerian degeneration

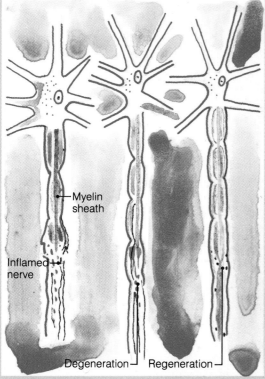

In GB, inflammation of axons in the PNS may cause wallerian degeneration. This breakdown of the axon's myelin sheath and sometimes of the axon itself decreases the muscle action potential. However, it leaves the axon's outermost layer (neurilemma) intact. This layer acts as a guide while the damaged axon and myelin sheath regenerate and function returns.

scribed with varying degrees of effectiveness. In ADEM, high doses of steroids may be helpful, but the course of the disease is still unpredictable. In MS and GB, corticosteroids may relieve acute symptoms but don't alter the disease's course.

In MG, anticholinesterases, such as neostigmine (Prostigmin) and pyridostigmine bromide (Mestinon), improve neuromuscular transmission. Unfortunately, these drugs become less effective as MG progresses. Corticosteroids and immunosuppressive drugs, such as cyclophosphamide and azathioprine, may produce remission and establish long-term control of symptoms.

**Thymectomy.** Removal of the thymus is often the second treatment of choice (the preferred treatment is anticholinesterase drugs) for patients with MG because of the proposed role of the thymus in the autoimmune response. Considered for all MG patients except those with nondisabling ocular myasthenia, thymectomy usually produces improvement and induces remission within 5 years.

**Supportive care.** In the acute stages of GB or MG, physical therapy including passive range-of-motion exercises can help some patients completely recover motor skills. Patients with ADEM, MG or GB may also require respiratory care—intubation and mechanical ventilation. Such care should include frequent suctioning and assessment of vital capacity and may involve a tracheostomy for prolonged mechanical ventilation. Nutritional support and general comfort measures are also required.

## NURSING MANAGEMENT

Because the patient's history and physical examination are key components in diagnosing immune-related neurologic disorders, your role in thorough data collection is critical. In addition, an ongoing neurologic examination to detect daily changes in status is an integral part of nursing care for these patients.

### Obtain history—present and past

Collect biographic data, keeping in mind that the patient's age and sex are significant. Both MS and MG, for example, affect women more often than men and usually strike in young to middle-aged adults.

Determine the patient's chief complaint. His symptoms may involve any area of neurologic function: cerebral, cerebellar, cranial nerve, motor, or sensory. For example, the patient with GB may initially seek help because of weakness and paralysis in the extremities; the patient with MS may complain of a visual disturbance from optic neuritis.

Next, get a history of the present illness, questioning the patient in detail about onset and quality of symptoms. For instance, intermittent muscle weakness with progressive fatigability that becomes more severe late in the day may indicate MG. Abrupt onset of flaccid weakness with lower leg paresthesia suggests GB.

Obtain a past history. Ask about any recent infections or immunizations. Remember that ADEM can occur simultaneously with measles, mumps, rubella, varicella, and influenza; following these illnesses; or following immunizations. Similarly, GB can follow infection— usually measles, infectious mononucleosis, hepatitis, upper respiratory infection, or exanthem—or immunization. Find out if the patient has a history of any other major illness,

## Diagnostic tests

Although diagnosis of immune-related neurologic disorders relies heavily on the patient's history and clinical features, clues to diagnosis can come from various analyses.

### CSF analysis
• May reveal mildly to moderately increased cell count (pleocytosis) and mildly increased total protein levels in ADEM
• May show progressively elevated protein levels in repeat spinal taps in GB
• May detect elevated IgG levels in MS, although levels often don't vary with chronic attacks

### Blood tests
• Reveal antibodies to acetylcholine receptors in 90% of patients with MG

### I.V. anticholinesterase
• Detects MG by markedly relieving symptoms within 1 minute after I.V. administration of 2 to 10 mg of edrophonium chloride (Tensilon), followed by recurrence of symptoms within 5 minutes

### X-ray
• X-ray of the mediastinum may reveal thymic hyperplasia or thymoma, often associated with MG

### Computerized tomography (CT)
• CT scan can show low-density lesions in more than one CNS site, indicating MS, although confirmation depends on two episodes of neurologic deficit.

## Signs and symptoms of immune-related neurologic disorders

### ADEM
Pain
Numbness
Paresthesia
Motor weakness
Incoordination
Dysarthria
Dysphagia
Pooling of pharyngeal se-
    cretions
Respiratory dysfunction
Spasticity
Abnormal reflexes
Visual defects
Stupor
Coma
Seizures

### MS
Visual problems (nystag-
    mus, diplopia, field
    cuts)
Slow, slurred speech
Muscular weakness
Incoordination
Paresthesia
Inappropriate emotional
    responses
Bowel and bladder dys-
    function
Increased deep tendon
    reflexes
Positive Babinski's sign
    and clonus
Cranial nerve involvement

### GB
Progressive weakness
Usually mild numbness
    and paresthesia
Cranial nerve involvement
    (especially facial nerve)
Decreased or lost tendon
    reflexes
Respiratory dysfunction
Autonomic dysfunction

### MG
Progressive muscular fa-
    tigue (may become
    generalized)
Bilateral ptosis of the eye-
    lids
Blurred or double vision
Impaired swallowing
Voice weakness
Difficulty maintaining head
    position
Respiratory dysfunction

especially autoimmune diseases (such as rheumatoid arthritis), thymoma, and thymic hyperplasia, which often accompany MG.

Make a systems review part of your history taking. Remember that a diversity of symptoms can accompany these neurologic diseases (see *Signs and symptoms of immune-related neurologic disorders*).

Ask about a family history of MS, since this disorder shows some genetic tendency and since the risk multiplies 10 to 15 times for first-degree relatives.

Also obtain a psychosocial history. Knowing the patient's current situation helps you anticipate the adjustments he'll have to make to a possibly chronic and debilitating disease. When appropriate, inform him and his family about supportive community agencies, such as the Visiting Nurse Association, the Myasthenia Gravis Foundation, and the Multiple Sclerosis Society.

### Assess neurologic function
During the physical examination, focus on the five areas of neurologic assessment: cerebral function, cranial nerve function, motor function, sensory function, and reflex status. (See Chapter 2.) Dysfunction may occur in one or all of these areas and may range from mild presentation to severe deficit. Also assess for ophthalmic and speech abnormalities and respiratory distress. (See *Signs and symptoms of immune-related neurologic disorders.*)

### Plan realistic goals
You'll find that caring for the patient with an immune-related neurologic disorder can be extremely complex, since these disorders affect multiple body systems. As the patient becomes unable to control neurologic function, he'll rely on your supportive nursing care to help him meet his needs. As the disease progresses, you may even have to monitor and care for involuntary movements such as respiration.

The widespread effects of these disorders call for nursing diagnoses that are equally wide-ranging. The following are among the most common.

**Ineffective breathing patterns related to respiratory muscle weakness.** To maintain adequate ventilation and to prevent retention of secretions, frequently assess the patient for changes in his breathing pattern and rate, color, and sensorium. Obtain arterial blood gases, as ordered and needed. Auscultate the lungs for atelectasis and pooling of secretions. Have the patient cough and breathe deeply at

least every 4 hours, if he's able, to eliminate retained secretions. During chest physiotherapy, avoid placing him in positions that could further compromise breathing by putting pressure on the diaphragm and abdominal contents. Give oxygen as prescribed, and suction as needed. If progressive muscle weakness necessitates mechanical ventilation, provide appropriate respiratory care.

You've met your goals if the patient maintains adequate ventilation and doesn't retain secretions.

**Sensory alterations related to decrease in neurologic function.** To prevent patient injury and to use compensatory measures satisfactorily, begin by identifying the patient's level of sensory impairment. Check him frequently, and notify the doctor of any changes. If diplopia develops, use an eye patch or occluder, switching the patch to the other eye every 4 hours. Notify the doctor of any changes in visual function. Instruct the patient to rest his eyes when he first notices fatigue. If the patient experiences numbness, examine the affected areas frequently for signs of injury. Encourage the patient to reposition the affected extremity on a consistent schedule to avoid pressure ulcers. When the patient is preparing to go home, instruct him in safety measures, such as testing bath temperature with the unaffected extremity, and in ways to overcome decreased touch and position sense. To ease anxiety, reassure him that paresthesia and visual symptoms frequently subside.

You've met your goals if the patient remains free of injury and learns to compensate for any sensory impairment.

**Impaired physical mobility related to neurologic dysfunction.** To maintain mobility and prevent injury, first determine the patient's current level of mobility. Instruct the patient in wheelchair safety and in the correct use of canes, walkers, and other devices, as needed. Encourage him to balance rest periods with activity and to avoid fatigue. If the patient has developed paralysis, perform range-of-motion exercises every 4 to 8 hours; reposition him every 2 hours; and take appropriate measures to prevent skin breakdown. Make referrals to the physical therapist and occupational therapist, as needed. Before discharge, determine the patient's and his family's understanding of these measures and of the effects of any drug treatment on mobility.

Your interventions are successful if the patient maintains his highest level of mobility without injury.

**Alterations in bowel elimination: Constipation related to decreased mobility.** To establish normal bowel movements and to prevent fecal impaction, determine the patient's normal bowel pattern, and ask about dietary habits and home remedies for constipation. Initiate a bowel-training program, as indicated, and educate the patient about the need for fluid intake (at least 8 to 10 glasses a day if not contraindicated) and for foods high in roughage (such as whole grains, fruits, and vegetables). Obtain a doctor's order for a suppository, laxative, or stool softener, as needed. Coordinate measures to combat bowel and bladder dysfunction, since treatment should encompass both areas. Evaluate bowel management daily or at outpatient visits.

You've reached your goals when the patient reestablishes a normal pattern of elimination.

**Alterations in patterns of urinary elimination related to neurologic impairment.** To establish adequate urinary elimination and prevent urinary tract infection, first identify symptoms of dysfunction and assess bladder function by obtaining volumes of voided and residual urine, with the doctor's approval. Monitor fluid intake and output. Encourage a fluid intake of at least 2,000 to 3,000 ml/day, if not contraindicated, to minimize precipitation of urinary crystals and stone formation and to prevent bacteria accumulation. To control enuresis, limit distribution of fluid intake to morning and afternoon hours.

Institute a bladder-training program with appropriate use of mechanical assistance, such as Credé's method, Valsalva's maneuver, or intermittent catheterization, as ordered by the doctor. Teach correct care of catheters when indicated, as with intermittent and indwelling (Foley) catheterization. Also teach symptoms of urinary tract infection (burning, frequency, urgency), and emphasize the need to report such infections promptly. Be sure to include a family member in your teaching session when preparing the patient for discharge.

You've met your goals if the patient is free of urinary tract infections and establishes adequate urinary elimination.

**Potential for impairment of skin integrity related to decreased mobility.** To maintain skin integrity, especially over bony prominences, and to reduce the size and depth of existing decubiti, assess the patient's understanding of personal skin care and his ability to care for his skin. Use digital circular massage on problem areas every 2 to 4 hours daily. Keep the patient's skin clean, dry, and lubricated with protective ointment. Turn the patient every 2 hours while he's in bed, and encourage him to shift his weight frequently when sitting. Tell him what types of clothing deter skin breakdown. For instance, tell him to wear cotton and to avoid nylon. Use sheepskin, a water mattress, or heel pads at pressure areas, and teach the patient to inspect these areas for redness. Evaluate skin condition daily.

Your interventions are successful if the patient understands how he can avoid trauma to his skin and if any existing decubiti are healing.

**Alterations in nutrition: Below body requirements related to muscle weakness.** To achieve an adequate fluid balance and sound nutrition, obtain a dietary history for evidence of imbalance, and determine the patient's dietary likes and dislikes. If muscle weakness is present, elevate the head of the bed during and after meals to prevent regurgitation and aspiration. Before beginning oral feeding, test the patient's swallowing reflex cautiously with a small amount of water; keep the patient upright; and have suction equipment handy. If oral feedings are not feasible, administer tube feedings as ordered. When the patient can swallow, begin oral feedings with soft foods. Because of diminished buccal sensation, pretest food and fluids to prevent burns. Encourage self-feeding as much as possible, even though it may prolong mealtimes and require rewarming of food. If necessary, provide several smaller meals a day to maintain adequate intake.

You've met your goals if the patient receives adequate fluid and nutritional intake and maintains an appropriate weight.

Other nursing diagnoses that may be used in the care of patients with these disorders include alterations in comfort, impaired verbal communication, disturbance in self-concept, ineffective coping of patient and his family, fear, self-care deficit, powerlessness, sexual dysfunction, and impaired home maintenance management.

### Looking ahead
One of the most frustrating aspects of these diseases is the unpredictability of their progression. You can help prepare the patient and his family to cope with their emotional impact by informing them about the patient's disease and teaching them how to cope with neurologic sequelae and with the possibility of later flare-ups.

**Points to remember**

- The major neurologic disorders believed to be caused by immune dysfunction include acute disseminated encephalomyelitis, Guillain-Barré syndrome (acute idiopathic polyneuritis), multiple sclerosis, and myasthenia gravis. The first three involve demyelination of central or peripheral nerves; myasthenia gravis involves destruction of acetylcholine receptor sites at the myoneural junction.
- Signs and symptoms of demyelination vary according to the location of lesions.
- A thorough assessment is important in the diagnosis of immune-related neurologic disorders because diagnosis is based primarily on clinical findings in the history and physical examination.
- Supportive therapy focuses on managing symptoms, from acute crisis in myasthenia gravis to chronic neurologic deficit.

# 14 CONTROLLING GASTROINTESTINAL DISORDERS

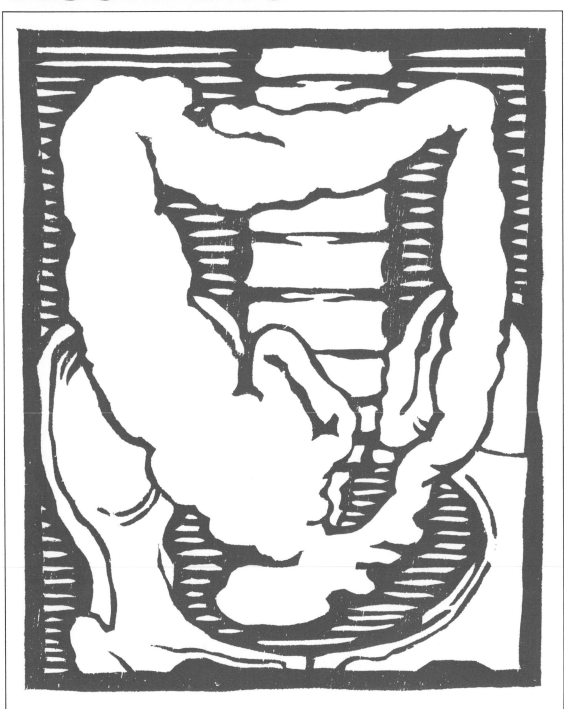

Ulcerative colitis

The immune system plays an important role in gastrointestinal (GI) homeostasis, so it's not surprising that certain GI and liver disorders appear to involve immune reactions. But little is known of their causes and underlying mechanisms and even less of effective treatment.

This being so, what *can* you do for a patient with, say, pernicious anemia or inflammatory bowel disease? You can assess him as thoroughly as possible, develop a good care plan based on your findings and the results of diagnostic tests, and then apply it to provide the best supportive care you possibly can for the patient and his family. Accomplishing these goals—assessment and support—is easier if you understand what's known about the pathology of these disorders.

## PATHOPHYSIOLOGY

The pathogenesis of such disorders as chronic atrophic gastritis, pernicious anemia, gluten-sensitive enteropathy (celiac sprue), inflammatory bowel disease, primary biliary cirrhosis, and alcohol- and drug-induced hepatitis is still unknown. However, each disorder exhibits identifiable immunologic features. For example, in pernicious anemia, destruction of glands found in the body of the stomach resulting in loss of intrinsic factor may be immunologically induced through antibody formation. (See *Immune-related gastrointestinal and liver disorders,* pages 174 and 175.)

## MEDICAL MANAGEMENT

Diagnosis of GI and liver disorders is based on test results, a detailed patient history, and a thorough physical examination.

### Tests help support diagnosis

Diagnostic tests of blood, electrolytes, stool, and tissue samples, along with endoscopic and contrast studies, help identify changes reflecting inflammation, ulceration, or tissue destruction.

**Complete blood count.** This test may reveal decreased hemoglobin and hematocrit levels, which commonly occur in anemia accompanying many GI and liver disorders.

**Fecal occult blood test.** Appearance of occult blood in the stool indicates GI tract bleeding, which may suggest ulcerative colitis or gastritis. However, further testing, such as endoscopic and contrast studies, is required to pinpoint the source of bleeding.

**Serum electrolytes.** Low levels of phosphate, calcium, potassium, and sodium may indicate malabsorption. Low levels of magnesium and phosphorus due to inadequate diet often accompany alcohol-induced hepatitis.

**Endoscopic studies.** Endoscopy may identify lesions or strictures often present in inflammatory bowel disease and may locate sources of GI bleeding. Examination of GI tissue helps confirm a diagnosis or detects associated complications in a known primary diagnosis. For example, a colonic biopsy often reveals premalignant changes in a patient with colitis.

**Liver biopsy.** This valuable test can distinguish between specific types of hepatitis. For example, in drug-induced hepatitis, a liver biopsy may reveal spotty liver-cell necrosis around central veins, whereas in chronic hepatitis, the biopsy may reveal inflammation of portal tracts with no significant piecemeal necrosis.

**Liver profile studies.** These tests help assess liver disorders by measuring the levels of alkaline phosphatase, serum glutamic-pyruvic transaminase (SGPT), serum glutamic-oxaloacetic transaminase (SGOT), lactic dehydrogenase (LDH), bilirubin, urobilinogen, prothrombin time (PT), serum proteins, blood ammonia, and total cholesterol.

Various combinations of test results indicate different disorders. For example, elevated alkaline phosphatase and bilirubin levels with only slightly elevated SGOT and SGPT levels indicate primary biliary cirrhosis. In drug-induced hepatitis, SGOT and SGPT levels may be as much as 50 times greater than normal; in alcohol-induced hepatitis, the level of SGOT is higher than that of SGPT.

Elevated direct or indirect bilirubin levels help distinguish one type of jaundice from another: hepatocellular jaundice may indicate cirrhosis; obstructive jaundice may indicate hepatic cholestasis from drugs, such as halothane; and hemolytic jaundice may reflect pernicious anemia.

Prolonged PT and hypoalbuminemia reflect poor hepatic synthetic function in alcohol-induced hepatitis or cirrhosis. An elevated level of ammonia, which the liver normally converts to urea, indicates liver failure. An elevated level of total cholesterol may suggest biliary obstruction.

**Immune response tests.** These tests include measurements of various antibodies and immune complexes to help diagnose immune reactions, which can directly involve the GI tract and liver.

*Antiparietal cell antibody (APA) test.* This

## Immune-related gastrointestinal and liver disorders

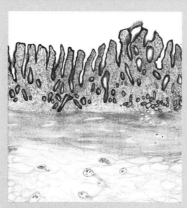

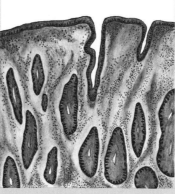

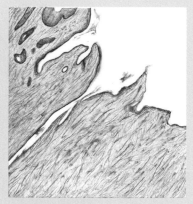

### Chronic atrophic gastritis and pernicious anemia

**Pathophysiology**
In pernicious anemia, destruction of normal glands of body of the stomach; partial or complete loss of acid, pepsinogen, and intrinsic factor secretion, resulting in inability to absorb vitamin $B_{12}$

**Immunologic features**
Humoral and cell-mediated immunity to gastric mucosal antigens; canaliculi and intrinsic factor antiparietal cell antibodies; autoantibodies in gastric mucosal plasma cells and in secretions (IgA)

**Signs and symptoms**
*In atrophic gastritis without pernicious anemia:* gastric lesion is usually asymptomatic.
*In pernicious anemia:* weakness, fatigue, appetite loss, weight loss, pallor, variable neurologic involvement

### Gluten-sensitive enteropathy (celiac sprue)

**Pathophysiology**
Distortion of columnar jejunal epithelial cells and microvilli; infiltration of lamina propria with inflammatory cells

**Immunologic features**
If untreated, infiltration of jejunal lamina propria with lymphocytes and plasma cells; production of IgM antigluten antibodies with possible local IgA deficiency; genetic association with HLA-Dw3 and -B8

**Signs and symptoms**
Malabsorption; stunted growth in children; weight loss; vitamin or mineral deficiencies; greasy, bulky stools; dermatitis herpetiformis

### Crohn's disease

**Pathophysiology**
Transmural ulceration of mucosa of any part of GI tract, but particularly the terminal ileum; if ulceration reaches serosa, perforation and fistulas may occur; two or more diseased segments may be separated by normal bowel

**Immunologic features**
Granulomatous response to intestinal lesions and regional lymph nodes; alterations in humoral immunity (not consistently demonstrated); abnormalities in cell-mediated immunity (may be secondary)

**Signs and symptoms**
Colic, diarrhea, malabsorption, weight loss, fever, vitamin or mineral deficiencies

test measures APAs—antibodies to canaliculi and antibodies to intrinsic factor. Detectable parietal canalicular antibodies indicate chronic gastritis. Antibodies to intrinsic factor indicate pernicious anemia.

*AGM test.* This test measures three of the five immunoglobulins (IgA, IgG, and IgM) normally found in the blood. Decreased IgA levels reflect malabsorption; increased IgG levels reflect liver disease; and increased IgM levels may accompany primary biliary cirrhosis.

*Antimitochondrial antibody (AMA) and antismooth muscle antibody (ASMA) tests.* These tests are usually performed together. Increased AMA levels commonly accompany primary biliary cirrhosis and, less often, chronic active hepatitis and drug-induced jaundice. Increased ASMA levels commonly accompany chronic active hepatitis and, less often, primary biliary cirrhosis.

*Circulating immune complex test.* This test detects circulating immune complexes, which are often present in liver disease as well as chronic inflammatory bowel disease. Since circulating immune complexes are present in many infections, positive test results must be cautiously interpreted.

### Treatment involves support
Treatments for most immune-related GI and liver disorders have been disappointing. However, in treating disorders caused by offending substances such as alcohol, drugs, or wheat gluten, their removal has resolved or at least halted the underlying pathology. (See *Hepatotoxicity: A formidable problem,* page 176.)

For the remaining disorders, the most effective treatment involves a combination of drug

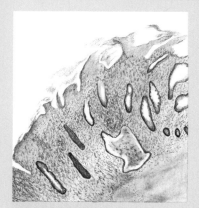

**Ulcerative colitis**

**Pathophysiology**
Ulceration and inflammation of colonic mucosa; ulcers may be superficial or may involve entire mucosa, resulting in mucosal loss and replacement by granulation tissue; submucosal inflammatory changes occur in chronic disease

**Immunologic features**
Increased turnover of IgG, IgM, and C3 levels in active disease; lymphocytes are cytotoxic for colonic epithelial cells; intestinal lipopolysaccharide antibodies cross-react with *Escherichia coli* 014

**Signs and symptoms**
Mild diarrhea without systemic upset or passage of more than 10 bloody stools daily, sustained fever, prostration, dehydration

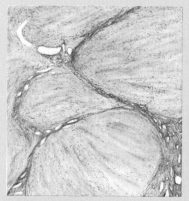

**Primary biliary cirrhosis**

**Pathophysiology**
Destruction of intrahepatic biliary tree due to chronic granulomatous inflammation

**Immunologic features**
Diminished suppressor cell function, increased polymeric and monomeric IgM serum concentrations, failure to convert from IgM to IgG production, complement-activating immune complexes, granulomatous infiltration of intrahepatic biliary tree; 99% of patients are antimitochondrial antibody–positive

**Signs and symptoms**
Inflammation, pruritus, pain, tenderness, rigidity of right upper quadrant; nausea, vomiting

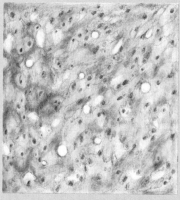

**Alcohol- and drug-induced hepatitis**

**Pathophysiology**
Liver necrosis due to toxic chemicals and drug; repeated episodes may lead to chronic liver disease

**Immunologic features**
Immunologically mediated response to altered or denatured membrane and intracellular antigens follows toxic damage; in alcohol-induced hepatitis, polyclonal hyperglobulinemia, particularly IgA; depressed cell-mediated immune response

**Signs and symptoms**
Similar to viral hepatitis; if chronic necrosis has developed, signs and symptoms similar to chronic liver disease

---

therapy, diet therapy, and, in extreme cases, surgery.

**Drug therapy.** Drugs are used to limit tissue destruction, to ease the patient's discomfort, and to correct electrolyte imbalances and vitamin deficiencies.

Experimental use of corticosteroids and immunosuppressive agents has not produced consistent benefits. In fundal gastritis, corticosteroids may enhance vitamin $B_{12}$ absorption and may encourage some parietal cell regeneration and intrinsic factor secretion.

*Sulfasalazine (Azulfidine),* an antimicrobial agent, is used in ulcerative colitis and Crohn's disease. There is no evidence that this drug alters intestinal microflora, and any beneficial effects may result from factors other than the drug's antibacterial activity.

*Hematinic drugs* correct anemia, which may accompany GI bleeding. However, oral iron is contraindicated because of decreased absorption in the bowel. Other drugs used to treat ulcerative colitis include sedatives to promote rest, anticholinergics to control abdominal cramps, and antidiarrheal drugs. Anticholinergic and antidiarrheal drugs must be administered cautiously to avoid causing toxic dilation (megacolon). Vitamin $B_{12}$ injections will be administered in pernicious anemia. Insoluble vitamin replacements correct insoluble vitamin deficiencies in primary biliary cirrhosis.

**Diet therapy.** Removing wheat gluten from the diet may restore small-bowel structure and function in gluten-sensitive enteropathy. Although clinical response to gluten withdrawal is immediate, histologic recovery could take weeks or months. Vitamins and other

## Hepatotoxicity: A formidable problem

Being aware of potentially toxic drugs is critical in treating patients with drug-induced hepatitis. Some common hepatotoxins are listed below:

Acetaminophen
Alcohol
Arsenic
Carbon tetrachloride
Chloroform
Gold compounds
Mercury
Phosphorus
Anabolic steroids
Halothane
Isoniazid (INH)
Propylthiouracil
Salicylates
Sulfonamides
Thiazide diuretics
6-mercaptopurine (6-MP)

nutrients may be administered if necessary.

In patients with chronic inflammatory bowel disease who are awaiting surgery or dehydrating from excessive diarrhea, administering intravenous hyperalimentation (IVH) restores nitrogen balance, reduces diarrhea, and rests the intestinal tract. A well-balanced, high-calorie, high-protein, low-residue diet may be introduced later. Well-balanced diets are also important in Crohn's disease and drug- and alcohol-induced hepatitis. If chronic liver disease develops, the patient's diet will have to be modified further.

**Surgery.** In Crohn's disease and ulcerative colitis, surgery may be done as a last resort. In Crohn's disease, surgery may correct complications such as obstructions and fistulas. In ulcerative colitis, colon resection with ileostomy may be necessary if the patient doesn't respond to medical management. Since patients with Crohn's disease and ulcerative colitis tend to develop malignancies in diseased areas, surgery may also be necessary to remove neoplastic lesions. In some patients, removal of precancerous lesions may prevent cancer development.

### NURSING MANAGEMENT

Because immune-related GI and liver diseases are chronic, and treatment is often a frustrating experience, maintaining optimal function demands skillful nursing management.

### Obtain a detailed patient history

Biographic data—particularly age and sex—may indicate that your patient runs a greater risk of having certain GI disorders. For example, although primary biliary cirrhosis affects both sexes and all ages, it most commonly affects females between ages 35 and 60; atrophic gastritis is more common in elderly patients; and ulcerative colitis occurs more often in young adult women.

Ask the patient about his past and present occupations. Was he ever exposed to hepatotoxic chemicals, such as carbon tetrachloride, arsenic, phosphorus, or mercury?

**Determine the chief complaint.** Ask the patient to describe it, giving as many details as possible. Patients with chronic inflammatory bowel disorders often have different symptoms. For example, diarrhea is almost always bloody in ulcerative colitis but is usually not bloody in Crohn's disease.

Ask the patient if he has abdominal pain. If so, what does it feel like? What other symptoms accompany the pain? In ulcerative coli-

tis, the pain is usually crampy and often subsides after a bowel movement. In Crohn's disease, pain is usually more persistent and may be aggravated by eating.

**Determine a past history.** Ask the patient if he's had any GI or liver disorders in the past, such as hepatitis, ascites, jaundice, cirrhosis, anemia, gastritis, diarrhea, constipation, malabsorption, or colitis? Was he ever hospitalized for the disorder?

Ask him about previous abdominal or rectal surgery. When was it done and for what condition? Also ask about postoperative complications and how these were treated.

Obtain an accurate drug history. Ask the patient what drugs he's taking now and what drugs he's taken in the past. Ask him to include over-the-counter drugs because many chemicals are potentially hepatotoxic. Anti-infectives, cytotoxic drugs, and many other drugs produce GI side effects, such as nausea, vomiting, diarrhea, or constipation. Also, ask the patient how much alcohol he consumes. Does he drink more or less than in the past?

Determine a family history of GI and liver diseases. Crohn's disease, ulcerative colitis, pernicious anemia, and gluten-sensitive enteropathy tend to be familial.

**Review other body systems.** This review may reveal extraintestinal complications such as arthritis, the most common complication of chronic inflammatory bowel disease. Ask the patient about skin and eye problems, which are also affected in inflammatory bowel disease for unknown reasons. For instance, uveitis can accompany ulcerative colitis and Crohn's disease. Also ask about cirrhosis or biliary tract carcinoma.

**Include a detailed nutritional assessment.** Has the patient gained or lost weight recently? Ask him about his eating habits. Does he eat very hot or spicy foods? Does he have any food allergies? What foods does he like, and what foods does he dislike?

### Perform the physical examination

Begin your examination by assessing the patient's overall appearance. Check for pallor, which may indicate possible anemia. Check for dermatitis herpetiformis, a sign of gluten-sensitive enteropathy. Look for dry, grayish skin; sunken eyes; jerky movements; and irritation—signs of electrolyte and fluid imbalance.

**Record vital signs.** Hypotension and tachycardia may reflect anemia. A sustained fever often accompanies ulcerative colitis.

**Inspect the abdomen.** Check for a hollow or

scaphoid abdomen, indicating possible malnutrition. Note any abdominal distention with an everted umbilicus, which may be a sign of ascites often accompanying liver disorders. Inspect the abdominal skin. Tense or glistening skin is also a sign of ascites. Check skin color for changes indicating bilirubin accumulation.

Auscultate the abdomen for abnormal bowel sounds. Rapid, high-pitched, tinkling sounds or loud, gurgling noises with visible peristaltic waves often accompany diarrhea in ulcerative colitis and Crohn's disease. If you suspect ascites, percuss the patient's flanks for shifting dullness (see Chapter 2). Palpate for tenderness, suggesting an inflamed colon in Crohn's disease or ulcerative colitis. If you palpate an enlarged liver, suspect liver disease.

### Formulate nursing diagnoses
Now that you've completed a detailed history and a thorough physical examination, you're ready to combine appropriate physical care with effective emotional support. Depending on the severity of symptoms, expect to incorporate the following nursing diagnoses in your care plan for the patient with GI or liver disease.

**Disturbance in self-concept related to altered body image.** Malnutrition, excessive weight loss, ileostomy, jaundice, or ascites may alter the patient's appearance, so he will need your understanding. To establish an open relationship with the patient, encourage him to talk about his feelings and daily activities. To allay his apprehension, explain all procedures and treatments.

Help the patient focus his attention on pleasant activities. If he isn't coping effectively, suggest psychotherapy.

Respect the patient's need for privacy. If he has inflammatory bowel disease and persistent diarrhea, ask him if he'd prefer a private room.

Consider your interventions effective when the patient discusses his feelings, understands the reasons for his body changes, and feels comfortable in his surroundings.

**Alteration in fluid and electrolyte balance due to diarrhea.** In acute phases, replace lost vitamins and electrolytes with intravenous fluids as ordered. To rest the bowel in patients with inflammatory bowel disease, expect to give IVH as ordered.

Record the patient's fluid intake and output, and check his weight daily. Provide oral care frequently. Determine the patient's food pref-

erences. To avoid depressing the appetite in the patient with chronic inflammatory bowel disease, remove his food tray when peristalsis is stimulated.

Before he's discharged, give him specific dietary instructions. For example, in the patient with gluten-sensitive enteropathy, stress the importance of avoiding even trace amounts of wheat gluten.

Consider your interventions effective when the patient is adequately hydrated and well nourished and understands the importance of dietary compliance.

**Alteration in skin integrity related to diarrhea, edema, ascites, or prolonged bed rest.** To prevent skin breakdown in the patient with diarrhea, pad the rim of his bedpan. Wash the perianal area after each bowel movement. To prevent skin breakdown from edema or ascites, provide an alternating air pressure mattress and change the patient's position at least every 2 hours. If ascites is present, support his abdomen with pillows. If he's confined to bed, teach him to perform range-of-motion exercises.

Consider your interventions effective when the patient's skin remains intact or begins to heal.

**Knowledge deficit concerning home-care procedures.** Since most patients with GI or liver disease will continue drug therapy after they leave the hospital, you'll need to incorporate specific drug instructions into your discharge planning. Involve family members in this planning so they can help support the patient at home. If the patient has had an ileostomy, teach him and his family how to care for the site and to replace the pouch. If he has had other surgery, give thorough instructions about appropriate postoperative wound care.

Consider your interventions effective when the patient and his family understand the purpose of, and comply with, the drug and treatment regimen.

### A sensitive task
Diagnosing and treating immune-related GI and liver disorders may or may not restore your patient to health. Current therapy is frequently ineffective, reflecting uncertain pathogenesis, and the chronicity of these disorders provokes frustration. Your task is to ensure that the patient takes his medication and is comfortable and to sensitively help him and his family understand his disorder and its distressing physical effects.

**Points to remember**

- Many immune-related GI and liver disorders have an unknown pathogenesis.
- Patients with alcohol- or drug-induced hepatitis usually have depressed cell-mediated immune reactions.
- Liver biopsy is a valuable diagnostic tool because it can differentiate between liver disorders.
- A thorough physical examination is essential to assess systemic effects caused by GI and liver disorders.
- To help the patient accept the chronicity of his immune-related GI or liver disorder, plan your care with sensitivity and understanding.

# Immunologic drugs

## Antihistamines

| Drug, dose, and route | Interactions | Side effects | Special considerations |
|---|---|---|---|
| **brompheniramine**<br>4 mg P.O. t.i.d. or q.i.d.; or timed-release 8 to 12 mg b.i.d. or t.i.d.; or 5 to 20 mg I.M., I.V., or S.C. q 12 hours | *Narcotics and other CNS depressants:* increased drowsiness and sedation | Drowsiness, dizziness, nausea, dry mouth, thickening of bronchial secretions | This drug causes less drowsiness than some other antihistamines. Tell patient that coffee or tea may reduce drowsiness, and sugarless gum, sour hard candy, or ice chips may relieve dry mouth.<br>    Administer the 10-mg/ml injection form diluted or undiluted very slowly I.V. Don't give the 100-mg/ml injection form I.V. |
| **chlorpheniramine**<br>2 to 4 mg P.O. t.i.d. or q.i.d.; or timed-release 8 to 12 mg P.O. b.i.d. or t.i.d.; or 5 to 40 mg I.M., I.V., or S.C. daily in divided doses | *Narcotics and other CNS depressants:* increased drowsiness and sedation | Drowsiness, dizziness, nausea, dry mouth, thickening of bronchial secretions | This drug causes less drowsiness than most other antihistamines. Tell patient that coffee or tea may reduce drowsiness, and sugarless gum, sour hard candy, or ice chips may relieve dry mouth.<br>    Administer I.V. injection over 1 minute.<br>    This drug is a common ingredient in cold remedies. |
| **clemastine**<br>1.34 to 2.68 mg P.O. once daily | *Narcotics and other CNS depressants:* increased drowsiness and sedation | Drowsiness, dizziness, nausea, dry mouth, thickening of bronchial secretions | Tell patient that coffee or tea may reduce drowsiness, and sugarless gum, sour hard candy, or ice chips may relieve dry mouth.<br>    Titrate the dose; response varies. |
| **cyproheptadine**<br>4 mg P.O. t.i.d. or q.i.d. | *Narcotics and other CNS depressants:* increased drowsiness and sedation | Drowsiness, dizziness, nausea, dry mouth, thickening of bronchial secretions | Tell patient that coffee or tea may reduce drowsiness, and sugarless gum, sour hard candy, or ice chips may relieve dry mouth.<br>    This drug is also prescribed to relieve pruritus. |
| **diphenhydramine**<br>25 to 50 mg P.O., I.M., or I.V. t.i.d. or q.i.d. | *Narcotics and other CNS depressants:* increased drowsiness and sedation | Drowsiness, dizziness, nausea, dry mouth, thickening of bronchial secretions | Administer I.M. injection deep into large muscle. Alternate injection sites to prevent irritation. Tell patient that coffee or tea may reduce drowsiness, and sugarless gum, sour hard candy, or ice chips may relieve dry mouth.<br>    This drug is one of the most sedating antihistamines. It is often used as a hypnotic. |
| **promethazine**<br>12.5 mg P.O. q.i.d., or 25 mg at bedtime; or 25 mg I.M. or I.V. rectally | *Narcotics and other CNS depressants:* increased drowsiness and sedation<br>*Phenothiazines:* increased phenothiazine effects; don't give together | Drowsiness, dizziness, nausea, dry mouth, thickening of bronchial secretions, photosensitivity | Administer I.M. injection deep into large muscle. This drug may be safely mixed with meperidine (Demerol) in the same syringe. Tell patient about possible photosensitivity and precautions to avoid it.<br>    This antihistamine belongs to the phenothiazine family. |
| **tripelennamine**<br>25 to 50 mg P.O. q 4 to 6 hours, or timed-release 100 mg b.i.d. or t.i.d. | *Narcotics and other CNS depressants:* increased drowsiness and sedation | Drowsiness, dizziness, nausea, dry mouth, epigastric distress, thickening of bronchial secretions | Administer this drug with food or milk to reduce GI distress. Tell patient that coffee or tea may reduce drowsiness, and sugarless gum, sour hard candy, or ice chips may relieve dry mouth. |

## Antimalarial antiarthritic

| Drug, dose, and route | Interactions | Side effects | Special considerations |
|---|---|---|---|
| **hydroxychloroquine**<br>400 to 600 mg P.O. daily; when good response occurs (usually in 4 to 12 weeks), continue with maintenance dose of 200 to 400 mg daily | None significant | Blood dyscrasias, visual disturbances and retinopathy, changes in skin pigmentation | Monitor periodic blood cell counts and liver function studies during prolonged therapy; if severe blood disorder appears that is not attributable to disease under treatment, inform doctor. He may discontinue this drug.<br>    Obtain baseline and periodic ophthalmologic examinations. Report blurred vision, increased sensitivity to light, or muscle weakness. Check periodically for ocular muscle weakness after long-term use. |

## Antimyasthenics

| Drug, dose, and route | Interactions | Side effects | Special considerations |
|---|---|---|---|
| **neostigmine**<br>15 to 30 mg P.O. t.i.d.; or 0.5 to 2 mg I.M. or I.V. q 1 to 3 hours, as needed | *Procainamide, aminoglycoside antibiotics, quinidine:* may reverse cholinergic effect on muscle; observe for lack of therapeutic effect<br>*Succinylcholine:* prolonged respiratory depression and possible apnea | Nausea, vomiting, diarrhea, muscle cramps, respiratory depression | Administer this drug with milk or food to reduce GI side effects. Document patient's response after each dose. Monitor his vital signs frequently, especially respirations. Keep atropine injection available to treat serious side effects. Show patient how to observe and record variations in muscle strength. |

## Antimyasthenics (continued)

| Drug, dose, and route | Interactions | Side effects | Special considerations |
|---|---|---|---|
| **pyridostigmine**<br>60 to 180 mg P.O. b.i.d. to q.i.d. with maximum dose of 1,500 mg; or 2 mg I.M. or very slow I.V. injection q 3 hours | *Procainamide, aminoglycoside antibiotics, quinidine:* may reverse cholinergic effect on muscle; observe for lack of therapeutic effect<br>*Succinylcholine:* prolonged respiratory depression and possible apnea | Nausea, vomiting, diarrhea, headache | Double-check all orders for I.M. or I.V. administration. Parenteral dose is 1/30 of oral dose. Adjust dose depending on patient response. |

## Glucocorticoids

| Drug, dose, and route | Interactions | Side effects | Special considerations |
|---|---|---|---|
| **beclomethasone**<br>*For rhinitis:* one spray (42 mcg) in each nostril b.i.d. to q.i.d.<br>*For asthma:* two to four inhalations t.i.d. or q.i.d. | None significant | Mild nasal burning and stinging (nasal form), hoarseness, fungal infections of mouth and throat | Warn patient not to exceed recommended dosage. This drug may suppress hypothalamic-pituitary-adrenal function.<br>Nasal inhaler is used when antihistamines or nasal decongestants fail. Tell patient to stop drug and notify doctor if symptoms don't improve within 3 weeks or if nasal irritation persists.<br>To prevent oral fungal infections, tell patient to follow oral inhalations with glass of water. Tell patient to keep inhaler clean and unobstructed. Instruct him to wash it with warm water and dry it thoroughly. |
| **flunisolide**<br>Two sprays (50 mcg) in each nostril b.i.d. If necessary, increase dose to two sprays in each nostril t.i.d. | None significant | Mild nasal burning and stinging (nasal form), hoarseness, fungal infections of mouth and throat | Explain that therapeutic effects of this corticosteroid, unlike those of decongestants, are not immediate. Most patients achieve benefit within a few days, but some may need 2 to 3 weeks for maximum benefit.<br>Patients with dryness and crusting of the nasal mucosa may prefer the liquid spray of flunisolide to the aerosolized powder of beclomethasone. If symptoms don't improve within 3 weeks or if nasal irritation persists, tell patient to stop drug and notify doctor. |
| **cortisone acetate**<br>25 to 300 mg P.O. or I.M. daily or on alternate days<br><br>**dexamethasone**<br>0.25 to 4 mg P.O. b.i.d. to q.i.d.<br><br>**hydrocortisone**<br>5 to 80 mg P.O., I.M., or I.V. b.i.d. to q.i.d.<br><br>**methylprednisolone**<br>2 to 250 mg P.O., I.M., or I.V. daily in single or divided doses<br><br>**prednisone**<br>2.5 to 15 mg P.O. b.i.d. to q.i.d. | *Amphotericin B, diuretics:* may increase potassium loss; monitor for hypokalemia<br>*Barbiturates, phenytoin, rifampin:* decreased corticosteroid effect; dose may need to be increased<br>*Indomethacin, aspirin:* increased risk of GI distress and bleeding; give together cautiously | Euphoria, insomnia, hypokalemia, hyperglycemia, peptic ulcer and GI irritation, fluid retention with possible hypertension, congestive heart failure | Give once-daily doses in the morning for better results and less toxicity. Give P.O. dose with food when possible. Unless contraindicated, give salt-restricted diet rich in potassium and protein. Potassium supplement may be needed. Corticosteroid doses are highly individualized, depending on patient and his condition.<br>Warn patient on long-term therapy about cushingoid symptoms. Teach him early signs of adrenal insufficiency (fatigue, muscle weakness, joint pain, fever, anorexia, nausea, dyspnea, dizziness, fainting). Instruct patient to carry a card indicating need for supplemental systemic glucocorticoids during stress, especially as dose is decreased. Monitor weight, blood pressure, and serum electrolytes. Patients with diabetes may need increased insulin; monitor urine for glucose. |

## Gold salts

| Drug, dose, and route | Interactions | Side effects | Special considerations |
|---|---|---|---|
| **aurothioglucose**<br>Initially, 10 mg I.M. followed by 25 mg for second and third doses at weekly intervals; then, 50 mg weekly until 1 g has been given<br><br>**gold sodium thiomalate**<br>Initially, 10 mg I.M. followed by 25 mg after 1 week; then, 50 mg weekly for 14 to 20 doses | None significant | Anaphylaxis, blood dyscrasias, dizziness, metallic taste, stomatitis, kidney toxicity, skin rash | Administer these drugs only under constant supervision of a doctor thoroughly familiar with their toxicities and benefits. Administer all gold salts I.M., preferably intragluteally. Color of drug is pale yellow. Don't use if it darkens.<br>Observe patient for 30 minutes after administration for anaphylactic reaction. Dermatitis is the most common side effect. Tell patient to report skin rashes or problems immediately. Stomatitis is the second most common side effect. Tell patient to report a metallic taste to the doctor immediately as this often precedes stomatitis. Most side effects are reversible if drug is stopped immediately.<br>Tell patient that therapeutic effects may not appear for 6 to 8 weeks or longer. |

## Immune globulins

| Drug, dose, and route | Interactions | Side effects | Special considerations |
|---|---|---|---|
| **immune globulin intramuscular**<br>1.2 ml/kg I.M. followed by 0.66 ml/kg q 3 to 4 weeks | *Live virus vaccines:* immune globulin may interfere with response; wait 3 months | Tenderness and stiffness at injection site, urticaria, anaphylaxis | Give cautiously to patients with a history of allergic reactions to human immunoglobulin preparations. Divide dose of more than 10 ml, and inject into different sites, preferably the buttocks. Don't inject more than 3 ml per injection site. Adequate serum levels occur in 2 to 7 days. |
| **immune globulin intravenous**<br>100 mg/kg I.V. infusion monthly; increase to 200 mg/kg if clinical response is not adequate | *Live virus vaccines:* immune globulin may interfere with response; don't administer within 3 months after administration of immune globulin | Anaphylaxis | Give cautiously to patients with a history of allergic reactions to human immunoglobulin preparations. Because anaphylaxis is more likely to occur when this drug is given I.V., keep epinephrine available.<br>This drug may be diluted with a solution of dextrose 5% in water. I.V. administration provides immediate antibody levels. |

## Immunosuppressants

| Drug, dose, and route | Interactions | Side effects | Special considerations |
|---|---|---|---|
| **azathioprine**<br>Initially, 3 to 5 mg/kg P.O. daily. Maintenance dose: 1 to 2 mg/kg daily depending on patient response | *Allopurinol:* impaired inactivation of azathioprine; decrease azathioprine dose to one quarter to one third of normal dose | Bone marrow depression (leukopenia, macrocytic anemia, pancytopenia, thrombocytopenia), risk of infection due to immunosuppression, nausea, vomiting | Give drug with meals to improve GI tolerance. Azathioprine is a potent immunosuppressive.<br>Tell patient to report even mild infections (coryza, fever, sore throat, malaise). Warn him that his hair may thin.<br>Obtain hemoglobin, white blood cell (WBC), and platelet counts at least weekly and more often at beginning of treatment. Avoid all I.M. injections when platelets are low. |
| **cyclosporine**<br>Before transplantation: 15 mg/kg P.O. After transplantation: continue dose daily for 1 to 2 weeks. Then reduce gradually to maintenance dose of 5 to 10 mg/kg daily. Or administer I.V. until patient can tolerate oral solution. | *Ketaconazole, amphotericin B:* possible increased blood levels of cyclosporine; monitor for increased toxicity | Tremor, hypertension, nephrotoxicity, gum hyperplasia, hirsutism | Cyclosporine and adrenal corticosteroids are given concomitantly. Measure oral doses carefully in an oral syringe. Mix with whole or chocolate milk or fruit juice to increase palatability. Use a glass container to minimize adherence to container walls. Give drug once daily in the morning. Tell patient to take drug at the same time each day.<br>Cyclosporine may cause nephrotoxicity up to 3 months after transplantation. Monitor blood urea nitrogen (BUN) and serum creatinine levels and report findings to doctor. He may reduce dose. Tell patient to use hair remover cream if hirsutism occurs. |

## Nonsteroidal anti-inflammatory drugs

| Drug, dose, and route | Interactions | Side effects | Special considerations |
|---|---|---|---|
| **aspirin**<br>2.6 to 5.2 g P.O. daily in divided doses<br><br>**choline salicylate**<br>870 mg (5 ml) to 1,740 mg (10 ml) P.O. q.i.d. | *Ammonium chloride (and other urine acidifiers):* increased blood levels of aspirin products; monitor for aspirin toxicity<br>*Antacids in high doses (and other urine alkalinizers):* decreased levels of aspirin products; monitor for decreased aspirin effect<br>*Corticosteroids:* increased salicylate elimination; monitor for decreased salicylate effect<br>*Oral anticoagulants and heparin:* increased risk of bleeding; avoid using together if possible | Prolonged bleeding time, tinnitus and hearing loss, nausea, vomiting, GI distress, occult bleeding, hypersensitivity | Give with food, milk, antacid, or water to reduce GI side effects. Tell patient to check with doctor or pharmacist before taking over-the-counter combinations containing aspirin. Warn that alcohol may increase GI blood loss. Don't give to patients with a GI ulcer, GI bleeding, or aspirin hypersensitivity.<br>The therapeutic blood salicylate level for arthritis patients is 20 to 30 mg/dl. |
| **fenoprofen**<br>300 to 600 mg P.O. q.i.d. | None significant | Headache, drowsiness, dizziness, nausea, epigastric distress, occult blood loss, skin rash | Give drug with milk or meals. Tell patient that full therapeutic effect may be delayed for 2 to 4 weeks.<br>Use drug cautiously in patients with a history of peptic ulcer disease. Check renal, hepatic, and auditory function periodically in long-term therapy. Stop drug if abnormalities occur. Fenoprofen decreases platelet aggregation and may prolong bleeding time. |
| **ibuprofen**<br>300 to 600 mg P.O. q.i.d. | None significant | Headache, drowsiness, dizziness, epigastric distress, occult blood loss, skin rash | Give drug with milk or meals. Tell patient that full therapeutic effect may be delayed for 2 to 4 weeks.<br>Use drug cautiously in patients with a history of peptic ulcer disease. Check renal and hepatic function periodically in long-term therapy. Stop drug if abnormalities occur.<br>Ibuprofen is available over-the-counter as Advil and Nuprin. |

## Nonsteroidal anti-inflammatory drugs (continued)

| Drug, dose, and route | Interactions | Side effects | Special considerations |
|---|---|---|---|
| **indomethacin**<br>25 to 50 mg P.O. b.i.d. or t.i.d.; or sustained-release capsule once or twice daily | *Beta blockers:* decreased effectiveness of beta blockers<br>*Diflunisal, probenecid:* decreased indomethacin excretion; watch for increased incidence of indomethacin side effects<br>*Furosemide:* impaired response to both drugs; avoid if possible<br>*Lithium:* possible lithium toxicity<br>*Triamterene:* possible nephrotoxicity; don't use together | Headache, dizziness, blood dyscrasias, blurred vision, nausea, vomiting, diarrhea, reversible renal failure, severe GI bleeding, hypersensitivity | Give this drug with meals because it is irritating to the patient's GI tract. Tell the patient to notify the doctor of any GI side effects. CNS side effects are more common and serious in elderly patients. The patient may experience a severe headache within 1 hour of administration. Decrease dose if headache persists.<br>    Periodically, test the complete blood count (CBC), renal function, and the eyes of patients receiving this drug long-term. Use drug cautiously in patients with a history of peptic ulcer disease. Don't use drug routinely as an analgesic or antipyretic because chronic use results in increased incidence of side effects. |
| **meclofenamate**<br>200 to 400 mg P.O. daily in three or four equal doses | None significant | Headache, dizziness, nausea, vomiting, diarrhea, hepatotoxicity, skin rash | Give this drug with meals to minimize GI side effects. Stop drug if rash or diarrhea develops.<br>    Use this drug cautiously in patients with a history of peptic ulcer disease. |
| **naproxen**<br>250 to 500 mg P.O. b.i.d. | None significant | Nausea, epigastric distress, occult blood loss, skin rash | Tell patient that full therapeutic effect may be delayed for 2 to 4 weeks. Use this drug cautiously in patients with a history of peptic ulcer disease.<br>    Naproxen is available in two forms: naproxen and naproxen sodium. Warn patients to avoid taking both forms at the same time because side effects are cumulative. |
| **oxyphenbutazone**<br>100 to 200 mg P.O. t.i.d. or q.i.d.<br><br>**phenylbutazone**<br>100 to 200 mg P.O. t.i.d. or q.i.d. | *Oral anticoagulants:* increased hypoprothrombinemic effect; monitor carefully<br>*Oral hypoglycemics:* possible hypoglycemia; monitor blood glucose<br>*Phenytoin:* possible phenytoin toxicity; monitor carefully | Bone marrow depression (fatal aplastic anemia, agranulocytosis, thrombocytopenia), cardiac decompensation, sodium retention, edema, nausea, vomiting, diarrhea, hepatotoxicity, skin rashes | Give these drugs with food or milk. Response to therapy should occur in 2 to 3 days. If not evident within 1 week, stop drug.<br>    Record the patient's weight, intake, and output daily. These drugs may cause sodium retention and edema. Tell the patient to stop drug and notify doctor immediately if fever, sore throat, mouth ulcers, GI discomfort, bruising, rash, or weight gain occurs.<br>    A patient over age 60 shouldn't receive either drug for more than 1 week. |
| **piroxicam**<br>20 mg P.O. once daily | None significant | Epigastric distress, nausea, dizziness, headache, occult blood loss, skin rashes | Give drug with milk or meals. Tell patient that full therapeutic effect may be delayed for 2 to 4 weeks.<br>    Skin rashes occur more often with this drug than with similar drugs. Use drug cautiously in patients with a history of peptic ulcer disease. This drug permits once-a-day administration because it has a longer duration of action than similar drugs. |
| **sulindac**<br>150 to 200 mg P.O. b.i.d. | None significant | Epigastric distress, nausea, dizziness, headache, occult blood loss, blood dyscrasias, edema, hepatoxicity | Administer this drug with milk or meals. This drug causes sodium retention. Tell the patient to report edema and to have his blood pressure checked regularly.<br>    Use this drug cautiously in patients with a history of peptic ulcer disease. |

## Sympathomimetics

| Drug, dose, and route | Interactions | Side effects | Special considerations |
|---|---|---|---|
| **ephedrine**<br>12.5 to 50 mg P.O. b.i.d. to q.i.d. | *Beta-adrenergic blockers:* blocked bronchodilating effect; monitor patient carefully<br>*Guanethidine:* may antagonize guanethidine's antihypertensive action<br>*MAO inhibitors, tricyclic antidepressants:* may cause hypertension; give cautiously with ephedrine<br>*Urinary alkalinizers:* may increase ephedrine's toxic effects | Insomnia, nervousness, palpitations, tachycardia, urinary retention, hypertension | To prevent insomnia, tell patient not to take this drug within 2 hours of bedtime. Warn him not to take over-the-counter drugs that contain ephedrine without informing doctor.<br>    Because effectiveness decreases within 2 to 3 weeks, dosage may need to be increased. Although tolerance develops, ephedrine isn't known to cause addiction. |
| **epinephrine**<br>0.1 to 0.5 ml of 1:1,000 S.C. or I.M. Repeat dose q 10 to 15 minutes p.r.n. | *Beta-adrenergic blockers:* blocked bronchodilating effect; monitor patient carefully<br>*Guanethidine:* may antagonize antihypertensive action<br>*Tricyclic antidepressants:* may cause hypertension; give cautiously with epinephrine | Nervousness, headache, palpitations, tachycardia, cardiac dysrhythmias, hyperglycemia, hypertension | After injection, observe patient closely for side effects. Massage injection site to counteract vasoconstriction and prevent necrosis. Repeated local injection can cause necrosis at site due to vasoconstriction. If blood pressure rises sharply, rapid-acting vasodilators, such as the nitrates or alpha-adrenergic blocking agents, can be given to counteract the marked pressor effect of large doses of epinephrine.<br>    Use drug cautiously in elderly patients and in those with a history of heart disease, hyperthyroidism, angina, hypertension, or diabetes. |

## Sympathomimetics (continued)

| Drug, dose, and route | Interactions | Side effects | Special considerations |
|---|---|---|---|
| **pseudoephedrine**<br>30 to 60 mg P.O. q 4 to 6 hours | *Guanethidine:* may antagonize guanethidine's antihypertensive action<br>*MAO inhibitors:* may cause hypertension; use together carefully<br>*Urinary alkalinizers:* may increase pseudoephedrine's toxic effects | Anxiety, nervousness, palpitations, insomnia | To prevent insomnia, tell patient not to take this drug within 2 hours of bedtime and to stop drug if he becomes unusually restless. Warn him not to take other over-the-counter products containing ephedrine or other sympathomimetic amines. |

## Xanthine derivatives

| Drug, dose, and route | Interactions | Side effects | Special considerations |
|---|---|---|---|
| **aminophylline (theophylline ethylenediamine)**<br>Loading dose: 5.6 mg/kg I.V.; maintenance dose by I.V. infusion: 0.3 to 0.9 mg/kg hourly; oral maintenance dose: 250 to 500 mg q 6 to 8 hours | *Beta-adrenergic blockers:* may antagonize pharmacologic effect of aminophylline; may cause bronchospasm; use together cautiously<br>*Erythromycin, cimetidine:* decreased hepatic clearance of aminophylline, causing elevated aminophylline levels; monitor for toxicity<br>*Phenytoin:* increased pharmacologic effects of both drugs possible | Restlessness, dizziness, insomnia, convulsions, palpitations, nausea, vomiting, anorexia | Before giving loading dose, make sure patient hasn't had recent theophylline therapy. Warn elderly patients of dizziness, a common side effect at start of therapy.<br>Individuals metabolize xanthines at different rates. Adjust dose by monitoring response, tolerance, pulmonary function, and aminophylline blood levels. Consider 10 to 20 mcg/ml a therapeutic level. Monitor carefully for GI symptoms, which usually accompany toxicity. Plasma clearance may be decreased in patients with congestive heart failure, hepatic dysfunction, or pulmonary edema. Smokers show accelerated clearance. Adjust dose as necessary.<br>Suppositories are unreliably absorbed. Avoid rectal administration or schedule after evacuations, if possible. |
| **oxtriphylline**<br>200 mg P.O. q 6 hours | *Beta-adrenergic blockers:* may antagonize pharmacologic effects of oxtriphylline; use together cautiously<br>*Erythromycin, cimetidine:* decreased hepatic clearance of oxtriphylline, causing elevated oxtriphylline levels; monitor for toxicity<br>*Phenytoin:* increased pharmacologic effects of both drugs possible | Restlessness, dizziness, insomnia, convulsions, palpitations, nausea, vomiting, anorexia | Ask patient whether he's using other drugs. Warn him that over-the-counter drugs may contain ephedrine in combination with theophylline salts. Concomitant use may cause excessive CNS stimulation. Tell patient to check with doctor before taking any other drugs.<br>Advise patient to report signs that may indicate excessive CNS stimulation: GI distress, palpitations, irritability, restlessness, nervousness, or insomnia.<br>Store this drug at 59° to 86° F. (15° to 30° C.). Protect elixir from light and tablets from moisture. |
| **theophylline**<br>100 to 200 mg P.O. q 6 hours or q 8 to 12 hours for timed-release form | *Beta-adrenergic blockers:* may antagonize pharmacologic effects of theophylline; use together cautiously<br>*Erythromycin, cimetidine:* decreased hepatic clearance of theophylline, causing elevated theophylline levels; monitor for toxicity<br>*Phenytoin:* increased pharmacologic effects of both drugs possible | Restlessness, dizziness, insomnia, convulsions, palpitations, nausea, vomiting, anorexia | Warn elderly patients of dizziness, a common side effect at the start of therapy.<br>Individuals metabolize xanthines at different rates. Adjust dose by monitoring response, tolerance, pulmonary function, and theophylline plasma levels. Consider 10 to 20 mcg/ml a therapeutic theophylline level.<br>Ask patient whether he's using other drugs. Warn him that over-the-counter drugs may contain ephedrine in combination with theophylline salts. Concomitant use may cause excessive CNS stimulation. Tell patient to check with doctor before taking other drugs.<br>Be careful not to confuse sustained-release with standard-release dosage forms. |

## Miscellaneous

| Drug, dose, and route | Interactions | Side effects | Special considerations |
|---|---|---|---|
| **cromolyn sodium**<br>*For asthma prophylaxis:* powder contents of 20 mg capsule inhaled q.i.d. at regular intervals<br>*For rhinitis prevention and treatment:* spray in each nostril three to six times daily at regular intervals | None significant | *Inhaled powder:* irritation of throat and trachea, coughing, esophagitis<br>*Nasal solution:* sneezing, nasal stinging and burning, nasal irritation | *Inhaled powder:* Tell patient not to swallow capsule. Tell him to insert it into the inhaler provided and then to follow the manufacturer's directions. Teach patient how to use a Spinhaler: insert capsule in device properly; exhale completely before placing mouthpiece between lips, then inhale deeply and rapidly with steady, even breath; remove inhaler from mouth, hold breath a few seconds, and exhale; repeat until you have inhaled all the powder. Advise patient to relieve esophagitis with antacids or milk.<br>*Nasal solution:* Instruct patient to clear his nasal passage before administering spray and to inhale through his nose during administration. Tell him to replace the pump device every 6 months. |
| **D-penicillamine**<br>Initially, 250 mg P.O. daily. Increase 250 mg q 2 to 3 months, if necessary | *Digoxin:* may reduce digoxin's serum levels; monitor carefully<br>*Oral iron:* decreased effectiveness of D-penicillamine; if used together, give at least 2 hours apart | Blood dyscrasias, nephrotic syndrome, glomerulonephritis, hepatotoxicity, hypersensitivity | Administer drug on an empty stomach to facilitate drug absorption. Tell patient to drink large amounts of fluid, especially at night. Also tell him that therapeutic effect may be delayed up to 3 months.<br>Monitor patient's CBC and renal and hepatic function regularly during therapy (every 2 weeks for the first 6 months and then monthly). Tell doctor if fever or other allergic reactions occur. |

## Selected immune disorders

| Disorder | Cause | Clinical features | Treatment |
| --- | --- | --- | --- |
| **Addison's disease** | Results from an autoimmune process | Postural hypotension, weight loss, anorexia, weakness, and hyperpigmentation of folds of the skin | Hormonal replacement |
| **Aplasia-thymoma, pure red cell** | May result from an autoimmune process | Fatigue, weakness, shortness of breath, hemorrhagic manifestations (possibly progressive), pallor, and possible myasthenia gravis symptoms | Thymectomy, splenectomy, immunosuppressive therapy, transfusions, corticosteroids |
| **Aspergillosis, allergic bronchopulmonary** | Results from hypersensitivity to *Aspergillus fumigatus* | Asthma-like symptoms (coughing, wheezing, dyspnea); intermittent fever; sputum with brown flecks or plugs | Corticosteroids, antiasthmatic drugs |
| **Cryoglobulinemia, essential mixed** | Unknown cause; related to immune complex disease | Polyarthralgia, palpable purpura, weakness, and glomerulonephritis associated with IgM-IgA cryoglobulinemia | Cytotoxic drugs, corticosteroids |
| **Dermatitis herpetiformis** | Unknown cause; may result from local activation of complement | Chronic pruritic vesicles on erythematous bases erupting in symmetrical clusters on extensor surfaces; and possible small intestinal lesions | Dapsone, sulfapyridine, gluten-free diet |
| **Diabetes mellitus (Type I)** | Unknown cause; may result from an autoimmune process | Hyperglycemia causing polyuria, polydipsia, polyphagia, and weight loss | Diet, insulin, exercise |
| **Dressler's syndrome** | Unknown cause; may result from formation of autoantibodies against an antigen from myocardial necrosis | Fever, chest pain, and pericarditis developing 2 to 10 weeks after a myocardial infarction | Corticosteroids, analgesics |
| **Erythema multiforme** | Unknown cause in 50% of patients; may result from drugs and radiation therapy | Flat, red maculopapules on the skin and possibly mucosa, increasing in 48 hours to 1 to 2 cm, or erythematous plaques with central bulla and ring of vesicles; malaise; myalgia | Corticosteroids, antibiotics |
| **Felty's syndrome** | Unknown cause; a variant of rheumatoid arthritis | Signs of rheumatoid arthritis, splenomegaly, generalized lymphadenopathy, recurrent infections from neutropenia, malaise, anorexia, and weight loss | Splenectomy |
| **Gardner-Diamond syndrome** | Results from autosensitization to red blood cells (RBCs) | Local sensations (tingling, burning) in extremities, face, and scalp, preceding purpuric lesions; affects only females | None |
| **Goodpasture's syndrome** | Unknown cause; may result from a virus or an autoimmune process | Pulmonary hemorrhage, hemoptysis, and necrotizing glomerulonephritis with hematuria | Bilateral nephrectomy, immunosuppressive therapy, cytotoxic drugs, corticosteroids |
| **Granulomatosis, Wegener's** | Unknown cause; may result from a hypersensitivity mechanism | Granulomatous inflammation of respiratory mucosa followed by necrotizing inflammatory skin lesions, pulmonary lesions with cavitation, diffuse vasculitis, and focal glomerulitis | Immunosuppressive therapy, cytotoxic drugs, corticosteroids |
| **Graves' disease** | Results from a serum thyroid-stimulating immunoglobulin | Hyperthyroidism marked by increased adrenergic activity, infiltrative ophthalmopathy, and infiltrative dermopathy | Surgery, antithyroid drugs, radioiodine |
| **Heavy-chain disease, alpha (Seligman's syndrome)** | Unknown cause | Severe malabsorption syndrome with chronic diarrhea, steatorrhea, weight loss, hypocalcemia, and lymphadenopathy | Cyclophosphamide, radiation, corticosteroids, antibiotics |
| **Heavy-chain disease, gamma (Franklin's disease)** | Unknown cause | Abrupt onset of lymphadenopathy without fever, and occasional edema and erythema of the uvula and soft palate | Chemotherapy, corticosteroids |
| **Heavy-chain disease, mu** | Unknown cause | Long-standing chronic lymphocytic leukemia with progressive hepatosplenomegaly; commonly fatal | Chemotherapy, radiation, corticosteroids |
| **Hemoglobinuria, paroxysmal nocturnal** | Unknown cause; may result from RBCs unusually susceptible to complement | Abdominal and lumbar pain, splenomegaly, intermittent hemoglobinemia, hemoglobinuria, and symptoms of severe anemia | Corticosteroids, transfusions, anticoagulants, oral iron therapy |
| **Hyperimmunoglobulinemia E syndrome (Buckley's syndrome)** | Results from elevated IgE | Lifelong recurrent staphylococcal abscesses of the skin, lungs, joints, and other sites; and pruritic dermatitis | Long-term therapy with antibiotics or antifungals |
| **Hypoparathyroidism, primary** | Unknown cause; may result from an autoimmune process | Muscle spasm, tetany, nervousness, weakness, blurred vision, headache, memory loss, and alopecia | Dihydrotachysterol, vitamin D |
| **Hypothyroidism, primary** | Unknown cause; may result from an autoimmune process | Dry skin; dry, coarse hair; constipation; cold intolerance; loss of vigor; slowed speech, mental processes, and reflexes | Thyroid hormone replacement |
| **Immunodeficiency with hyper-IgM** | Unknown cause; possible X-linked inheritance | Recurrent pyogenic infections; occasionally, recurrent neutropenia, hemolytic anemia, or aplastic anemia | Immunoglobulin replacement therapy, antibiotics |

## Selected immune disorders (continued)

| Disorder | Cause | Clinical features | Treatment |
|---|---|---|---|
| **Keratitis, herpes simplex** | Unknown cause; may result from a hypersensitivity response to the virus | Lacrimation and photophobia, possibly leading to deep, disk-shaped corneal inflammation with iritis | Idoxuridine, trifluridine, vidarabine; topical corticosteroids |
| **Leukemia, hairy-cell** | Unknown cause | Fatigue; malaise; infection; abdominal discomfort; pancytopenia; splenomegaly; and, at times, lymphadenopathy | Splenectomy, chemotherapy |
| **Leukoencephalopathy, progressive multifocal** | Results from a virus; associated with immunosuppression | Ataxia, spasticity, visual disturbances, difficulty with speech and swallowing, and rapid progression to coma and death | None |
| **Lymphadenopathy, angioimmunoblastic** | Unknown cause; may result from abnormal immune state | Weight loss and generalized lymphadenopathy | Corticosteroids, immunosuppressive therapy |
| **Monoclonal gammopathy, benign** | Unknown cause; may result from proliferation of a B-cell or a plasma cell | Monoclonal protein in serum or urine | None |
| **Nezelof's syndrome** | Results from cellular immunodeficiency with abnormal immunoglobulin synthesis | Recurrent fungal, protozoal, viral, and bacterial illnesses, often marked by chronic pulmonary infections, candidiasis, diarrhea, skin infection, and failure to thrive | Thymus implantation, gamma globulin, antibiotics, transfer factor therapy |
| **Ophthalmia, sympathetic** | Results from hypersensitivity to uveal pigment after eye trauma, possibly through an autoimmune mechanism | Inflammation of the second eye after penetrating injury to the other eye; uveal tract irritation marked by photophobia, lacrimation, transient blurring of vision, neuralgic pain, and eye tenderness | Corticosteroids, immunosuppressive therapy |
| **Pemphigoid, bullous** | Unknown cause; may result from local activation of complement | Self-limiting, subepidermal, tense bullae usually in flexor areas (axillary and inguinal folds and sides of the neck) | Corticosteroids, immunosuppressive therapy |
| **Pemphigoid, cicatricial** | Unknown cause; related to bullous pemphigoid | Subepidermal blisters of the oral and ocular mucous membranes with extensive conjunctival scarring and adhesions; may result in blindness | Artificial tears, protection of the cornea from trauma or infection |
| **Pemphigoid, IgA bullous** | Unknown cause | Subepidermal bullae on glabrous skin | Sulfones |
| **Pemphigus vulgaris** | Unknown cause; may result from an autoimmune reaction | Tense or flaccid bullae on mucous membranes, eventually rupturing and leaving chronic, often painful erosions | Corticosteroids, antibiotics, immunosuppressive therapy |
| **Pneumonia, eosinophilic** | Unknown cause; may result from a hypersensitivity reaction | Low-grade fever, minimal respiratory symptoms, and symptoms of bronchial asthma (coughing, wheezing, and dyspnea at rest) | Corticosteroids |
| **Pneumonitis, hypersensitivity** | Results from an allergic (Type III) response to various inhaled organic dusts | Acute: fever, chills, cough, dyspnea, and GI distress. Chronic: progressive exertional dyspnea, productive cough, fatigue, and weight loss; may progress to respiratory failure | Corticosteroids, avoidance of exposure to dust |
| **Polyendocrinopathy, autoimmune** | Unknown cause; may result from an autoimmune process | Effects of endocrine hypofunction on the adrenals, parathyroid, pituitary, and pancreas | Hormonal replacement |
| **Postpericardiotomy syndrome** | Unknown cause; may result from formation of autoantibodies against an antigen from damaged myocardium | Fever, pleuropericardial pain, pericardial friction rub, and pleural or pericardial effusion | Corticosteroids, analgesics |
| **Sarcoidosis** | Unknown cause; may result from a hypersensitivity mechanism, genetic disposition, or chemical exposure | Initially, fever, weight loss, and arthralgias; also, peripheral lymphadenopathy, mediastinal adenopathy, pulmonary infiltration, skin lesions, hepatic granulomas, uveitis, angina, congestive heart failure, conduction disorders, variable CNS involvement, diabetes insipidus, and calcium imbalance | Corticosteroids |
| **Sclerosis, amyotrophic lateral** | Unknown cause; may result from a viral process | Weakness, atrophy, and fasciculations, especially in the muscles of the forearms and hands | Symptomatic, such as baclofen (Lioresal) for spasticity |
| **Serum sickness** | Results from an adverse response to an allergen | Fever, myalgias, arthralgias, arthritis, urticaria, lymphadenopathy, and splenomegaly | Epinephrine, antihistamines, salicylates, corticosteroids |
| **Stevens-Johnson syndrome** | Unknown cause | Vesiculobullous lesions of the skin and two or more mucous membrane sites, malaise, mild pruritus, burning sensation, arthralgia, myalgia, and fever | Antibiotics, corticosteroids |
| **Thyroiditis, Hashimoto's** | Results from an autoimmune reaction | Goiter; neck pain with upward radiation; and, occasionally, hypothyroidism with dry skin, coarse hair, and myxedema | Thyroid hormone replacement |
| **Vogt-Koyanagi-Harada syndrome** | Unknown cause; may result from an autoimmune process | Uveal inflammation of one or both eyes, with acute iridocyclitis, patchy choroiditis, and serous detachment of the retina | Corticosteroids, immunosuppressive therapy |

# Glossary

## A

**Aeroallergens:** airborne particles, such as pollen or house dust, that cause respiratory, cutaneous, or conjunctival allergy.

**Agglutination:** the clumping together of antigens due to their interactions with specific antibodies (agglutinins).

**Agglutinin:** an antibody that promotes antigen agglutination.

**Aggressin:** a diffusible substance produced by a bacterium that interferes with normal defense mechanisms and enhances the organism's ability to establish itself in host tissues. Also known as a virulence factor.

**Allele:** one of a pair of genes, or of multiple forms of a gene, occupying the same locus on homologous chromosomes and controlling a particular characteristic.

**Allergen:** an antigenic substance capable of inducing an allergic response.

**Allergy:** an alteration in immune reactivity resulting in an untoward physiologic response.

**Alloantigen:** an antigen obtained from different individuals or an inbred line of the same species, such as histocompatibility antigens.

**Allogenic:** of the same species but not genetically identical.

**Allograft:** a tissue or organ graft between two genetically different members of the same species. Also known as a homograft.

**Alternative complement pathway:** a complement activation pathway involving factor B, factor D, and C3b interaction, eventually leading to C3 activation and C5 cleavage, then progressing as in the classical complement pathway.

**Anaphylatoxin:** a substance produced by complement activation that functions in inflammation.

**Anaphylaxis:** an immediate hypersensitivity reaction resulting from sensitization of tissue-fixed mast cells by certain antibodies to a previously encountered antigen.

**Anergy:** a diminished or absent reaction to an antigen or panel of antigens.

**Antibody:** a protein that is produced in response to an antigen and that has the ability to combine with that antigen.

**Antigen:** a substance that elicits a specific immune response.

**Antigen presenting cell (APC):** a cell, such as a macrophage, that captures, processes, and presents the antigen to immunocompetent B and T cells, thus activating them.

**Antiserum:** animal or human serum containing antibodies against a specific antigen.

**Arthus reaction:** an acute local antigen-antibody reaction to injection of an antigen into a previously immunized host. This reaction may progress to a lesion marked by edema, hemorrhage, and necrosis.

**Atopic allergy:** a hereditary tendency to develop a hypersensitivity reaction to commonly encountered antigens.

**Autoantibody:** an antibody that reacts with an antigen that is a normal constituent of the body (a self antigen).

**Autoantigen:** a normal body constituent that stimulates autoantibody production. Also known as a self antigen.

**Autograft:** a tissue transplanted from one part to another part of the same body.

**Autoimmunity:** immunity to autoantigens.

## B

**Bacteriolysis:** destruction of bacteria induced by antibody and complement in the absence of cells.

**Bacteriophage:** any virus that destroys bacteria in the host.

**B cells:** a class of lymphocytes derived from a stem cell and believed to mature in the bone marrow. When activated, they differentiate into plasma cells (which produce antibodies) and memory cells.

**Blast cell:** a large, immature cell with a nucleus containing loosely packed chromatin, a large nucleolus, and a large amount of cytoplasm.

**Bradykinin:** a 9-amino-acid peptide that causes contraction of smooth muscle, increased vascular permeability, and increased mucous gland secretion.

**Bulla:** a vesicle on the skin or mucous membranes greater than 1 cm in diameter.

## C

**Cell-mediated immunity:** the specific immune response that occurs when T cells react to antigens.

**Chemotaxis:** a process in which phagocytes are attracted to the pathogenic invasion site.

**Classical complement pathway:** a complement activation pathway involving various enzymes and proteins that cause cleavage of C3 and C5 and ultimately, with binding of other components, cause cell lysis.

**Cleavage:** the act of splitting a complex molecule into two or more simpler molecules.

**Clone:** a group of cells derived from a single ancestral cell.

**Cold agglutinin:** an antibody that agglutinates bacteria or erythrocytes better at temperatures below 37° C. (98.6° F.).

**Complement:** the primary humoral mediator of inflammation, consisting of approximately 20 proteins that interact with each other, with antibody, and with cell membranes. Complement plays a role in various biologic mechanisms, including lysis, opsonization, and inflammation.

**Cryoglobulin:** an abnormal plasma protein that forms a gel or a precipitate at low temperatures.

## D

**Delayed hypersensitivity:** a delayed inflammatory reaction mediated by T cells and macrophages.

## E

**Endotoxin:** a lipopolysaccharide present in the cell walls of some microorganisms (primarily gram-negative bacteria) that has toxic and pyrogenic effects.

**Enhancement:** improved survival of tumor cells in animals that have been previously immunized with the tumor antigens. This may occur because these antigens are coated with antibodies that protect them from lymphocytes.

**Exotoxin:** a diffusible toxin formed by certain gram-positive and -negative microorganisms.

## G

**Gammopathy:** an immune disorder characterized by abnormalities of immunoglobulins.

**Gene:** the biologic unit of heredity.

**Genome:** the complete set of hereditary units in the chromosomes of a cell.

**Genotype:** the total genetic composition of an organism.

**Granulocytes:** includes neutrophils, eosinophils, and basophils. Granulocytes are derived from the stem cell and participate in immune reactions.

## H

**Haplotype:** one half of the genotype (each person has a maternal haplotype and a paternal haplotype).

**Hapten:** substances of small molecular weight (less than 10,000 daltons) that are not capable of eliciting an immune response. After combining with a carrier molecule, usually a serum protein, the hapten-carrier complex is able to elicit an immune response.

**Hemolysin:** a substance capable of lysing red blood cells.

## Glossary (continued)

**Heterograft:** a tissue graft transplanted from one species to another. Also called a xenograft.

**Histamine:** a vasoactive amine that is an important mediator in anaphylactic reactions. Found in mast cell and basophil granules and platelets, histamine causes increased capillary permeability, smooth muscle contraction, and increased secretion by nasal and bronchial mucous glands.

**Histocompatibility antigens:** the genetically determined cell-surface antigens that stimulate graft rejection in organ transplantation.

**Homograft:** an allograft.

**Human leukocyte antigen (HLA):** the major histocompatibility complex.

**Humoral immunity:** the specific immune response that occurs when B cells react to antigens by producing antibodies.

**Hypogammaglobulinemia:** an immunodeficiency characterized by a decrease in all of the major classes of serum immunoglobulins.

### I

**Immediate hypersensitivity:** an immune response to an antigen that occurs within minutes after the antigen combines with the specific antibody.

**Immune complexes:** antigen-antibody complexes.

**Immune response genes:** genes within the major histocompatibility complex that control immune responses to specific antigens.

**Immunity:** resistance to possible invasion by an infectious agent.

**Immunoelectrophoresis:** a test that combines electrophoresis and immunodiffusion techniques to distinguish between proteins and other materials.

**Immunofluorescence:** a technique used to identify an antigen by observing its antigen-antibody reaction with known antibodies tagged with fluorescent dye.

**Immunoglobulin:** a protein molecule composed of light and heavy polypeptide chains linked together by disulfide bonds. All antibodies are immunoglobulins.

**Inflammation:** the complex of protective responses caused by infection, injury, or intrusion of foreign substances. These responses help to eliminate dead tissue, toxins, microbes, and inactive foreign substances.

**Interferon:** a class of small, soluble proteins, produced by infected host cells, that interfere with viral multiplication.

**Isograft:** a graft between genetically identical individuals, such as monozygotic twins.

### L

**Lymphokine:** a soluble mediator, produced by lymphocytes, that regulates macrophage, lymphocyte, and non-lymphoid cell interactions.

**Lysosomes:** granules, occurring in the cytoplasm of many cells, that contain hydrolytic enzymes and participate in localized intracellular digestion.

### M

**Macrophage:** the chief cell of the mononuclear phagocyte system, derived from the stem cell. Primarily engaged in phagocytosis, this cell also plays a role in antigen processing and presentation, the release of various mediators, and the production of fever. Macrophages are also known as mononuclear phagocytes.

**Major histocompatibility complex (MHC):** a group of genes, located on the short arm of chromosome 6, that code for surface antigens. The MHC is critical in the recognition of self versus nonself, since it defines what is self. Also known as human leukocyte antigen.

**Mast cell:** a tissue cell, resembling a basophil, with granules containing serotonin and histamine. Mast cells are essential for the antibody (IgE) response, important in anaphylactic reactions.

**Monoclonal antibody:** a homogeneous group of a single type of antibody made against a specific antigen.

**Mononuclear phagocyte:** a macrophage.

**Mononuclear phagocyte system:** the reticuloendothelial system.

### N

**Neutralization:** the interaction in which antibody or antibody in complement counteracts the infectivity of a pathogen.

### O

**Oncogene:** an altered version of a normal gene.

**Opsonin:** a substance that enhances phagocytosis.

**Opsonization:** the coating of foreign particles with opsonins, making them more susceptible to phagocytosis.

### P

**Phagocytes:** cells that are able to ingest particulate matter. Examples of phagocytes are macrophages and neutrophils.

**Phagocytosis:** engulfing and ingesting of bacteria, fungi, dead tissue, antigen-antibody complexes, and tumor cells by macrophages and neutrophils.

**Phenotype:** the sum total of physical, physiological, and biochemical makeup of an individual as determined by genetic and environmental factors.

**Plasma cell:** a cell derived from B cells that secrete large amounts of immunoglobulin.

**Precipitation:** formation of interlocking aggregates caused by interactions between soluble antigens and antibodies.

### R

**Radioallergosorbent test (RAST):** a test that measures IgE antibodies in serum that are directed at specific allergens.

**Rejection:** an immune response directed against transplanted tissue. Rejection can be classified according to the time span between transplantation and rejection; namely, hyperacute (occurring within minutes to hours); accelerated (occurring after about 5 days); acute (occurring within days to months); and chronic (occurring 6 months to years later).

**Reticuloendothelial system (RES):** the system of cells distributed throughout the body that removes microorganisms from the blood and tissues and responds to activated lymphocytes to participate in immune responses. The chief cell is the macrophage. Also known as the mononuclear phagocyte system.

**Rheumatoid factor (RF):** anti-immunoglobulin antibodies formed in response to altered IgG. RF is often found in the serum of patients with rheumatoid arthritis and other rheumatoid disorders.

### S

**Sensitization:** immunologic activation of cells in response to an antigen.

**Syngraft:** an isograft.

### T

**T cells:** a class of lymphocytes that is derived from the stem cell and matures in the thymus. When activated, they differentiate into various cells, including helper cells, suppressor cells, lymphokine-producing cells, cytotoxic cells, and memory cells.

**Toxoid:** a toxin that is altered to reduce its toxic effect but that retains its antigenic properties.

**Transfer factor:** an extract of sensitized lymphocytes that transfers cell-mediated immunity from one individual to another.

### V

**Vaccination:** immunization with antigens to prevent infectious diseases.

**Vesicle:** a small blister containing a serous fluid.

**Virulence factor:** aggressin.

### X

**Xenograft:** a heterograft.

# Selected References and Acknowledgments

## Selected References

Benacerraf, Baruj, and Unanue, Emil. *Textbook of Immunology.* Baltimore: Williams and Wilkins, 1979 (reprint 1981).

♦

Blacklow, Robert S., et al. *MacBryde's Signs and Symptoms: Applied Pathologic Physiology and Clinical Interpretation,* 6th ed. Philadelphia, J.B. Lippincott Co., 1983.

♦

Brandt, B. "A Nursing Protocol for the Client with Neutropenia," *Oncology Nursing Forum* 11(2):24-28, March/April 1984.

♦

Brunner, Lillian, and Suddarth, Doris. *The Lippincott Manual of Nursing Practice,* 3rd ed. Philadelphia: J.B. Lippincott Co., 1982.

♦

Brunner, Lillian, and Suddarth, Doris. *Textbook of Medical-Surgical Nursing,* 5th ed. Philadelphia: J.B. Lippincott Co., 1984.

♦

Buckley, R.H. "Immunodeficiency," *Journal of Allergy and Clinical Immunology* 72(6):627-41, December 1983.

♦

Campbell, Claire. *Nursing Diagnosis and Intervention in Nursing Practice,* 2nd ed. New York: John Wiley & Sons, 1984.

♦

Centers for Disease Control. "General Recommendations on Immunization: Recommendations of the Immunization Practices' Advisory Committee." *Ann. Intern. Med.,* 98:615-622, 1983.

♦

Christensen, Mary L. *Microbiology for Nursing and Allied Health Students.* Springfield, Ill.: Charles C. Thomas Pubs., 1982.

♦

Devita, Vincent T., Jr., and Hellman, Samuel. *Cancer: Principles and Practice of Oncology.* Philadelphia: J.B. Lippincott Co., 1982.

♦

Delp, Mahlon H., and Manning, Robert T. *Major's Physical Diagnosis: An Introduction to the Clinical Process,* 9th ed. Philadelphia: W.B. Saunders Co., 1981.

♦

Fidler, R. "Complement Assays... Deciphering Diagnostic Studies," *Nursing83* 13(3):65-67, March 1983.

♦

Greenberger, Norton J. *Gastrointestinal Disorders.* Chicago: Year Book Medical Pubs., 1980.

Henry, John B., ed. *Todd-Sanford-Davidsohn: Clinical Diagnosis and Management by Laboratory Methods,* 17th ed. Philadelphia: W.B. Saunders Co., 1984.

♦

Hoeprich, Paul D., et al, eds. *Infectious Diseases: A Modern Treatise of Infectious Processes,* 3rd ed. Philadelphia: J.B. Lippincott Co., 1983.

♦

Jett, M., and Lancaster, L. "The Inflammatory-Immune Response: The Body's Defense Against Invasion," *Critical Care Nurse* 3(5):64-86, October 1983.

♦

Kaye, Donald, and Rose, Louis F. *Fundamentals of Internal Medicine.* St. Louis: C.V. Mosby Co., 1983.

♦

Malasanos, Lois. *Health Assessment,* 2nd ed. St. Louis: C.V. Mosby Co., 1981.

♦

Maser, Henry. "The Acquired Immunodeficiency Syndrome," *Disease a Month* 30(1), 1983.

♦

Melchers, et al. "Mechanisms of B cell Neoplasia." *Immunology Today* 5:214-217, February 1984.

♦

Middleton, Elliott, Jr., et al, eds. *Allergy: Principles and Practice,* 2 vols., 2nd ed. St. Louis: C.V. Mosby Co., 1983.

♦

Newmark, Peter. "Cell and Cancer Biology Meld," *Nature* 307:499, February 1984.

♦

Oppenheim, Joost J., Rosenstreich, David L., and Potter, Michael (eds.). *Cellular Functions in Immunity and Inflammation.* North Holland/New York: Elsevier, 1981.

♦

Paul, W.E. (ed.). *Fundamental Immunology.* New York: Raven Press, 1984.

♦

Petersdorf, Robert G., and Adams, Raymond D. *Harrison's Principles of Internal Medicine,* 10th ed. New York: McGraw-Hill Book Co., 1983.

♦

Rodman, G.P., and Schumacher, H.R., eds. *Primer on the Rheumatic Diseases,* 8th ed. Atlanta: The Arthritis Foundation, 1983.

♦

Rutman, Roanne, and Miller, William V., eds. *Transfusion Therapy: Principles and Procedures.* Rockville, Md.: Aspen Systems Corp., 1982.

♦

Salvaggio, John E., et al, eds. "Primer on Allergic and Immunologic Diseases," *Journal of the American Medical Association* 248(20), November 26, 1982; special edition prepared by the American Academy of Allergy and Immunology.

♦

Stiehm, E. Richard, and Fulginiti, Vincent A. *Immunologic Disorders in Infants and Children,* 2nd ed. Philadelphia: W.B. Saunders Co., 1980.

♦

Stites, D.P., et al, eds. *Basic and Clinical Immunology,* 5th ed. Los Altos, Calif.: Lange Medical Publications, 1984.

♦

Weir, Donald M. *Immunology: An Outline for Students of Medicine and Biology,* 5th ed. New York: Churchill Livingstone, 1983.

## Acknowledgments

♦ p. 41 Illustration adapted with permission from Noel R. Rose and Herman Friedman, *Manual of Clinical Immunology* (Washington, D.C.: American Society for Microbiology, 1980), p. 203.

♦ p. 45 Chart adapted with permission from D.P. Stites, et al., eds. *Basic and Clinical Immunology,* 5th ed., p. 501. © 1984 by Lange Medical Publications, Los Altos, Calif.

♦ p. 48 Photo courtesy of Maurice Barcos, MD, Roswell Memorial Institute, Buffalo, N.Y.

♦ pp. 62, 63 Tables courtesy of Roy Patterson, MD, and Philip S. Norman, MD, "Immunotherapy—Immunodulation," *Journal of the American Medical Association* 248(20):2763 and 2765, November 26, 1982.

♦ pp. 64-65 Adapted with permission from Fenwall Laboratories, Deerfield, Ill.

♦ pp. 74, 80, 81 Adapted with permission from AIDS Activity, Center for Infectious Diseases, Centers for Disease Control, Atlanta, Ga., December 31, 1984.

♦ p. 100 Adapted with permission from G.P. Rodman and H.R. Schumacher, *Primer on the Rheumatic Diseases,* 8th ed. (Atlanta: The Arthritis Foundation), 1983, p. 36.

♦ p. 106 X-rays courtesy of John Mosher, MD, Department of Orthopedic Surgery, University Hospital, Syracuse, N.Y.

♦ p. 135 Charts adapted from *New England Journal of Medicine* 292:838-39, 1975, with permission from the publisher.

♦ p. 164 Courtesy of Tito Cavallo, MD, "Immune Aspects of Renal Diseases," *Journal of the American Medical Association* 248(20):2701-02, November 26, 1982. © 1982, American Medical Association.

# INDEX

i = illustration; t = table

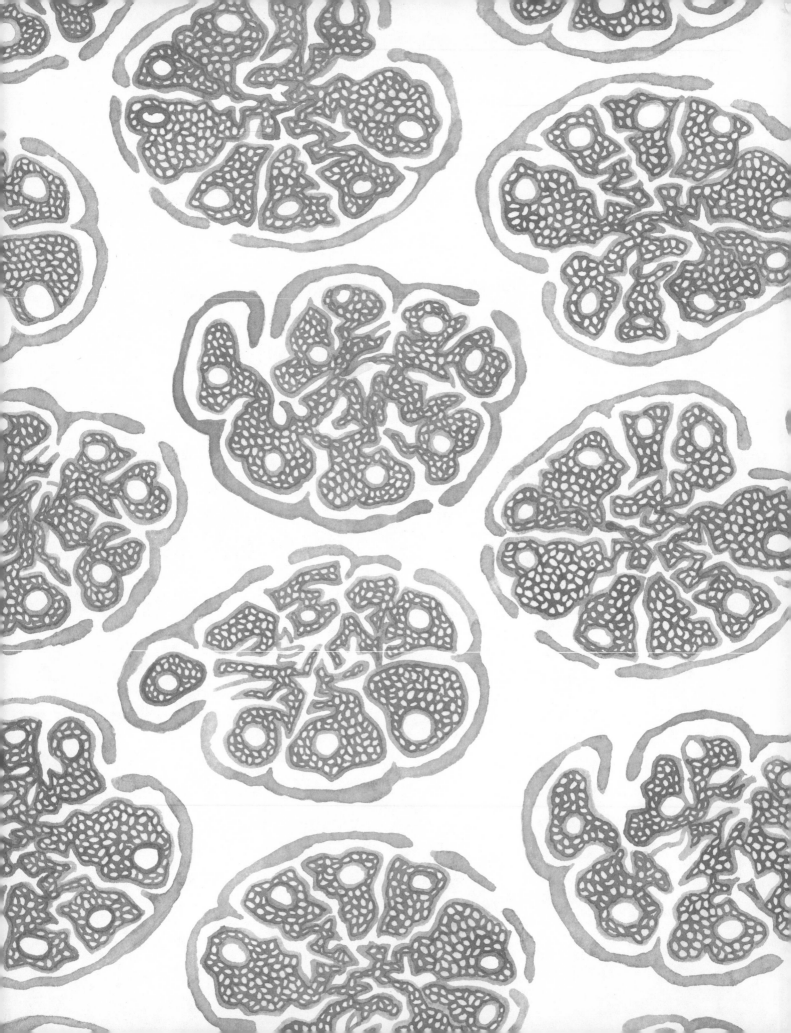